Men'sHealth

THE BOOK OF MUSCLE

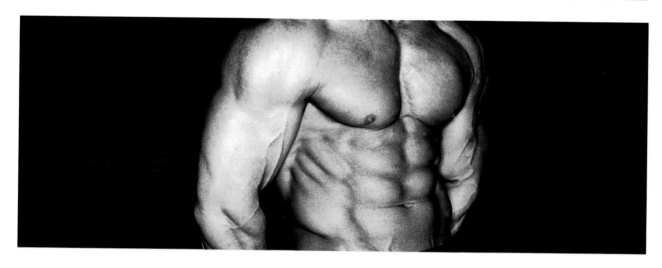

THE WORLD'S MOST AUTHORITATIVE GUIDE TO BUILDING YOUR BODY

IAN KING

AND LOU SCHULER

RODALE

Book design by Susan P. Eugster

Library of Congress Cataloging-in-Publication Data

King, Ian, date.
Men's health the book of muscle : the world's most authoritative guide
to building your body / by Ian King and Lou Schuler.
            p.   cm.
            Includes index.
        ISBN 1–57954–768–0 hardcover
        ISBN 1–57954–769–9 trade hardcover
    1. Bodybuilding.   2. Physical fitness.   I. Schuler, Lou.   II. Men's
            health (Magazine)   III. Title.
            GV546.5.K52   2003
613.7'1—dc21   2003010825

Distributed to the book trade by St. Martin's Press

8 10 9   trade hardcover
8 10 9 7   direct-marketing hardcover

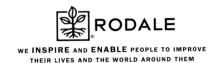
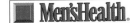

CONTENTS

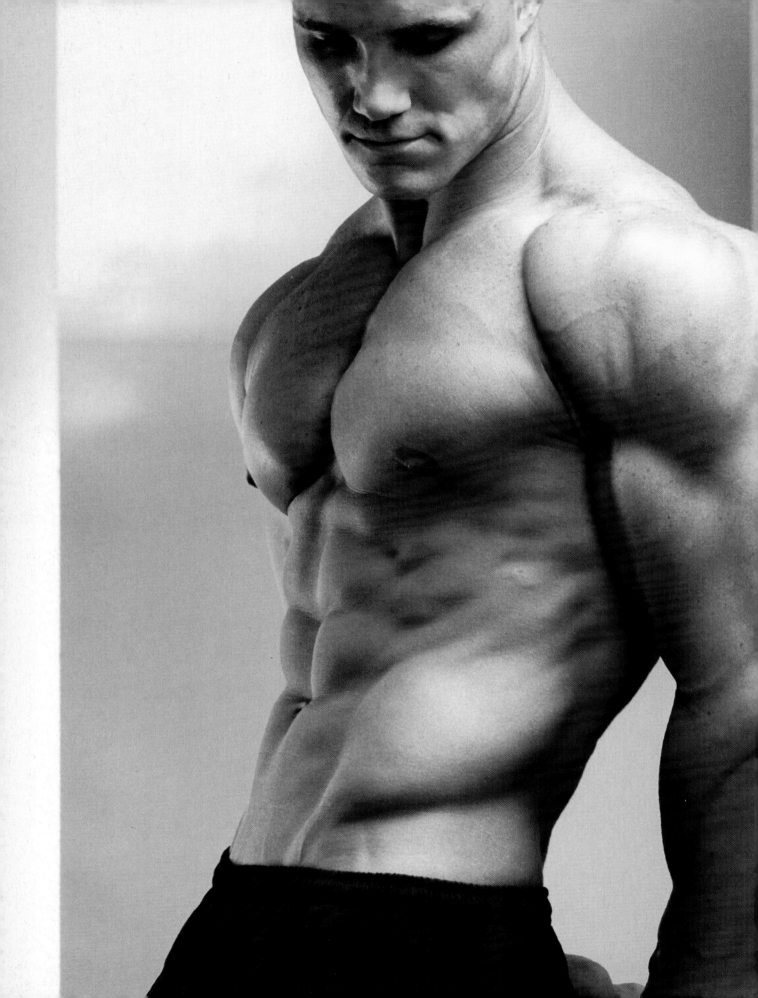

PART 1

THE PHYSIOLOGY

ALL MUSCLES, GREAT AND SMALL

YOUR BODY HAS ABOUT 650 MUSCLES. No matter that you care about just four or five of them, all of which can be sculpted with maybe a half-dozen strength-training exercises. You still need all of them to perform the normal functions of everyday life—breathing, eating, walking, sucking in your stomach at the beach.

Fortunately, you don't need to spend a lot of time thinking about most of your muscles. The ones involved in breathing, eating, and walking will do the job whether you monitor them or

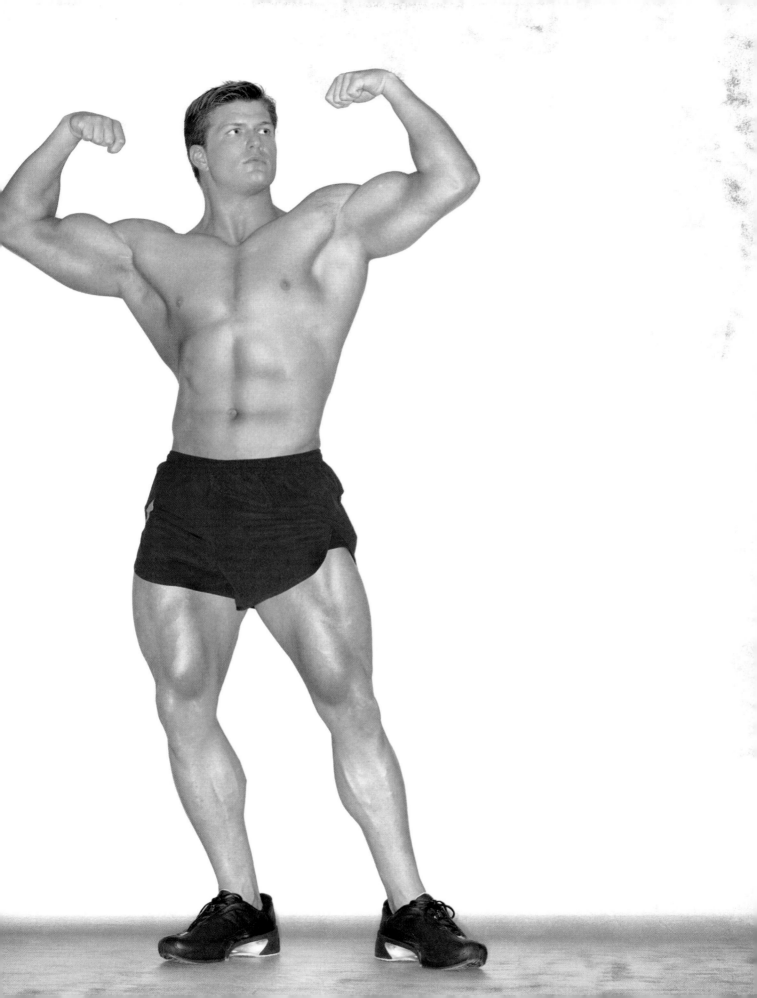

not. You couldn't bulk up the 50 muscles in your face even if you wanted to. You can always try to impress your friends with your intellectual muscle by telling them that the gluteus maximus is the body's strongest muscle, that the latissimus dorsi in your middle back is the largest, or that a middle-ear muscle called the stapedius is the smallest. But it probably won't work . . . unless you have some really unusual friends. Muscle trivia can never begin to capture the wonder of muscles themselves—the brilliance of coordinated muscles in motion, the magnificence of strong, well-developed muscles at work.

We hope, in the following chapters, to explain (briefly) what your muscles are and how they work, and then show you (in great detail) how to make them bigger, stronger, and more powerful. Our exercise programs include 6 months' worth of workouts each for beginner, intermediate, and advanced lifters, with those skill designations determined by Ian King's training-age system. These programs are biased toward exercises that work multiple muscle groups, as opposed 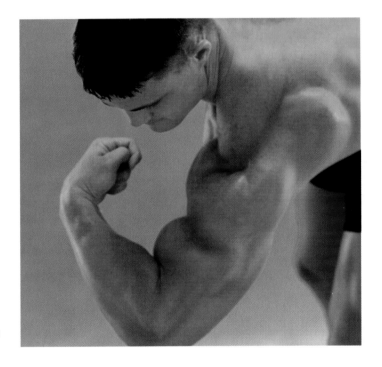 to those that isolate muscles and muscle groups. We want to ensure that your bigger, stronger, more aesthetically balanced muscles are also functional muscles.

Don't fret, however, if you're one of those guys who like to isolate muscle groups. There's plenty here for absolitionists, pectoralists, and biceptologists. We do want your muscles to work well together, but we also understand that you want your favorite muscles to really stand out and look as good as possible.

A LITTLE MORE DEFINITION

Muscles make up about 45 percent of a man's body weight. (By comparison, bones account for just 12 percent.) They're about 80 percent water. Most of the rest of muscle tissue is protein, although there's also some carbohydrate, fat, and salt.

Your body has three different types of muscle tissue:

1. SKELETAL muscles are the ones you check out in the mirror. These are also called *voluntary* muscles since you can move them at will. Conveniently, they're able to work without your thinking about them. They maintain a state of slight readiness—called *muscle tone*—whether you consciously tighten them or not. If they didn't, you'd collapse in a gelatinous heap. The only time they lose this tone entirely (in the absence of muscular diseases) is when your body is completely unconscious because of either trauma or medication.

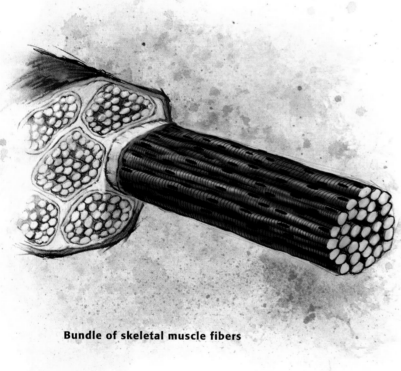

Bundle of skeletal muscle fibers

2. SMOOTH muscles surround your blood vessels and internal organs in thin layers. Whereas skeletal muscles can resemble steel cables (we like to think ours do, anyway), smooth muscles look like interesting bedsheets.

3. CARDIAC muscle has fibers that look like those of skeletal muscle. The crucial difference is that skeletal muscle is made up of individual fibers that, like the wires of a cable, work closely together, side by side, but aren't attached to each other. Cardiac muscle fibers are attached to each other, which allows them to send information from cell to cell in the form of electrical signals. Imagine walking

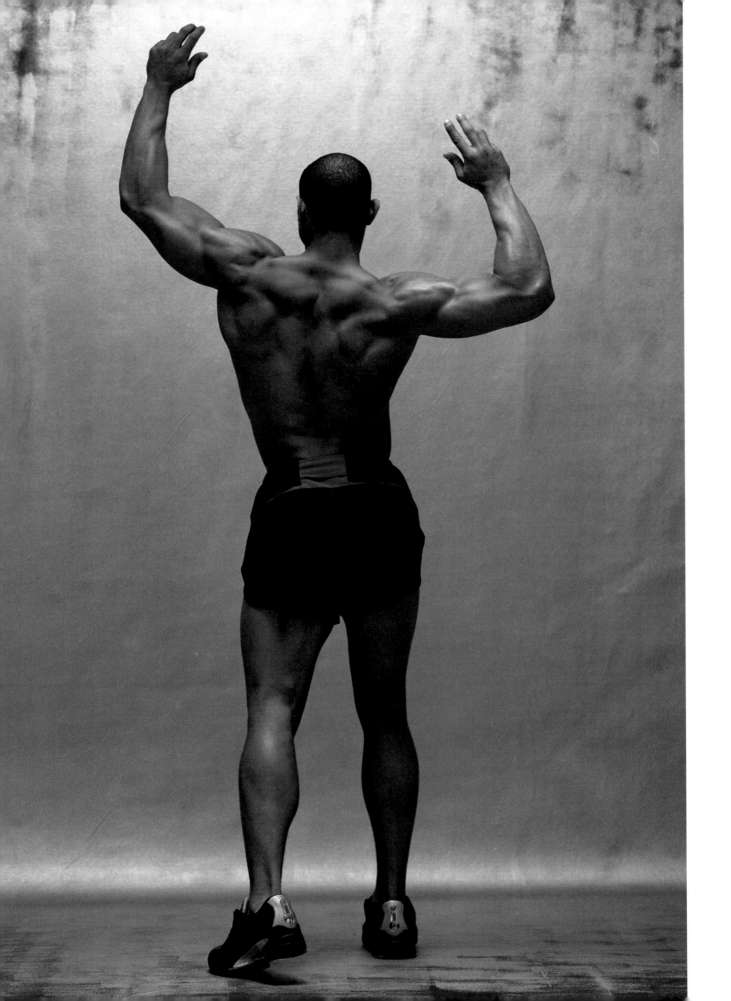

through a forest in which each tree sends a branch directly into the trunk of an adjacent tree, and you get the idea.

Now that we've defined the three types of muscle, let's forget about the second and third and take a closer look at skeletal muscles.

TYPECASTING

Your body has approximately a quarter-billion skeletal muscle fibers, all of which can be categorized as one of two main types. **TYPE I** fibers, also called **SLOW-TWITCH** fibers, are used for endurance activities, or tasks that don't require maximum strength. **TYPE II**, or **FAST-TWITCH,** fibers come into play when a task utilizes more than 25 percent of your maximum strength.

You have two subcategories of fast-twitch fibers, IIa and IIx. IIx fibers are the biggest and strongest, but they're incapable of sustaining effort for more than a few seconds. IIa fibers not only are used for strength-and-power activities but also keep going longer—for up to 3 minutes, in the most highly trained athletes.

It's easy to remember the types if you see them as part of a continuum: Type I are the smallest and most endurance-oriented; IIa are bigger and have limited endurance; and IIx are the biggest, with almost no endurance beyond what it takes to perform a single maximal effort. (There are other subtypes of fibers, creating even more of a continuum effect, but it's simplest to focus on the big three.)

A task doesn't have to be "slow" to use your slow-twitch fibers as the prime movers. It just has to be an action that doesn't require much of your fast-twitch strength. And an effort doesn't have to be "fast" to call your fast-twitch fibers into play. For example, even though a guy going for a personal record on the bench press isn't going to be able to move the barbell very fast, he will be using every fast-twitch muscle fiber his body can possibly recruit for the task (plus all the slow-twitch fibers, too, as we'll explain later in this chapter).

Skeletal muscles have a mix of fast- and slow-twitch fibers, and that mix can vary from person to person and from muscle to muscle. Some people are simply

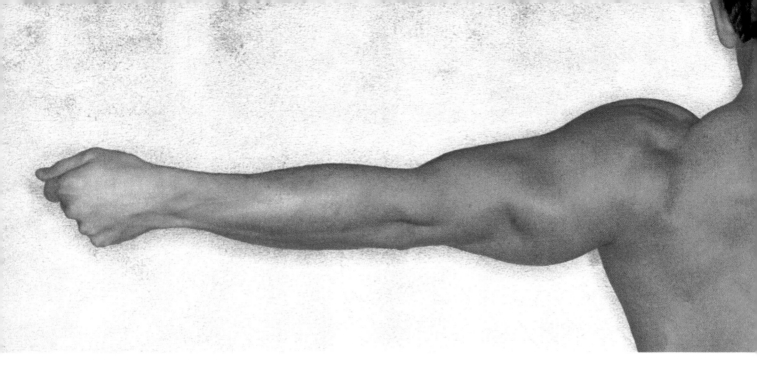

born with more slow-twitch fibers, which makes them genetically suited for endurance sports. Marathoner Joan Benoit Samuelson is said to have about 80 percent slow-twitch fibers. Those born with a predominance of fast-twitch fibers have a huge advantage in sports involving quick bursts of speed and power that don't have to be sustained for more than a minute or two. For example, Olympic-champion sprinter Carl Lewis is thought to have more than 70 percent fast-twitch fibers.

Some individual muscles, because of their function, are mostly one type or another. The soleus muscles in your calves are a good example. They're postural muscles, meaning their job is to keep you from falling over. So for that long-term, minimal-effort task, they're composed mostly of slow-twitch fibers.

On the other hand, your triceps (the muscles on the backs of your upper arms) are more fast-twitch since there aren't many jobs they'll be called to do that require a sustained, low-intensity effort. They're your push-the-car-out-of-a-snow-bank muscles, designed for maximum power.

We're not telling you this to prepare you for a career in exercise physiology. If you want to build your muscles, you have to target the right ones. The fast-twitch fibers are bigger than the slow-twitch fibers and have more potential for growth. We'll hit on this key concept in the workout sections of this book: The more experienced you are in the weight room, the more you have to target the fibers that have the most potential for getting bigger and stronger.

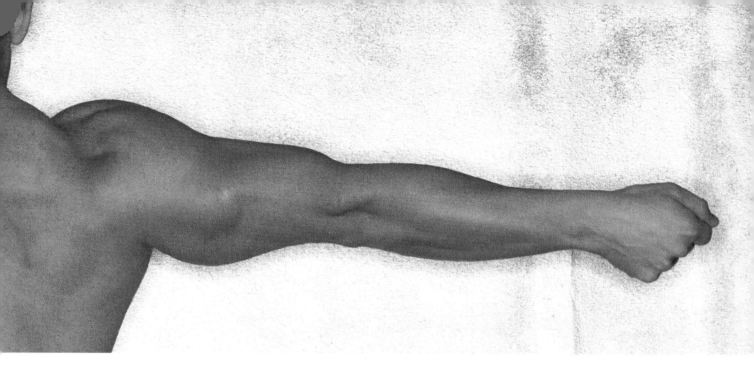

ROLE-PLAYING

It isn't completely sexist to say that a woman marries a man with the idea that she can change him into what she really wants. (In our experience, most women will admit this, and it rarely takes more than three beers to get them to do so.) Most guys do try to change, and with enough work we manage small transformations. Eventually, we all figure out that it makes more sense to play up our strengths than to waste a lot of effort minimizing our weaknesses.

Your muscle fibers undergo a similar transformational process when you exercise. When you first start training, your IIx fibers quickly remake themselves into IIa fibers, with the ability to perform more work. That's why some exercise scientists call IIx the couch-potato fibers: People who don't exercise have a lot of them, whereas people who are in shape don't have many.

In men, the transformation of IIx to IIa can happen in about 4 weeks. In one well-known study, 2 months of heavy, twice-weekly strength training decreased the number of IIx fibers to about 7 percent of the body's total number of fibers.

There's no evidence that type II fibers ever transform themselves into type I, or vice versa. This footnote in the giant tome of exercise science is actually crucially important for exercisers to understand.

Here's why: If you're genetically suited for endurance exercise—that is, if you were born with a high percentage of slow-twitch fibers—you probably find it easy to get or stay lean, but you may have a devil of a time trying to add a significant amount of muscle to your frame. Your abundant type I fibers have some potential to get bigger and stronger with dedicated strength training, and of course your relatively scarce type IIs can get bigger and stronger, too. But muscle growth will always be harder for you than for a guy who's genetically suited for strength-and-power sports.

Now let's say you're that strength-and-power guy. You're naturally pretty strong, probably wide-shouldered, possibly thick-waisted (unfortunately). When you exercise with weights, you get stronger fast, and you put on weight so quickly it scares you. It's a good bet that you were born with a preponderance of type II fibers. So although you're good at sports or exercises that require strength and power, you struggle to keep up with other guys on the jogging track. Over time, you can train your body to get better at endurance activities. Still, you'll probably be continually frustrated by poor finishes in any races you enter.

Most of us fall somewhere between the gifted endurance athlete and the guy who gets as strong as an ox just by inhaling the chalk dust in the weight room. All of us can get better at the sports and exercise activities we care about most. But it's foolish to think that powerlifters can be transformed into marathoners or that gazelles can be bulked up into oxen.

The reason is a slow-twitch fiber can't become a fast-twitch fiber, even if it's made bigger and stronger through resistance exercise. And although a fast-twitch fiber can be shrunk down to slow-twitch size with endurance exercise, it's never truly a type I fiber that will help you improve your 10-K time.

SIZE, AND WHY IT MATTERS

Here's the part where we show you how to apply everything we've just explained about muscle fibers.

When you begin a task, whether it's as simple as getting out of a chair or as complicated as swinging a golf club, your muscles operate on two basic physiological principles.

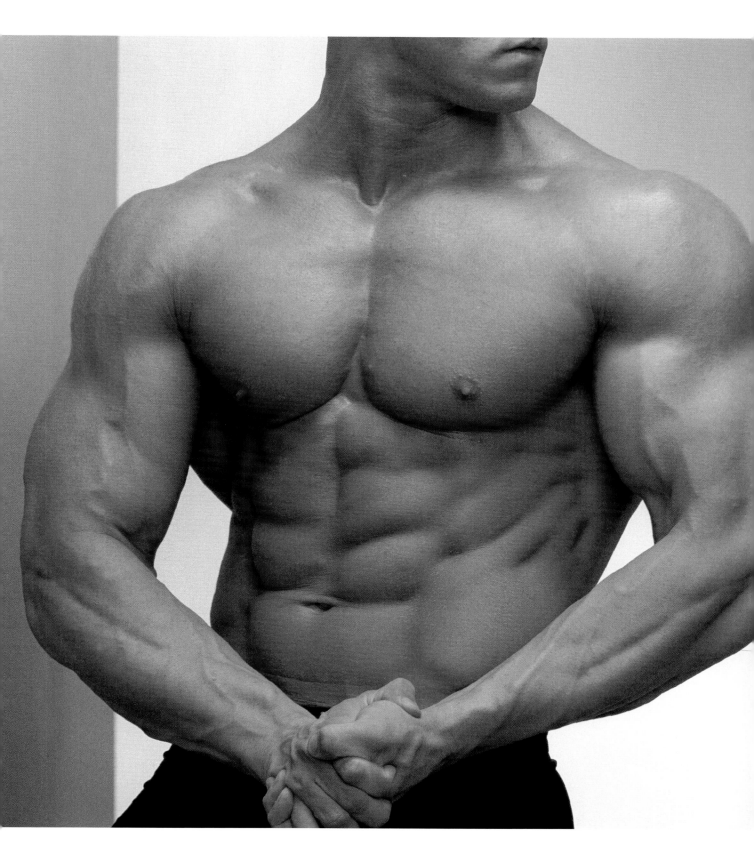

ALL MUSCLES, GREAT AND SMALL

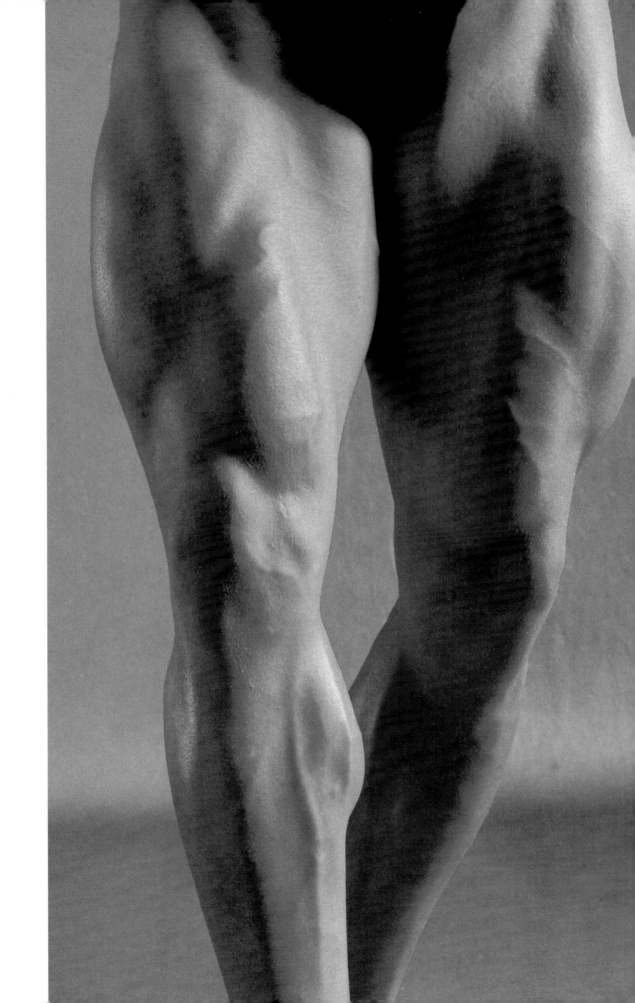

1. *THE ALL-OR-NOTHING PRINCIPLE.* A muscle fiber either gets into the action or doesn't. If it does, it performs an all-out effort. So the next time you get out of your chair to walk to the men's room, remind yourself that, somewhere in your body, a small percentage of your muscle fibers are working as hard as they can to get you there.

2. *THE SIZE PRINCIPLE.* In any task, the first muscle fibers pulled into action are the smallest ones. Since the smallest fibers on your body are most likely your slow-twitch fibers, they go in first. (In women and highly trained endurance athletes, some type I fibers may actually be larger than some type II fibers. This is why you should avoid estrogen and high-volume aerobic exercise when you're trying to build bigger muscles.) When your body realizes that the effort needed exceeds about 25 percent of your total strength, it activates your IIa fibers. And when it sees that the effort requires more than about 40 percent of your strength, it calls up the IIx fibers.

All this happens faster than you can think about it. Still, it's useful to know how it happens.

Think of muscle fibers as soldiers in an army. Just as individual soldiers are members of platoons, muscle fibers are arranged in groups called *motor units*. A motor unit consists of one nerve cell and any number of muscle fibers, from a few to thousands. Motor units, like the fibers that comprise them, have capabilities ranging from low threshold to high threshold.

Your body keeps the highest-threshold motor units in reserve for the toughest tasks. That's why a guy who's trying to build as much muscle as possible must eventually work with weights that require an all-out effort. Otherwise, the highest-threshold motor units would never get used. And those are the fibers that are not only the biggest ones on your body but also the ones with the most potential to get even bigger.

We'll make a better case for this idea in the coming chapters, and then the workout programs will show you how to train your body to the point where it's ready to make these all-out efforts without injury.

CHAPTER TWO

USING 'EM . . . AND LOSING 'EM

HAVE YOU EVER LOOKED AT A MUSCULAR ATHLETE or bodybuilder and asked yourself, "What does it take to look like that?" As we've already hinted, a big part of the answer is having the right parents.

Your genes determine three important pieces of the muscle-building puzzle.

1. YOUR MAXIMUM NUMBER OF MUSCLE FIBERS. Here's something to contemplate the next time you stumble across one

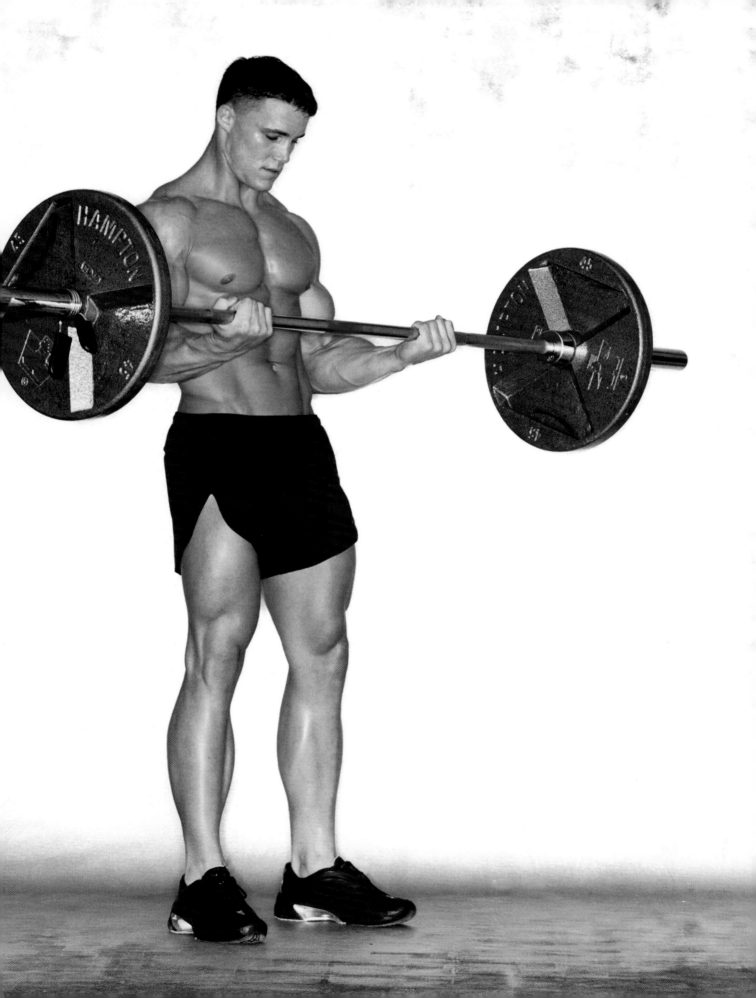

of your baby pictures: The squishy little diaper-loading machine in the photo already had all the muscle fibers you're ever going to possess. Those fibers became bigger as you grew, and they can become bigger still if you give them sufficient exercise. Conversely, if you don't exercise them enough, they may become smaller—and possibly disappear altogether. It's generally believed, though, that they can't increase in number. (Some scientists think there's a caveat or two, as we'll discuss in the next chapter.)

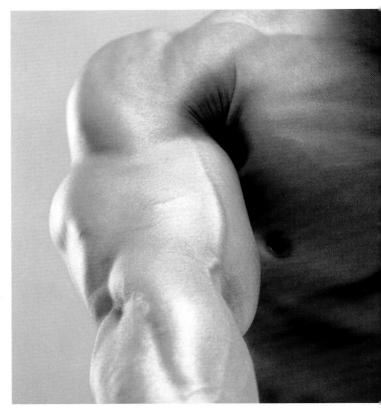

However many muscle fibers you're born with, it's too many to count, so there's no way to know exactly how you compare with other guys.

2. YOUR PERCENTAGE OF FAST-TWITCH AND SLOW-TWITCH FIBERS. As we said in chapter one, a fast-twitch fiber can't turn into a slow-twitch fiber, and a slow-twitch fiber can't become fast-twitch. Because you're born with all the fibers you're ever going to have, you're also born with a predisposition toward either endurance-type activities or strength-and-power sports, depending upon which type of fiber is predominant.

3. THE SHAPE OF YOUR MUSCLES WHEN THEY'RE FULLY DEVELOPED. If your father or mother had beautifully rounded biceps after a few years of strength training, chances are you can develop some nice-looking, beach-friendly muscles, too. If Dad trained diligently for years only to look like a big ol' dump truck with teeth . . . well, maybe you can do something about the "dump" part. The idea that muscles can be shaped—as opposed to developed to their full genetic potential—is

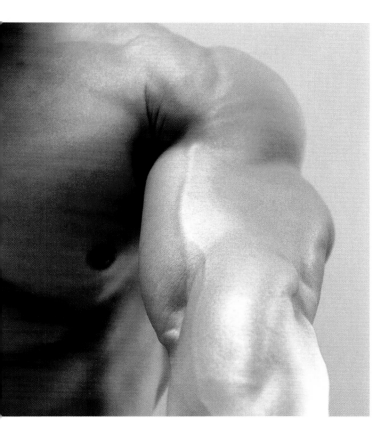

yet another topic for the next chapter. Until then, let's just say that the eventual shape of a muscle is determined by sperm and egg first, barbell and dumbbell second.

Genetics aside, in order for those tiny baby muscles to turn into the adult muscles you now flex in front of the mirror, you need a little something special—special with a capital S.

We're talking about steroids—the natural kind.

NATURE'S JUICE MACHINE

Steroids are hormones that take chemical signals directly to the DNA in the nuclei of cells. The particular steroid that we're concerned with—the one that shuttles messages telling your muscle cells to grow—is testosterone.

Testosterone is present in everybody—babies, little girls playing with tea sets, grandparents—but no one has testosterone increases from one year to the next like a maturing male. In boys, testosterone levels increase tenfold during puberty, starting sometime between ages 9 and 15. When it happens, a boy is catapulted from childhood to adolescence, leaving discarded G.I. Joes and outgrown clothes in his wake. He grows so fast—especially around age 14—that he's at increased risk for injuries such as broken bones and strained joints. His muscles and connective tissues tighten, and his bones lengthen. Meanwhile, his once-cherubic voice cracks like an inner-city sidewalk, and hair and strange odors sprout from his body's dark places.

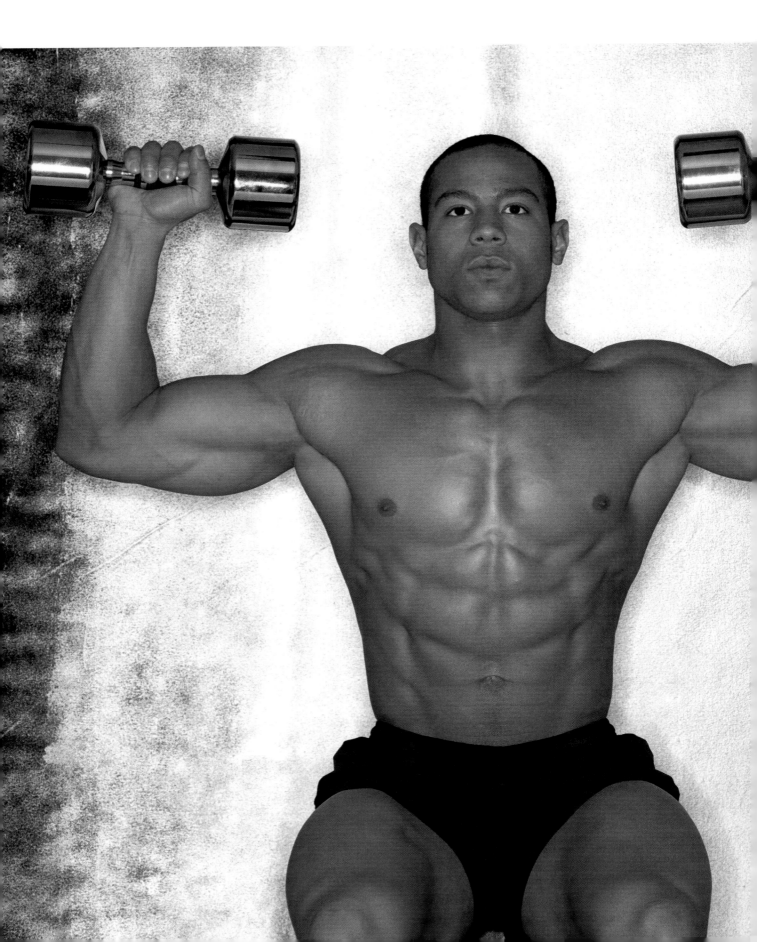

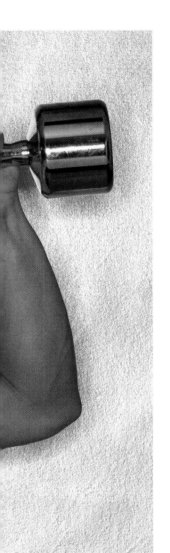

He hits near-peak testosterone production in his late teens, with levels slowly climbing until about age 30. Not coincidentally, a man reaches a number of other peaks at about that same time. Sexual desire tops out in his early thirties. Muscle mass peaks between the ages of 18 and 25—unless you throw strength training and dietary interventions into the mix. With weights and the right food, mass and strength can increase at any age—which, of course, is the reason you bought this book.

Among elite athletes, performance usually peaks in the late twenties and starts to decline in the thirties. One study of Olympic weightlifters showed that peak performance occurred at age 30 and declined by 1 to 1½ percent a year after that. At age 70, weightlifting performance started falling even faster, although we have to say we admire any man who's still doing snatches and clean-and-jerks when he's old enough to collect Social Security checks.

Testosterone declines slightly and gradually between the ages of 30 and 50, and then falls by about 1 percent a year until death. A man has 30 to 40 percent less testosterone at 70 than he had at 30. And, again, his testosterone levels seem to correlate to his muscle mass. Studies have shown that between the ages of 40 and 70, a man loses 12 to 20 pounds of muscle and about 15 percent of his bone mass. His libido does a swan dive during the second half of his life. About 25 percent of all men are impotent by 70. Some 50 percent of men over 75 have their daubers down, although that isn't necessarily related to falling testosterone levels; most men of this age who are impotent have diabetes or other severe, disabling diseases.

If all this were inevitable, we wouldn't bother warning you about it. Life can be depressing enough without reminders about how much worse it's going to get. Thankfully, neither muscle mass nor athletic performance has to decline so precipitously with age—nor, for that matter, does sexual potency. Yes, an elite athlete who's in peak condition for most of his life will hit a performance ceiling in his late twenties before experiencing declines starting in his thirties. Few men, however, qualify as elite athletes. A man who's never been in peak condition can start working out seriously in his forties and soon find himself stronger, more muscular and healthier than ever.

We now have evidence that muscles can get bigger and stronger at any age. The improvements are often startling. In one study, a group of men in their sixties and seventies did exercises for their knee flexors (hamstrings) and extensors (quadriceps). Their knee-flexor strength increased by 227 percent, and their knee-extensor strength jumped by 107 percent. The type I muscle fibers in those areas increased in size by 33½ percent, and the type II fibers grew by 27½ percent.

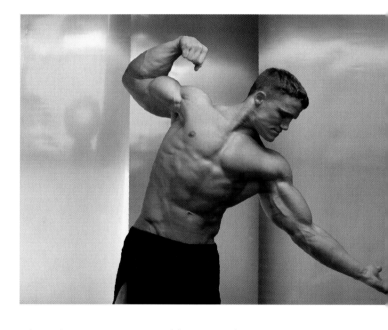

An interesting side note: If you're reading carefully, you've probably been surprised to learn that the type I fibers gained more bulk than the type IIs, since in young men you'd expect the opposite to occur. The muscle loss that accompanies aging—called *sarcopenia*—is literally a loss of muscle fibers, particularly type II fibers. (This loss is thought to be caused by disuse, rather than by hormonal shifts, so it isn't considered inevitable. But we're a long way from knowing this for certain.) In fact, if you look at the muscles of frail, older women, you may have trouble finding any type II fibers at all. Strength training can't make fibers regenerate—once they're gone, that's it. But, as demonstrated by the aforementioned study and many others, strength training can increase the strength and size of the remaining fibers.

NEVER TOO YOUNG OR OLD

The world of athletic training is governed as much by myth and tradition as by science. One of the most pernicious myths is that children don't benefit from strength training. In fact, the opposite is true. Studies have shown that children as young as age 6 make strength gains, with increases of 30 to 40 percent typical in preadolescents and one study showing improvements of up to 74 percent. Kids tend not to see large gains in muscle mass, due to low levels of circulating testosterone—a situation that's quickly rectified when testosterone goes ballistic in the teenage years.

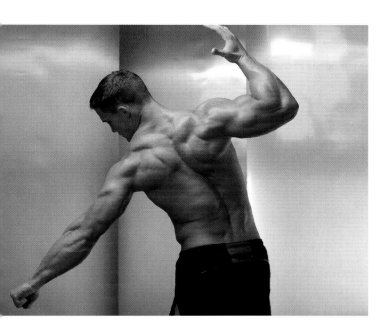

A bigger question, though, is whether strength training is a good idea for children. After all, an active child should be getting plenty of other intense exercise. A kid who jumps off a step to the floor is doing a type of exercise called *plyometrics* that's used to train elite athletes in almost every sport. A single pushup in gym class may be the equivalent of an adult's bench-pressing maximum weight. One chinup on the monkey bars could equal an adult's doing a lat pulldown with as much weight as he can manage. (Most adults can't do a single chinup.)

When kids play, whether it's a game of tag at recess or a Saturday-morning soccer contest watched by their camcorder-toting parents, they sprint, stop, and change directions quickly—all intense activities that the world's best strength coaches incorporate into programs for the world's best athletes.

The problem nowadays, as any parent will tell you, is that children don't do as much jumping, climbing, and sprinting as they used to. Those of us who are old enough to remember a simpler, safer world fondly recall daily after-school sports competition. We played baseball, football, and soccer with friends—no uniforms or referees required—until our parents called us home for dinner.

Today, kids rarely play sports outside formal, adult-organized practices and matches. That means they have fewer chances for intense, maximum-effort exercise. So parents step in and give them structured weight workouts—just as they've structured everything else in their children's lives.

This is a new world, and researchers aren't sure what to expect as kids are introduced to formal strength-building and muscle-developing programs at an early age. Will these young athletes be more likely to pursue structured exercise as adults, and thus go through life more fit and healthy than their parents and grandparents? Or will they burn out on exercise and, as adults, retreat to the comforts of a sedentary life in front of the television?

All we really know about preadolescent strength training is that it helps kids get stronger. Although there's debate about whether it improves athletic performance, no one believes it harms performance.

Like any type of intense exercise, strength training increases bone density in children. That should mean healthier bones in adulthood, unless the adult stops exercising. And it makes sense to introduce children to exercise early, just as we teach them proper study habits at a young age. Most jobs are sedentary now, so we don't imagine that exercise will be any less necessary for tomorrow's adults than for today's.

Further, we can speculate that formal strength training can help combat the plague of obesity. Just a decade or two ago, it was unheard of for a child to develop type II diabetes. This disease was called adult-onset diabetes because it afflicted sedentary, overweight people who were physically mature. Today, prepubescent children do develop this illness, and trend lines show children getting fatter faster than ever before—just like their parents. Since strength training is a weapon against obesity and diabetes in adults, it seems logical that it would help children, too.

Once a kid hits puberty (or maybe we should say, once puberty hits a kid), the questions about the efficacy or advisability of muscle-building exercise tend to resolve themselves. Because pubescent boys are drowning in testosterone, they see quick

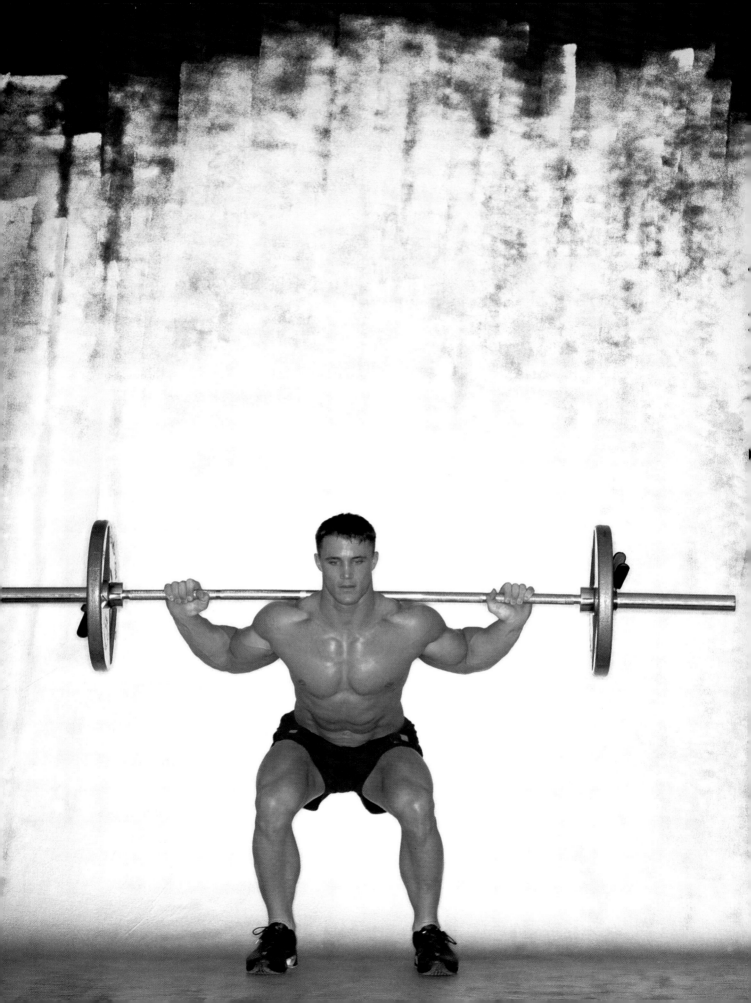

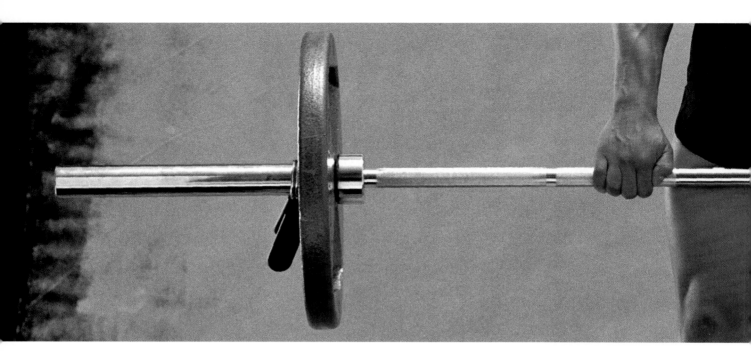

improvements in strength and muscle mass, even if their high-speed metabolic rates make it difficult to pack as much muscle on their frames as they'd like. And because teen society is driven by appearance, it isn't hard to convince girls to pick up weights either. They have estrogen surging through their systems, making their shapes more womanly but also giving them incentive to sculpt their growing curves.

The trickiest age for strength training is probably 14 for boys and 12 for girls. That's when children hit their peak "height velocity," meaning they're growing like well-fertilized weeds. Their bones are suddenly longer but not yet thicker, so they're more vulnerable to injury. It's a good time to emphasize flexibility (connective tissues tighten rapidly around this time) and correct any strength imbalances, since muscles on one side of a joint may get stronger than those on the other side, making the area more vulnerable to injury.

Once adolescents pass the "weed" stage, the benefits of strength training are obvious and easily understood: increased strength, increased muscle mass, increased muscular endurance, increased resting metabolic rate (which makes it easier to maintain weight), and decreased body fat.

We now know that these benefits apply to men and women of all ages, not just those in their twenties and thirties. Strength training can't remove wrinkles from aging skin, but it can make the muscles and bones beneath that skin stronger and

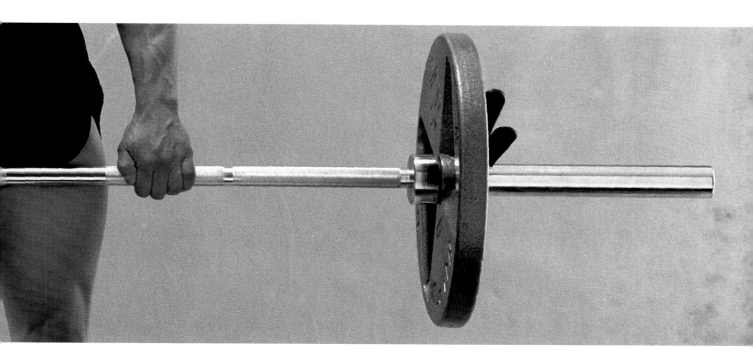

more resistant to injuries. Research on elderly subjects has shown that 2 months of strength training can reverse 2 *decades* of strength and muscle loss. And for the oldest adults, an increase in bone mineral density can be the difference between active, independent lives and the permanent disabilities that can be caused by hip fractures.

A pervasive myth about seniors is that they have to train differently than the rest of us. Certainly, many older adults have preexisting injuries, strength imbalances, and limited flexibility—but so do many younger adults. Many older people often need a longer period of initiation to strength training: more time spent learning the movements, discovering pain-free ranges of motion, and developing flexibility in conjunction with proper exercise technique. Once a person has conquered those hurdles, anything goes. Researchers have used all types of programs with older people, including intense exercises such as those normally used to train Olympic athletes, and they've found that not only did the seniors not break, they enjoyed and benefited from the challenge.

The most important difference between young and old is an older exerciser's need for additional recovery time. Whereas a young adult may need 48 hours to recover from a workout, an older adult may need 72 hours. And whereas a 30-year-old who's new to strength training could start with a Monday-Wednesday-Friday workout schedule, a senior may be better off with a Monday-Thursday schedule, at least at first.

CHAPTER THREE

ROOM
TO
GROW

AS WE'VE JUST DISCUSSED, muscle growth begins as part of the normal physical-maturation process. Once you've reached full maturity, growth happens as a result of the specific tasks you give your muscles. The scientific term for those tasks is **TRAINING STIMULUS**. You probably call it *pumping iron.*

So how does it work, exactly? You pick up a barbell, you lift it this way and that, and the next time you pick it up, 2 days later, your muscles are bigger and stronger, right?

It's a lot more complicated than that, as you probably guessed when you saw the size of this book. So let's look at what happens inside your muscles when you pick up that trusty barbell.

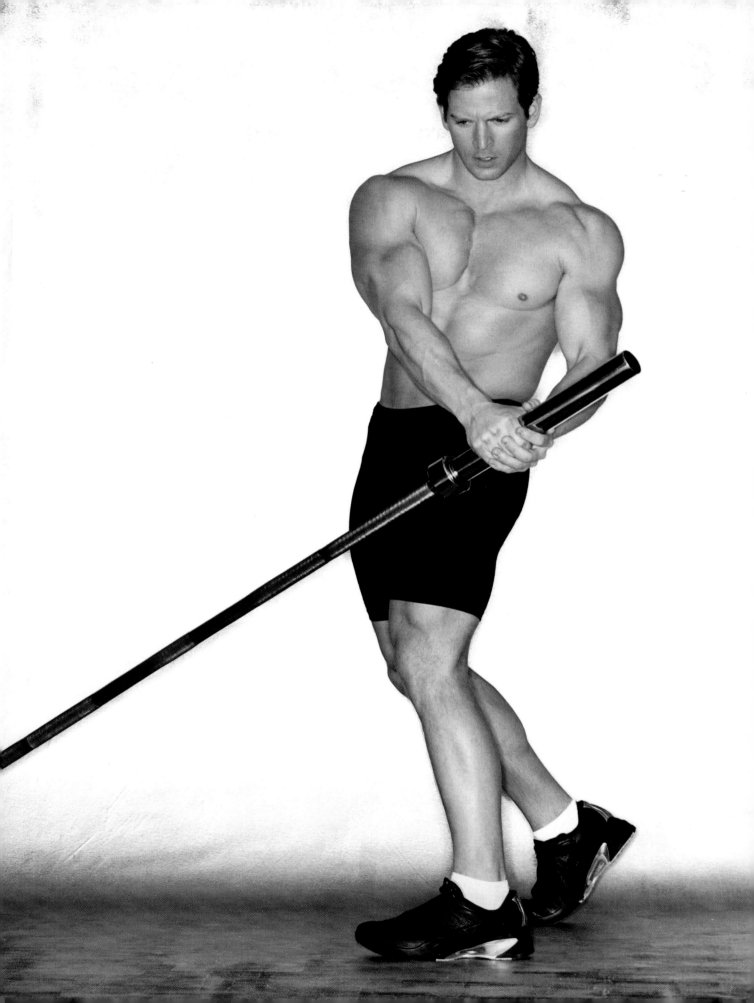

MUSCLE HYPERTROPHY

HYPERTROPHY (hy-PURR-truh-fee) is one of those great words that means nothing to 95 percent of the population and everything to the dedicated muscle enthusiast. It refers to the process by which muscles grow in response to a specific stimulus—such as mechanical work performed by the muscles, an infusion of testosterone, an increase in calories in general or protein calories in particular—or combination of stimuli. An easy way to remember the word: It's the opposite of *atrophy*, or a loss of muscle due to disuse, injury, malnutrition, disease, stress, heavy drug or alcohol use, or watching too many Meg Ryan movies.

To understand hypertrophy, you have to understand the structure of muscle itself. Individual muscle fibers can extend the length of the entire muscle or a fraction of it. They can be a few millimeters long or a few inches. But all skeletal muscle fibers are the same structurally. Each is a bundle of protein strands called **MYOFIBRILS**. These strands are so small that 100 of them equal the diameter of a human hair.

Within each myofibril are even smaller protein filaments called **ACTIN** and **MYOSIN**. The myosin filaments are the big boys here, even though each is about $\frac{1}{10,000}$ the diameter of a hair. Each one is surrounded by six actin filaments. A muscle contracts when structures on the myosin filaments called **CROSS-BRIDGES** grab hold of the actin filaments and pull. This shortens the muscle, creating a lot of force at first and less later, after most of the actin and myosin filaments have already overlapped each other.

Scientists call this sequence *the sliding-filament theory of muscle contraction*. We assume they hedge their bets and term it a "theory" because the protein structures are too small for us to know for sure if this is exactly what happens or if some as-yet-undiscovered process also contributes to muscle contraction.

Strength training with heavy loads increases both the number of myofibrils and the number of myosin and actin filaments within each myofibril. We've just used a lot of syllables to make a rather simple point: When you lift heavy weights, your muscle fibers get bigger. Lift weights diligently and systematically, and at some point the fibers will grow enough for you to notice the change.

MUSCLE TONE,
MUSCLE STRENGTH, MUSCLE SIZE

During the first few days of a strength-training program, your muscles feel tighter. They've responded to training by maintaining a heightened state of readiness, like a rope that you've pulled taut before using it to tie a boat to a dock. This slight increase in muscle tone may help you sit up straighter, or it may make you feel as stiff as the results of Dr. Frankenstein's transplantation experiment.

The next adaptation is an increase in strength that can be noticeable and dramatic from week to week—and even from workout to workout—in the first few weeks of strength training. Your body learns to do the exercises by assigning more and more motor units (groups of muscle fibers, each with its own nerve cell) to the movements; each time it sends more motor units into the fray, you get stronger. When you get stronger, you do the exercises with heavier weights, which prompts your brain to dispatch even more motor units to the task. You get even stronger, then you increase the weights again, and the process continues. This is called **NEURAL ADAPTATION**, and it's a type of motor learning.

Eventually, your body has recruited all its motor units to lift the weights, so it starts adding protein filaments to your muscle fibers to make them grow. Thicker and more numerous protein filaments allow your muscle fibers to generate more force. At this point, probably 4 to 6 weeks into your training program, you finally see an increase in muscle size to accompany your growing strength.

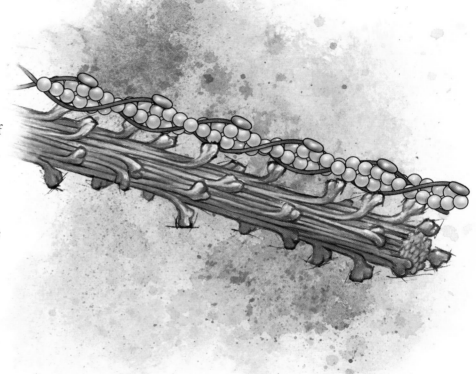

A myosin filament (bottom) and one of its six actin filaments. Protrusions on the myosin filament are cross-bridges that attach to and pull the actin filaments to produce muscle contraction.

Alas, your strength increases now slow down because strength development has become dependent on muscle growth, and muscle growth is a slow process. Your body has little interest in creating or maintaining large muscles, because big muscles require more than their fair share of resources for repair, refueling, and enlargement. Your body perceives this as wasteful, since it knows you don't really need much muscle to power daily activities such as typing or driving your riding lawn

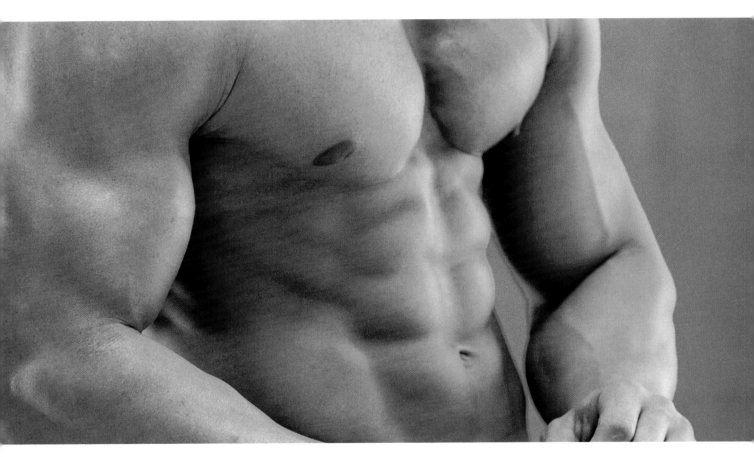

mower. So it sheds muscle tissue at the slightest provocation—illness, injury, malnutrition, or even just fixed or decreased activity. This is why, in most circumstances, if you don't continually give your muscles heavier loads to lift, or force them to lift the same loads faster, you won't grow bigger, more metabolically expensive muscles to display at the community pool. (Ironically, though, if you don't have more muscle than you need for sitting in front of your computer or on top of that John Deere, your slowing metabolism will allow your body to put on unhealthy quantities of fat.)

EARTH TO SATELLITE CELLS: WE NEED BIGGER MUSCLES HERE

We said in the previous chapter that you're born with your maximum lifetime allotment of muscle fibers. Though you can lose fibers as you age, mainstream science holds that you can't gain any. However, some people outside the mainstream believe you can gain new muscle fibers through a process called *hyperplasia*.

Here's the theory: Given a sufficient challenge to muscle fibers—one that verges on producing severe injury—the body produces more fibers by either splitting muscle cells or converting other types of cells into muscle fibers.

Scientists have proven that hyperplasia occurs in animals. In one experiment, researchers hung a weight from one of a bird's wings for an extended period of time, put the bird out of its misery, and then examined the muscle fibers in the weighted wing, comparing them with those of the unweighted one. The muscle fibers in the weighted wing were larger in number as well as size.

In other animal studies, scientists found small muscle fibers within bundles of hypertrophied fibers. At first, the scientists thought these small fibers must be atrophied cells, though it doesn't make much sense that some fibers would have shrunk while the rest grew. So another explanation is that these small fibers were new ones forming in response to the training stimulus.

You can't replicate these studies in humans for two very good reasons. First, in humans even relatively small and simple muscles have too damned many fibers to count. The biceps, for example, could have more than a half-million fibers. Second, even if they could easily count the fibers, scientists wouldn't be allowed to dissect a human after a training study. (Can you imagine getting the proposal for that research through a university's human-subjects committee?)

So we're left to guess whether hyperplasia occurs in humans. Some researchers have observed that bodybuilders' muscle fibers aren't any bigger than the fibers of untrained individuals. (Scientists can measure the size of muscle fibers via biopsy—sticking a needle into a muscle and pulling out a small chunk to be measured in cross section.) Even if you accept that genetically gifted bodybuilders have *more* muscle fibers than average schmoes, why would lifters' years of dedicated training fail to make those fibers bigger than average?

One intriguing theory is that fibers reach a maximum size and then split when they reach it. This certainly happens with human fat cells: You're born with a certain number, and the cells can fill up like balloons. Also like balloons, they can hold only so much before they burst. Rather than literally bursting, fat cells divide, splitting off into separate cells. Is it impossible that this process could happen in muscle cells as well?

A second hypothesis is that hyperplasia is caused by satellite cells, semiformed cells on the outside of muscle fibers that become new fibers when a mysterious physiological switch is turned on. This transformation has been shown to happen when young tissue grows and when muscle is injured. So far, no one has proved that exercise can lead satellite cells to become new fibers.

We'd be remiss if we didn't mention the real wild card in strength training: steroid use. When you look at a bodybuilder who's 5 foot 8 and weighs 260 pounds, with little visible body fat, you have to wonder whether something happened to

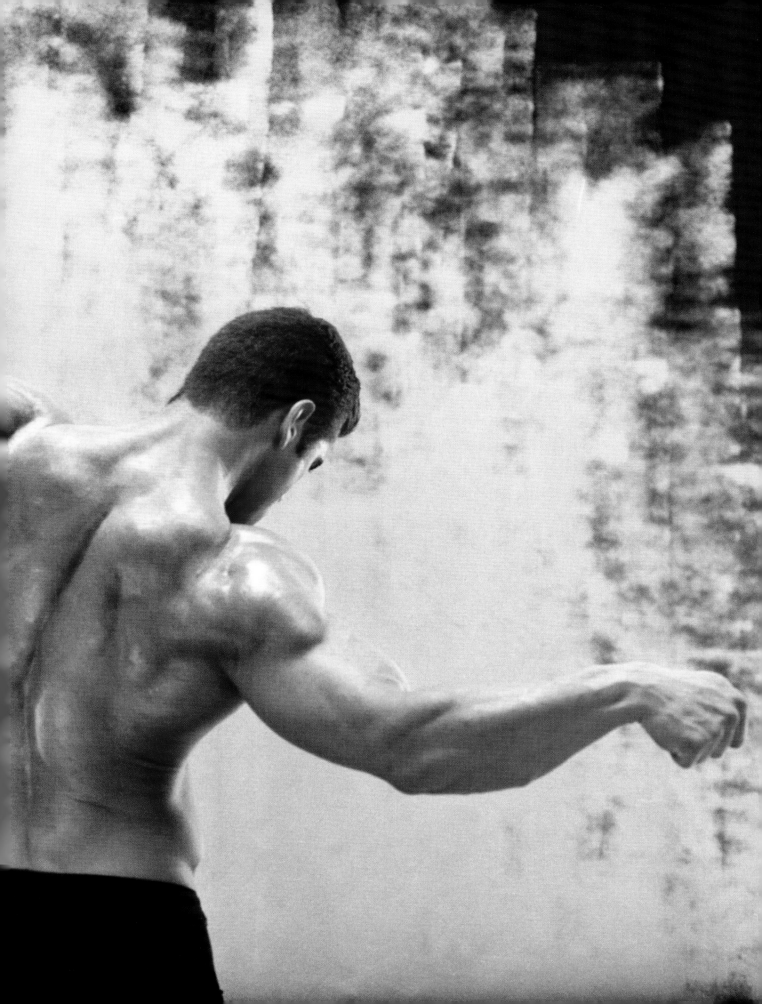

his muscles beyond what we currently understand about hypertrophy and training effects.

THE SHAPE OF MUSCLES TO COME

Scientists concede that hyperplasia is theoretically possible—and maybe even probable—in athletes who train long enough and hard enough. (The caveat is it's thought to account for only 5 to 10 percent of total training-induced muscle growth.)

A concept that's further afield is that dedicated bodybuilders can induce regional hypertrophy, making one part of a muscle bigger by selectively exercising it harder than other parts. It's fun to scoff at trainers who allege that a particular exercise can develop the "inner" or "outer" chest, or the "upper" or "lower" biceps. You can look at anatomical illustrations of human muscles—such as the ones in part two of this book—and see that these muscle classifications simply don't exist. Fibers in the pectoral muscle, for example, run latitudinally, so it should be impossible to selectively develop one end without also developing the other.

Before discounting regional hypertrophy, we should note that there's a tiny shred of truth behind bodybuilders' belief that they can "shape" their muscles. Some muscles are broken up into compartments, with different motor units given specific tasks within each compartment. In some muscles, compartmental divisions are obvious. For example, the pectoral muscle clearly has upper, middle, and lower segments, with some of the fibers in the upper portion attaching to the clavicle (collarbone) and some in the lower portion attaching to connective tissue that in turn connects to the upper abdominals. So it makes sense that these regions respond differently to various exercises, and every lifter in every gym knows that doing chest presses on an incline bench works the upper pectorals harder than other regions of the muscles, and that doing decline presses and dips works the lower portion the hardest.

The trapezius is another muscle with clear divisions between upper, middle, and lower portions, and it's indisputable that these regions have separate functions. The upper portion elevates the scapula (shoulder blade), whereas the middle portion retracts, or pulls back, the scapula, and the lower portion depresses it. So a

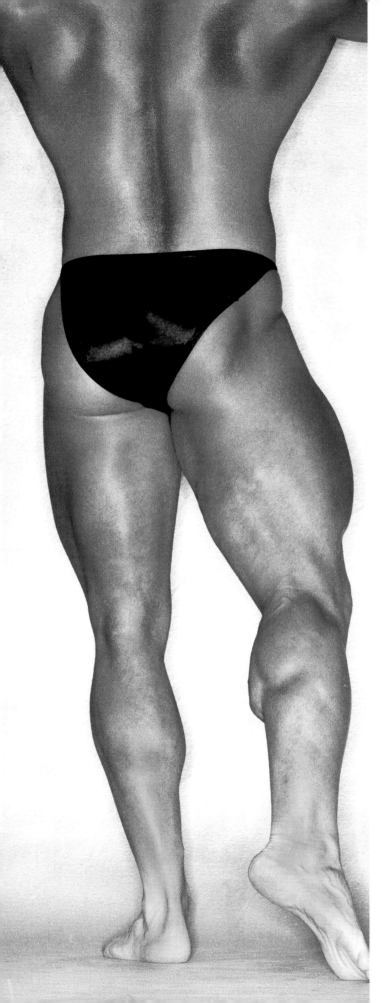

shoulder shrug or upright row works the upper trapezius, a bent-over or horizontal rowing movement uses the middle part, and a pullup or lat pulldown hits the lower part the hardest.

The biceps, on the front of the upper arm, has two separate portions that diverge at the top of the arm and thus have slightly different functions. The outer portion, also called the long head, works harder when your hands are closer together during a biceps curl and also helps lift your upper arm in front of your torso, as when you do a shoulder exercise called a front raise. The inner portion, or short head, works harder on a wide-grip biceps curl, when your hands are farther apart.

Most intermediate- and advanced-level bodybuilders understand this, and electromyographic studies have confirmed it. The million-dollar question, for those most interested in the aesthetic benefits of strength training, is whether you can change the shape of the biceps. For example, can a genetically short muscle belly (the part that bulges upward) be made longer with exercises that specifically target the lower quarter or third of the muscle?

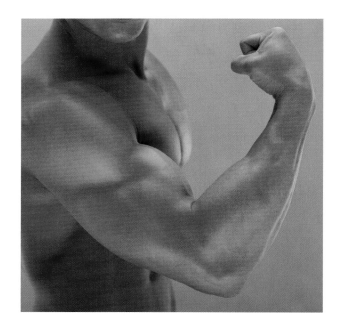

Exercise physiologist Jose Antonio, Ph.D., an adjunct professor at Florida Atlantic University in Boca Raton, has proposed a couple of mechanisms by which this may be possible. First, because the muscle fibers are bound more tightly by connective tissue on the ends of a muscle, those fibers may sustain more damage during heavy strength training, and with more damage may come more growth to defend the muscle against further damage. Second, type I and type II fibers aren't always distributed evenly throughout a muscle. In the case of the biceps, the lower end of the muscle, near the elbow, contains more type II fibers than does the top, near the shoulder. So it's possible that intense weight training would produce more growth in the lower part of the muscle, since type II fibers have more growth potential than type I fibers.

None of this means that a specific exercise will preferentially target the "lower" biceps. It just means that the muscle-building process remains mysterious in many ways, and that muscle growth doesn't occur predictably or uniformly.

HORMONAL HARMONY

A component of the muscle-building process that is on solid scientific ground is the work performed by testosterone and your other hormones—primarily growth hormone, but also including insulin, various stress hormones, and others. Your hormones start working during exercise in response to the intensity and duration of your effort. If your exercise intensity is high enough, your blood will be flooded with

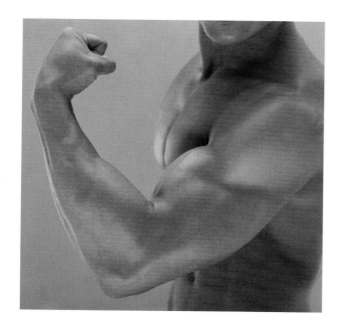

hormones at 10 to 20 times their resting levels. These hormones then keep working after exercise to repair and remodel your muscle tissue so you'll be better prepared for your next workout.

TESTOSTERONE. The mechanism by which testosterone helps your muscles grow isn't well-understood, though the hormone is thought to interact directly with DNA. In any case, all you care about is that you can increase the amount of testosterone your body releases in response to strength training. Here's how.

- Do the exercises that use the most muscle mass, such as squats, deadlifts, and power cleans.

- Use heavy weights: at least 85 percent of the most weight you can lift once on any given exercise.

- Do a lot of work: multiple exercises, multiple sets, multiple repetitions.

- Keep rest periods fairly short: 30 to 60 seconds.

- Train consistently for at least 2 years.

Of course, you can't do all these things at the same time. For example, when you exercise a lot of muscle mass using really heavy weights, you can't do a high volume of exercise, nor can you train effectively with short rest periods. (This is among the many reasons why you must periodize workout programs—that is, why you have to change your exercises, sets, repetitions, and rest periods systematically over a period of time. It's impossible to get all the benefits by training one way indefinitely.)

Testosterone levels don't have to stay elevated to build muscle. In fact, testosterone spikes during and immediately after your workout, then dips dramatically. That means, for hours after exercise, you walk around with testosterone levels lower than when you walked into the gym.

Has your principal muscle-building hormone abandoned you? Hardly. More likely, the acute increase in testosterone in response to your workout helps you get the desired results from the exercise, and the subsequent dip means the hormone has done its job.

However, your resting testosterone level—the chronic level in your bloodstream, separate from the rise and fall in response to training—does seem to increase after 2 years of serious training. This could be your body's way of ensuring that you continue to make gains even though your body is getting close to its genetic limits for strength and muscle size.

Diet has a profound effect on your chronic, resting testosterone level. A vegetarian diet lowers your level, whereas a meat-rich, omnivorous diet raises it. Likewise, a low-fat diet is also a low-testosterone diet. Your testosterone level is raised by two types of fat: saturated (found mostly in meat and other animal products) and monounsaturated (found in meat as well as in olives, peanuts, and avocadoes).

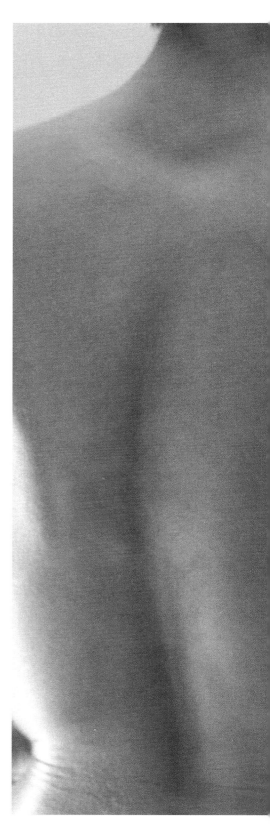

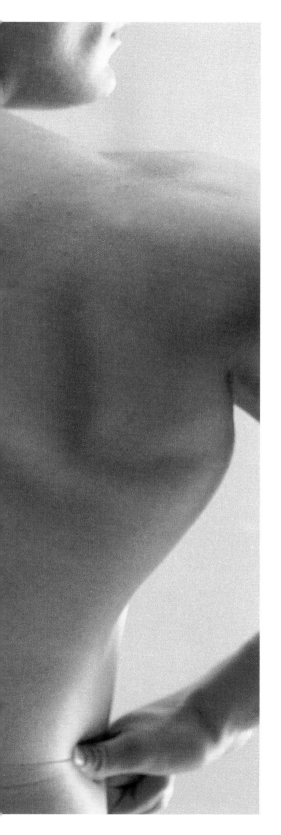

GROWTH HORMONE (GH). If testosterone is the primary hormone for building strength, growth hormone is perhaps most important for body composition—burning body fat for energy and ensuring that protein is transported to muscle cells for synthesis.

Your pituitary gland releases GH in spurts, the biggest of which occurs during sleep. All you need to do to prompt this spurt is fall asleep at a reasonable hour, reasonably sober. (Alcohol interferes with GH release.)

The next-biggest GH release comes in response to exercise. A few ways to manipulate GH to serve your goals:

- Exercise with vigor and intensity. Using unchallenging weights for garbage reps won't trigger a major GH release.

- Moderate repetitions (10) and short rest periods (1 minute) produce higher GH concentrations than fewer repetitions and longer rest periods. When you pump out sets of 10 reps with short rest periods, your muscles generate a waste product called lactate that produces a telltale discomfort. Lactate may trigger GH release, or your body may produce GH and lactate in response to the same stimuli. Either way, when you feel the burn, GH isn't far behind.

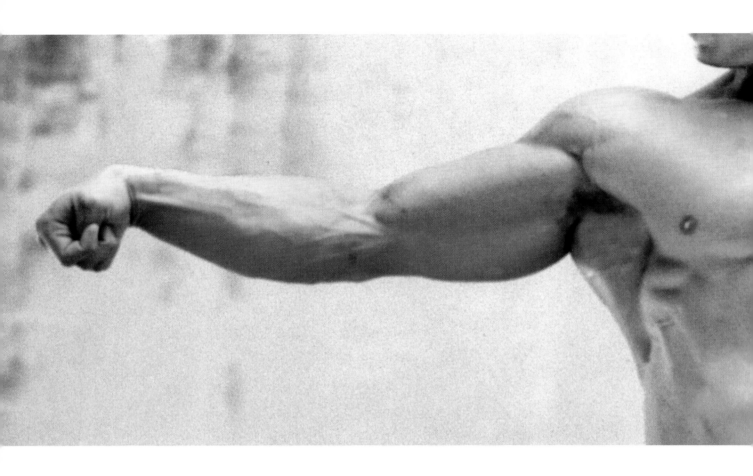

In addition to burning fat and transporting protein, GH also increases your body's production of connective tissues, including collagen and cartilage. This could explain why, compared with other strength and power athletes, bodybuilders have a lot of extra connective tissue inside their muscles. Their lifting protocols involve lots of sets and repetitions, generating buckets of lactate and, therefore, GH.

Interestingly, GH decreases with a high-carbohydrate diet, which helps explain why a diet featuring equal amounts of carbohydrate and fat seems to produce better body composition in response to strength training than a high-carb, low-fat diet does.

Eating fat immediately after a workout can blunt GH release. So it seems best to restrict post-workout snacks to just protein and carbohydrate, avoiding fat until at least an hour after a workout.

INSULIN. This hormone produced by your pancreas is crucial to helping your body recover from strength training. If you look at strength training as a war movie starring your muscles, insulin is the courageous soldier who delivers ammo to the front lines under heavy fire. The protein in your muscles is always breaking down

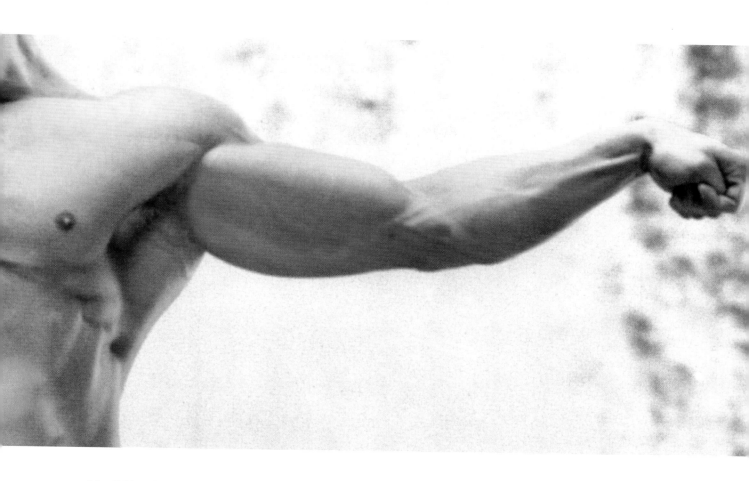

and building back up, but after exercise, it's *really* breaking down, and it won't stop until it has the carbohydrate and protein that only insulin can deliver.

Though insulin is capable of heroism in the heat of battle, it's nothing but trouble after the shooting ends. Once your muscles have begun recovering, insulin tells your body to do two bad things: burn carbohydrate for energy and store fat (since you don't need to use fat for energy post-exercise).

The last thing you want is for your body to store fat. So your ideal strategy is somewhat obvious here: Eat carbohydrate and protein before and after exercise, and perhaps at the start of the day, but minimize carbs at other times so your body is forced to burn fat instead. This strategy seems to work well with all the hormones we've discussed so far.

Conveniently, strength training improves your body's sensitivity to insulin, making just a little of the hormone go a longer way. This not only helps minimize body-fat storage but also prevents insulin resistance, a condition in which your body, for unknown reasons, doesn't use the hormone effectively. If you develop in-sulin resistance, your pancreas cranks out more and more insulin in an attempt to force your body to respond to the hormone. Eventually, this process poops itself out: Your pancreas gives up and stops producing any insulin at all, at which point you have type 2 diabetes and are unable to properly metabolize carbohydrate. Strength training can help prevent this vicious circle.

INSULIN-LIKE GROWTH FACTORS (IGFs). Whereas testosterone and growth hormone go to work immediately during and after exercise, IGFs are released as part of a long and complicated chain of events triggered by GH release. IGFs are produced by the liver but are stored in fat and muscle cells, from which they seem to do their muscle-building work. And they don't start this work until 8 to 29 hours after the initial stimulus.

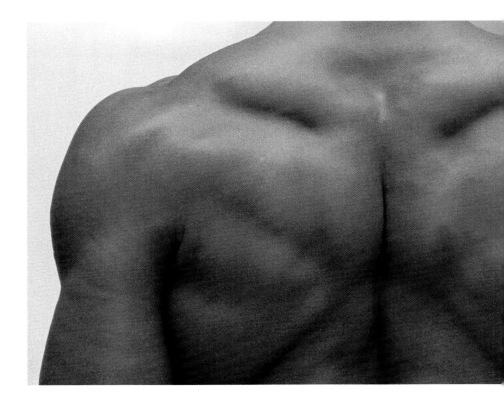

If you already have a high level in your blood, your cells may not release any IGFs in response to exercise. The converse also seems to occur: When your blood's IGF level is low, your cells release more.

IGFs—the best-known of which is IGF-I—may also respond better with pre- and post-exercise carbohydrate-protein supplements. This makes sense, of course, since IGF action is so closely linked to GH release.

ADRENAL HORMONES. One group of stress hormones produced by the adrenal gland is called the *catecholamines*. The most important of these, *epinephrine*—which you know as *adrenaline*—may be the first hormone to respond to exercise, and its actions make the other hormonal responses possible. It stimulates your nervous system, allowing you to do more work, and dilates blood vessels, allowing blood to flow more freely into your muscles. These two effects help your muscles contract faster and allow more nutrients to reach your muscles through the bloodstream. A companion hormone, *noradrenaline*, increases blood pressure, which is why you don't want this level of neural stimulation going on all day, every day. An hour or two a day is great; 12 hours a day could be deadly.

The catecholamines don't seem to have a direct muscle-building effect. Rather, they help increase the secretion rates of other hormones, primarily testosterone. And the same stimuli that increase GH—heavy exercise volume, with little rest between sets—also lead to a bigger catecholamine response.

The most famous stress-induced adrenal hormone is *cortisol*, a compound that preserves the carbohydrate energy stores (or glycogen) in your muscles. You stimulate cortisol release by doing lots of sets and lots of repetitions with short rest periods, depleting glycogen. In an attempt to conserve your remaining glycogen, cortisol converts muscle protein to carbohydrate for energy. This muscle breakdown—a type of stress—is important to the muscle-building process in that you have to disrupt the normal functions of your muscles to convince them they need to grow. Cortisol is the tough drill sergeant who breaks you down before you build yourself back up.

We can't say that the drill sergeant is personally responsible for building you back up, because then the metaphor falls apart; cortisol also inhibits protein synthesis, preferring to convert the dietary protein in your bloodstream to carbohydrate energy before it's synthesized, rather than going to all the trouble of pulling protein out of muscle tissue.

MUSCLE CHOW

Despite the fact that carbohydrate metabolism and protein synthesis are vital to the muscle-building process, many guys don't pay enough attention to the food they eat. So let's look at the role each of the three macronutrients—protein, carbohydrate, and fat—plays in muscle growth.

PROTEIN. The mythology surrounding protein and muscle building could fill a book on its own, even though the science is fairly straightforward. Researchers have determined that a person trying to build muscle needs between 1.5 and 2 grams of protein per kilogram of body weight each day. A kilogram is 2.2 pounds, so a 180-pound man who's training hard in the weight room can probably use, at most, 164 grams of protein a day. Many nutritionists like to use the lower number of 1.5 grams of protein per kilogram of body weight. Trainers and other gym rats tend to round the number up to 1 gram of protein per pound of body weight daily.

So the 180-pound guy who's lifting weights with some intensity three or four times a week is told he needs anywhere from 123 to 180 grams of protein per day. That's a pretty big range.

The minimalist reasoning goes like this: Your body isn't going to build more muscle just because you eat more protein. So you should fill up on other types of foods—carbohydrates and healthy fats—to provide energy. Besides, warn the minimalists, too much protein can be dangerous if you have preexisting liver or kidney disease.

The maximalist camp doesn't want to miss any opportunity to build muscle, and research shows that your body synthesizes more protein—turns it into lean body tissue, in other words—in the 24 to 48 hours following a strenuous resistance workout than it does normally. So this group recommends ingesting lots of protein at every meal. Since there's no evidence that protein is dangerous to healthy human organs, in any quantity, it's better to err on the high side. If you lose the excess through your urine, or if a little gets converted to carbohydrate for energy, or even to fat, so what? They claim that it's better than not getting enough protein to fully exploit the muscle-building stimulus you get in the gym three or four times a week.

We tend to agree with both sides. If you're young, lean, and trying to gain weight, a lot of extra protein—more than 2 grams per pound of body weight—may not help. Protein has two qualities that help weight loss and may curtail weight gain. First, protein is metabolically expensive for your body to process. Your body burns about 20 percent of each protein calorie just digesting that protein. (It burns about 8 percent of carbohydrate and 2 percent of fat during digestion. This phenomenon is called *the thermic effect of feeding*, and it accounts for about 10 percent of the calories you burn each day.)

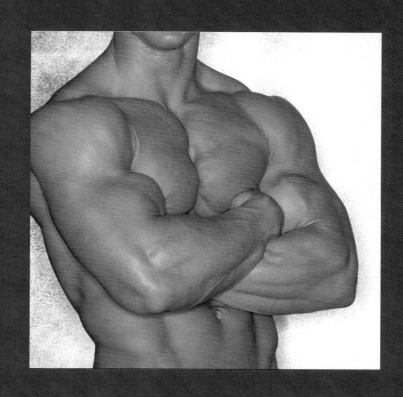

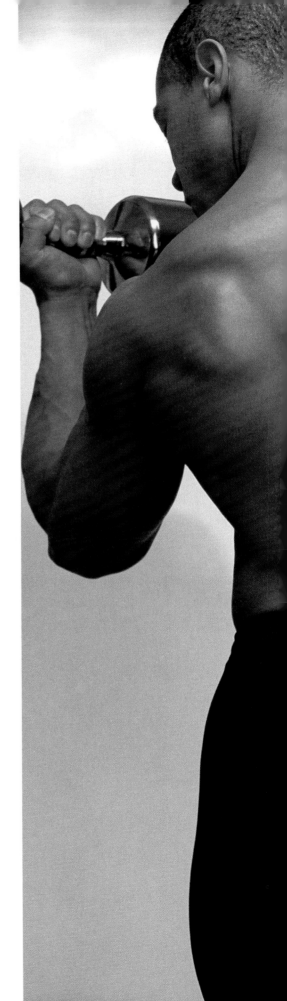

Second, protein creates a high level of satiety, both during meals and between them. In other words, it makes you feel fuller faster and keeps you feeling full longer between meals. Once more, this is a great tool for weight loss but perhaps not advisable when you're trying to gain. (This effect does wear off as you get used to a higher-protein diet, however, so it may not affect long-term weight gain or weight loss.)

On the other hand, if you're trying to lose weight via serious strength training, you may need to take in more than the recommended upper limit of protein while cutting back on fat or carbohydrate. Without extra protein, your body could lose muscle mass along with fat, and lost muscle means a slower metabolism. A slower metabolism means your weight loss stalls and you regain weight faster.

The highest-quality protein is found in animal foods: meat, fish, eggs, and milk and other dairy products. And the use of whey-protein and meal-replacement powders seems to be gaining grudging support among nutritionists because of the convenience, the high quality of the protein, and the emerging research showing that these supplements are safe and useful when you don't have time to bake a chicken breast or whip up an omelet.

The timing of protein intake has gotten more attention recently. Intriguing research at the University of Texas Medical Branch shows

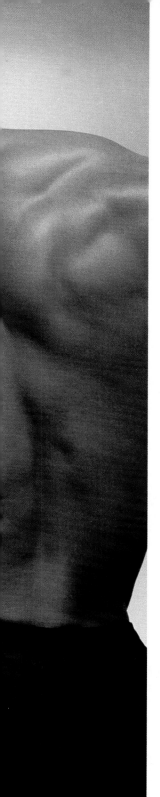

that ingesting a protein-carbohydrate supplement before doing strength training leads to more protein synthesis than a post-workout supplement does. The most likely reason: Bloodflow increases during exercise, so if you have more protein in your blood during exercise, more protein goes to your muscles.

CARBOHYDRATE. The arguments about optimum protein intake are mild compared to the bellowing over carbohydrate. Many nutritionists—perhaps most—remain stuck on the idea that because carbohydrate is the primary source of energy during exercise, it should make up the majority of an exerciser's diet (as well as a nonexerciser's diet, for that matter, since they also think that most everyone should eat less fat and protein).

This recommendation, although well-intentioned, doesn't seem to work particularly well in men who are trying to build muscle without gaining fat or trying to lose fat while retaining muscle. True, carbohydrate is your body's fuel of choice during intense, short-duration exercise, including strength training. However, strength training itself may not burn all that much fuel—perhaps 300 to 500 calories in a 1-hour workout, depending on your size and ambitions. (In the 24 to 48 hours following a hard workout, you do burn more calories than usual, but that seems to occur regardless of the composition of your diet.) You can get 300 calories from just 75 grams of carbohydrate, and you can eat that amount of carbs without really thinking about it. If you have 2 cups of Kellogg's raisin bran for breakfast, that's 74 grams of carbohydrate right there, before you add a drop of milk.

Carbohydrate is crucial at two points in the muscle-building process: the pre- and post-exercise meals, when carbs and protein combine to stimulate insulin, the hormone that drives nutrients to your muscles. Until recently, this carb-and-protein infusion was considered most important after exercise. Since the latest

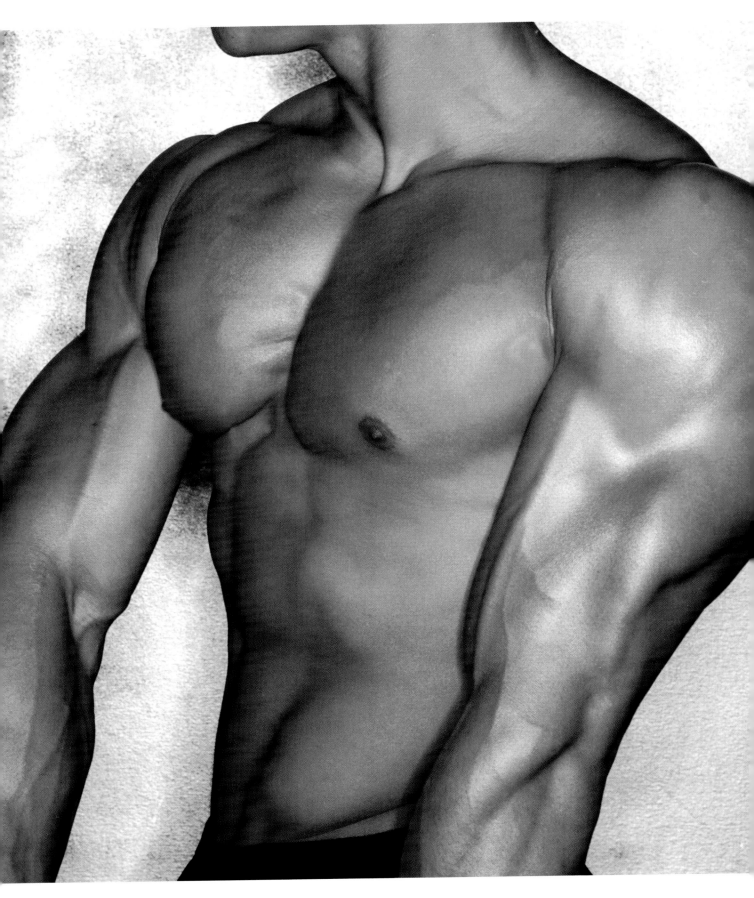

research shows the significance of pre-exercise nutrition, many experts now advise lifters to eat carbs and protein within an hour before exercise and again immediately after.

For men trying to build muscle, it's hard to say whether carbohydrate matters at all at other times of the day, especially if three or four weekly weight workouts constitute all the exercise they get. Some experts recommend very low carbohydrate diets for strength trainers who are most interested in aesthetics—having the most muscle with the least fat. Other authorities recommend the modern bodybuilding diet: one that is high in carbohydrate, moderate to high in protein, and very low in fat.

We wish we could tell you there's a rule, such as "Eat 100 grams of carbohydrate per hour of exercise each day." There isn't any such rule. (Although our hypothetical one might not be too bad, now that we've thought of it.) If you're struggling to gain weight, you may want to consider adding more carbohydrate to your diet. If you're fighting to lose fat, it makes sense to cut carbs from your diet since they're easily converted to fat when they aren't needed for immediate energy and there's no room in your muscles to store them. Plus, without carbohydrate for energy, your body shifts to using fat, which is the metabolic equivalent of a state of grace. That's why *lean, mean, carb-burnin' machine* has never become a catch phrase.

FAT. Fat's reformation in the late 1990s and early '00s has been stunning. After a solid 2 decades of low-fat everything, accompanied by skyrocketing obesity throughout the world, weight-loss researchers and practitioners are coming back to an old idea: Dietary fat, in the absence of carbohydrate, does not make you fat. As we've just discussed, it's excess carbohydrate that makes you fat.

In muscle building, fat plays two roles. First, it helps preserve nitrogen. Protein is 16 percent nitrogen, so nitrogen balance is the most reliable indicator of whether your body is building muscle (denoted by positive nitrogen balance, or an *anabolic state*) or breaking it down (signaled by negative nitrogen balance, or a *catabolic state*). Second, fat increases testosterone levels.

The next chapter will give you practical guidelines for planning healthful meals that include all three macronutrients to maximize muscle growth.

FEEDING YOUR MUSCLES

TO BUILD YOUR MUSCLES, you must give them extra calories—that is, you must eat more calories than you burn off. We don't believe there's any magic ratio of protein, carbohydrate, and fat that will optimize muscle gain. Simply eat enough food while performing the workouts in this book, and you will gain weight.

Some newcomers to strength training will find that their bodies respond so rapidly to the muscle-building workout stimulus that they build muscle and lose fat simultaneously, with a gain or no change in overall body weight. Most guys aren't so lucky. If you've been training consistently for at least 1 year, you'll have to accept that when you increase your calorie intake to gain muscle, you'll also gain some fat. So at some point, you'll need to concentrate on pure fat loss by creating a calorie deficit.

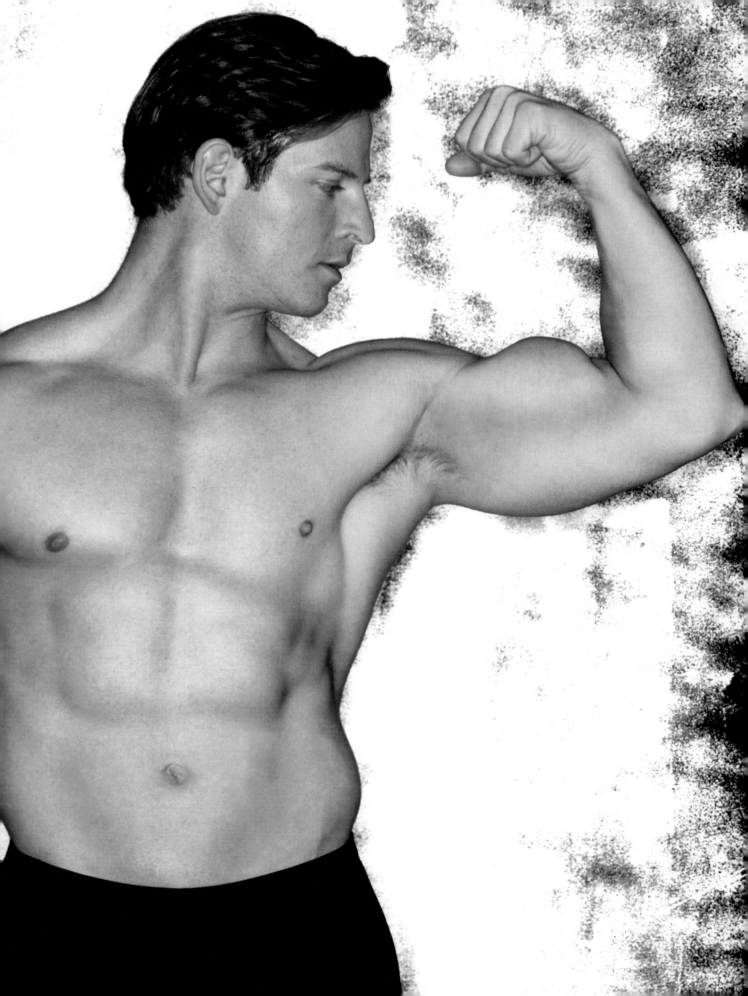

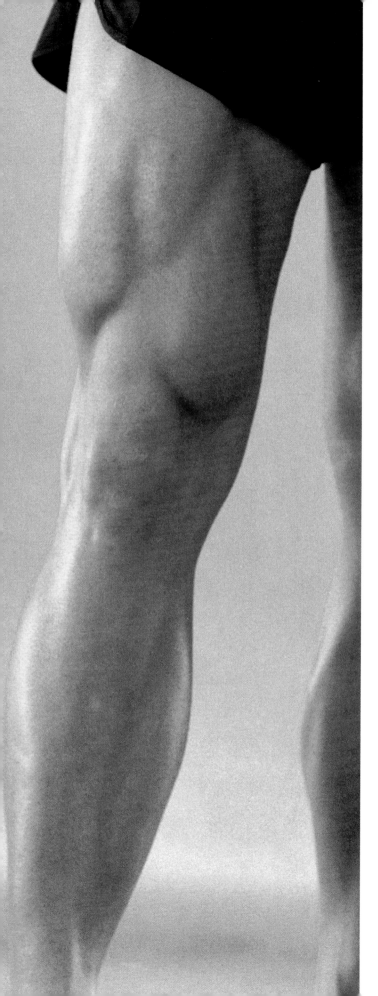

You decide how to schedule your muscle-building and fat-loss phases. You can do a full 6-month workout program while eating more, switching to a fat-loss phase only after completing that program. Or you can eat less during the program, to cut weight throughout. A third option is to jump-start fat loss by cutting calories when you first start a program, increase calories in the second and third (hypertrophy and strength) stages to bulk up a bit, and then cut again in the fourth, power phase.

HOW MUCH TO EAT

It's easy for us to say "Eat more to gain muscle" and "Eat less to lose fat." That still leaves you with a big question: more or less than what? You need a baseline number to start with.

So whip out the calculator, and let's figure out that magic number.

STEP 1: YOUR WEIGHT IN POUNDS ___ × 11 = ___ YOUR BASIC CALORIE NEEDS
This calculation tells you the amount of energy you'd burn without eating or exercising. It reveals your basic calorie needs—the caloric cost of being you.

STEP 2: YOUR BASIC CALORIE NEEDS ____ × CALORIC COST OF YOUR ACTIVITY LEVEL ___ % (FROM FOLLOWING CHART) = ___ YOUR METABOLIC RATE

Since you do eat and exercise, the total number of calories your body burns in a day is higher than your basic calorie needs. How much higher depends on your age, the amount of muscle you have, and the intensity at which you make that muscle work. Multiply your basic calorie needs by one of the following percentages to estimate the number of calories you burn metabolically. (Note that these percentages are averages; your actual metabolism may be faster or slower than these typical rates.)

ACTIVITY LEVEL	AGE		
	<30	30–40	>40
Mostly sedentary	30%	25%	20%
Moderately active	40%	35%	30%
Dedicated exerciser or athlete	50%	45%	40%

STEP 3: YOUR BASIC CALORIE NEEDS ___ + YOUR METABOLIC RATE ___ = ___ YOUR MAINTENANCE TOTAL

This sum reveals how many calories you need just to maintain your current body composition, without growing muscle or shedding fat.

STEP 4: YOUR MAINTENANCE TOTAL ___ + 500 = ___ TO GAIN MUSCLE

To build muscle, increase your daily calorie intake by 500 calories.

STEP 5: YOUR MAINTENANCE TOTAL ___ − 500 = ___ TO LOSE FAT

To lose weight, subtract 500 calories a day.

The amount of energy in a pound of fat equals 3,500 calories, so in a perfect world, creating a daily surplus or deficit of 500 calories would allow weight gain or weight loss of 1 pound a week. This equation is most accurate when you try to lose weight. Muscle gain is less predictable than fat loss, because adding calories and moving a heavier body both speed up your metabolism.

Let's run an example. Say you weigh 165 pounds, you're under 30, and you're extremely active, lifting 3 days a week and playing sports or doing some other type of intense exercise on other days. You want to gain some solid muscle mass.

Step 1: 165 × 11 = 1,815

Step 2: 1,815 × 0.5 = 907.5

Step 3: 1,815 + 907.5 = 2,722.5

Step 4: 2,722 + 500 = 3,222.5

In other words, you need to eat more than 3,200 calories a day to gain muscle mass.

Now say you're a 45-year-old, 230-pound guy who's mostly sedentary and wants to lose weight aggressively—2 pounds a week.

Step 1: 230 × 11 = 2,530

Step 2: 2,530 × 0.2 = 506

Step 3: 2,530 + 506 = 3,036

Step 4: 3,036 − 1,000 = 2,036

WHAT TO EAT

While you're doing the workouts in this book, your first dietary consideration is to get enough protein, either to build muscle or maintain muscle while shedding fat. We recommend close to a gram of protein per pound of body weight.

If you're a lean, very active guy trying to pack on muscle, you should hedge your bets with more than a gram of protein per pound, since extra dietary protein increases protein synthesis in the body.

At the same time, you need plenty of easily available fuel in the form of carbohydrate. (The more intense the activity, the more carbohydrate your body uses for energy.) Without a lot of carbs, you run the risk that your body will dip into your protein reserves for the energy it needs. Those protein reserves are in your muscles—the last place from which you want to donate energy.

Finally, you need enough fat to help produce testosterone and other anabolic hormones. And the fat can be used for energy, too, especially during any low-intensity activities—shooting hoops, playing golf, riding a bike.

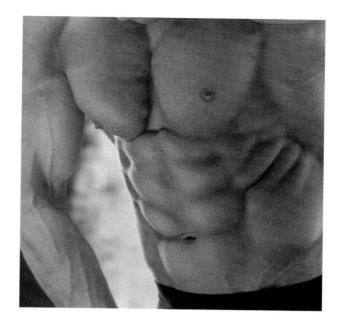

When trying to shed fat, you have a slightly different set of concerns. You need protein to maintain your muscle even though you can't expect to gain muscle mass while trying to lose 2 pounds a week. You want those pounds to come entirely from your fat stores, so you shouldn't eat a lot of carbohydrate. Eating carbs signals your body to burn carbs. Eat fat, though, and your body will be more willing to use fat for energy.

However, you shouldn't completely forgo carbohydrate. You need some for energy during exercise; you need fruits, vegetables, and whole grains for health reasons; and you don't want to feel deprived of the foods that comprise the vast majority of the available calories in the food chain. You're already cutting out a large chunk of your daily calories—don't pile on needless suffering by eating like a freak.

Does all this mean you have to follow a formal diet, counting every calorie? We think the answer is yes. If you're trying—and failing—to grow muscle or lose fat, you probably do need to follow a carefully calculated diet, at least for a while. Start by determining your actual food intake: Keep a 3-day food diary, making a list of everything you eat during that 72-hour period. Use a good calorie-counting Web site, such as www.usda.gov, to figure out your average daily calorie intake. Then you'll be able cut or add calories as necessary to reach the total you calculated back on page 53.

A simpler strategy is to examine your diet for less healthful foods and replace those with better ones. Here's a chart that's specially designed to make this easy.

Bad Foods	They're Bad Because . . .	Except . . .	Better Foods
PROTEIN			
Beef or pork ribs Brisket Ground beef Pork sausage	Very high in saturated fat, which is linked to heart disease; goes down so fast your body doesn't have time to activate its appetite-controlling mechanisms		Eggs Fish, including water-packed canned tuna Lean cuts such as sirloin, flank, or tenderloin 90% lean ground beef or turkey, chewed slowly Reduced-fat lunchmeats (roast beef, turkey, ham) Skinless chicken or turkey breast Turkey sausage Whey-protein or whey-and-casein-protein supplements
STARCHES			
Pasta Potatoes	Quickly digested, leaving you feeling hungry again soon after	Immediately before or after a workout, when you can combine them with good protein such as eggs or low-fat dairy products	Rye bread Sweet potatoes Whole grain breads, pastas, rice Whole wheat baked tortillas Whole wheat pitas
Sugar-laden or low-fiber breakfast cereals	Best to eat carbohydrate that packs some fiber, because fiber slows the emptying of food from your stomach, making you feel fuller longer; fiber is also linked to a lower risk of heart disease		All-Bran Fiber One Grape-Nuts Plain old-fashioned oatmeal (not instant) Raisin bran Shredded Wheat Shredded Wheat 'N Bran
White bread White rice			
DAIRY			
Whole milk and other full-fat dairy products	High in saturated fat		2%, 1%, or fat-free milk and other dairy products

Bad Foods	They're Bad Because . . .	Except . . .	Better Foods
FRUITS			
Dried fruit, such as raisins and prunes	Too easy to eat too much at one sitting		Apples Bananas Blackberries Blueberries Cherries Grapefruit Kiwifruit Oranges Pears Plums Raspberries Strawberries
VEGETABLES			
Carrots Corn	Relatively high in sugar and low in nutrients		Asparagus Avocado Broccoli Brussels sprouts Cauliflower Eggplant Green beans Lettuce (the darker the better) Mushrooms Onions Peas Peppers Spinach Tomatoes Zucchini
NUTS AND SEEDS			
Macadamia nuts			Almonds Brazil nuts Peanuts (technically a vegetable, but usually included in this category) Pecans Sunflower seeds Walnuts

Bad Foods	They're Bad Because . . .	Except . . .	Better Foods
SNACKS			
Chips, pretzels	Even low-fat chips are nothing but extra carbohydrate, usually laden with salt that causes your body to retain water and look fatter than it actually is	At a party, a few chips can go a long way if you dip them in guacamole, which is rich in monounsaturated fat (the same good fat found in olive oil)	Apples, peanut butter, string cheese—foods with as many (if not more) calories but with fat and protein to help you feel fuller, longer
BEVERAGES			
Apple juice Flavored ice tea Juice drinks	Apple juice is high in fructose, the one sugar that doesn't trigger an insulin response, meaning it doesn't shut off your appetite; plus, fructose is more easily stored as fat		Coffee (limited amounts) Crystal Light Diet soda Herbal tea Pure fruit juice (limited quantities) such as orange juice or grape juice
Soda	Most sodas are sweetened with high-fructose corn syrup		Tea Unsweetened seltzer Water
FATS AND OILS			
Butter Coconut oil Corn oil	High in saturated fat High in omega-6 fatty acids, which can trigger inflammation	Used sparingly, butter can turn a slice of whole grain toast into a decent snack since it's flavorful and the fat helps you feel full longer	Benecol spread Canola oil Flaxseed oil Olive oil Peanut oil Sesame oil Smart Balance spread
Margarine Vegetable shortening	High in trans fats, thought to be even more unhealthy than saturated fat		

WHEN TO EAT

The benefits of eating the right foods diminish if you don't get the frequency and timing right. These two factors can be summed up pretty easily: Eat five or six small meals throughout the day, whether your goal is pure muscle growth (without significant fat accumulation) or pure fat depletion (without significant muscle loss).

Think of your body as a fireplace, suggests Douglas Kalman, R.D., a spokesperson for the American College of Sports Medicine who helped compile the preceding charts. Would you expect a fireplace to burn consistently throughout the day, keeping your living room at a steady temperature, if you threw logs into it two or three times a day and left it alone the rest of the time? Hell, no. If you wanted the room to remain at a consistent, comfortable temperature, you'd replenish the tinder every couple of hours. And you'd never throw a huge stack of wood on the fire at any one time—the room would get too hot.

Now you know why it seems that lean, muscular people are always eating. When you're trying to build muscle, frequent small feedings allow you to get enough calories throughout the day without ever wolfing down 1,000-calorie meals. When you're trying to lose fat while sparing muscle, five or six small meals and snacks at regular intervals let you eat less overall without feeling ravenous and deprived.

Here's the best, simplest way to schedule your meals.

- ■ Eat your first meal as soon as you can after getting up in the morning—you want your fire to start burning as quickly as possible.

- ■ Try to eat every 3 hours after that.

- ■ Have a pre-workout snack or drink about an hour prior to exercise and a post-workout snack or drink within 1 hour of completing your exercise.

You'll recall that chapter three mentioned the need for carbohydrate and protein right before a workout and then again soon after. Most research shows that a carbohydrate-protein ratio of between 2-to-1 and 4-to-1 works best. You don't need fat in your pre- or post-exercise meals or drinks, since it could blunt the fat-burning, muscle-building effects of growth hormone.

You can eliminate macronutrient guesswork with the prepackaged powders and bars you find in GNC and other sports-supplement outlets—these products are formulated to the proper ratios. You just have to read (and understand) the nutrition information on the labels. Here's a quick tutorial: The first number in the chart is always fat, and the last is protein. Carbohydrate is listed in the middle, and total calories are listed to the left or above the chart.

A post-workout shake is one of the great pleasures of the muscle-building process—provided, of course, that your shake tastes like something other than chalk. Here are a few recipes we like, courtesy of Kalman. Each has a 2-to-1 carbohydrate-protein ratio, with just enough fat to provide some flavor and texture.

THE BASIC BODYBUILDER (187 calories)

1 teaspoon protein powder in the flavor of your choice

1 cup 1% milk

1 banana

THE GRAPEFUL BLEND (330 calories)

1 scoop vanilla-flavor Met-Rx Protein Plus

1 teaspoon flaxseed oil

½ cup fat-free, sugar-free plain or vanilla yogurt

1 cup grape juice

THE PB SHAKE (245 calories)

1 teaspoon protein powder

1 teaspoon natural peanut butter

1½ cups fat-free milk

1 banana

SAMPLE MEAL PLANS

Here's an example of a 1-day muscle-building meal plan featuring the healthful foods and schedule that we recommend, again provided by Kalman. Its 3,271 calories include about 44 percent carbohydrate (a whopping 358 grams per day), 24 percent protein (an aggressive 192 grams), and 33 percent fat (a reasonable 119 grams). Note that it doesn't include a pre- or post-workout shake, so if you choose to take advantage of those, you'll have to cut back on some of the other food.

BREAKFAST

Omelet made with one whole egg and three egg whites, ½ cup diced
mushrooms and peppers, and 1 ounce reduced-fat cheese

2 slices whole grain toast

6 ounces orange juice

Water

MID-MORNING SNACK

1 cup reduced-fat yogurt

LUNCH

Grilled skinless chicken breast

½ cup brown rice

1 cup steamed mixed Italian-blend vegetables

Small side salad with 1 tablespoon olive oil–and-vinegar salad dressing

Water

DINNER

8 ounces grilled sirloin steak

1 baked sweet potato

1 cup steamed mixed vegetables, such as broccoli and cauliflower

Small mixed-green salad with 1 tablespoon olive oil–and-vinegar salad dressing

Water

NIGHTTIME SNACK

1 apple

1 tablespoon natural peanut butter

Here's a day's worth of fat-trimming, muscle-maintaining meals totaling 2,039 calories, with 30 percent carbohydrate (150 grams), 40 percent protein (209 grams), and 30 percent fat (67 grams, which will help you stay fuller longer and maintain your testosterone levels).

BREAKFAST

Scrambled eggs made with one large egg and four egg whites

2 links turkey sausage

1 cup 1% milk

MID-MORNING SNACK

1 packet Meso-Tech meal-replacement supplement

1 apple

LUNCH

Sandwich made with 2 slices multigrain bread, 6 ounces fat-free turkey lunchmeat, 1 tablespoon mustard, 2 slices tomato, and ½ cup spinach or other dark green leafy vegetable

1 cup fat-free milk

MID-AFTERNOON SNACK

3 pieces string cheese

1 cup 1% milk

DINNER

Hamburger made with ½ pound 90% lean ground sirloin on multigrain roll with 1 teaspoon mustard, 1 teaspoon ketchup, 2 slices dill pickle, and 1 large slice tomato

Water

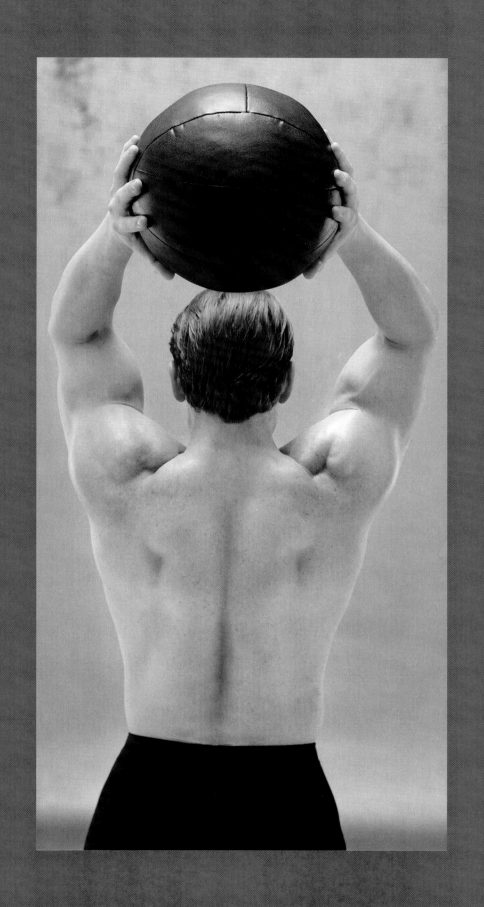

CHAPTER

FIVE

THE SUPPORTING CAST

FOR EVERY PERSON you see up on a movie screen, there are at least a dozen others working behind the scenes to make sure the actor looks good, sounds right, and isn't killed by falling light towers. Your anatomy is analogous to a movie production. Your muscles are the stars: You feed them, you exercise them, you admire them, and you generally aren't aware of the tissues supporting them—tendons, ligaments, cartilage. You rarely think about the nerves that tell them when to go into action and when to knock off for the day. And bones? They get your attention only when they break.

All these crew members are vital, if underappreciated, so let's discuss what they do.

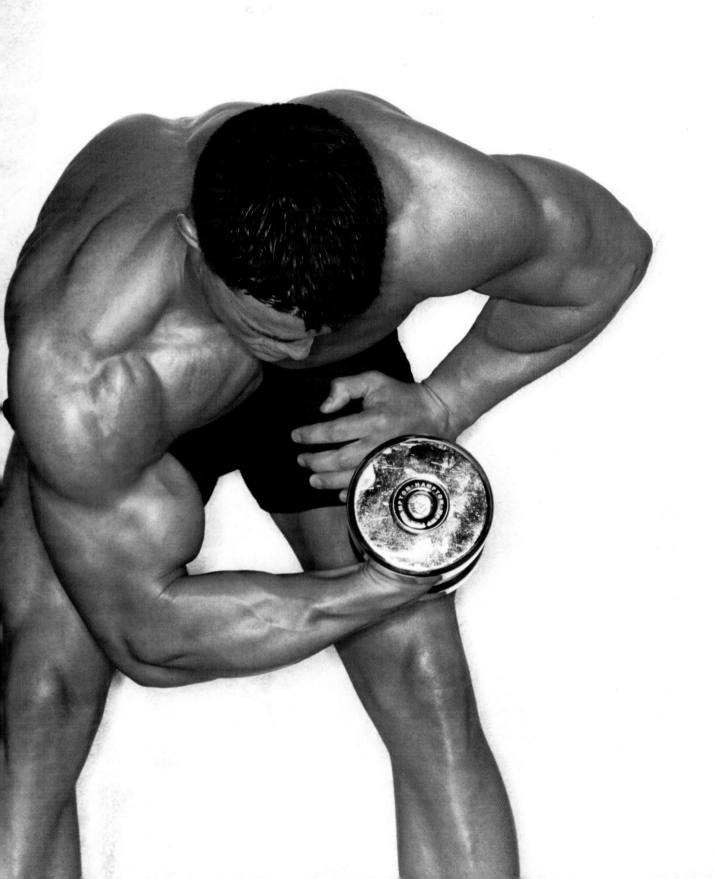

MAKING THE CONNECTIONS

If you ever read scientific literature relating to strength training, you come across odd terms such as *elbow flexion* and *hip extension*. If you're lucky, you figure out that the academics are referring to biceps curls and deadlifts. Odds are, though, that you have no idea what those eggheads are going on about.

There's a good reason why fitness professionals use such jargon. The average gym rat probably knows a dozen variations on the biceps curl. To the scientist, they're all just elbow flexion because the joint action is the key to the movement, and the muscles used are just details. (The Hollywood equivalent would be when a screen-

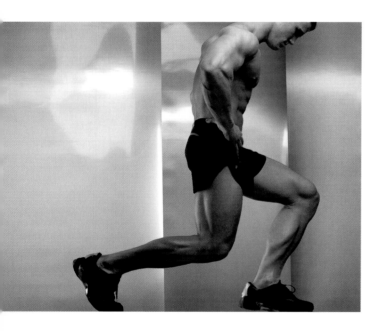

writer gets rave reviews for a script performed by a cast of B-list actors.) And as you'll see in part two, even though we're muscle guys, not mind guys, we decided that the best way to organize the exercises in this book is indeed by joint action.

Muscles can't move their respective joints without the help of intermediaries. **TENDONS** connect muscle to bone, and **LIGAMENTS** connect bone to bone. Sometimes muscle connects to muscle with tissues called **FASCIA** that form sheaths over and around all muscles. **CARTILAGE** is a fourth type of connective tissue, mainly used to protect bones from rubbing against each other.

Perhaps the most important lesson an entry-level personal trainer learns is that connective tissues develop more slowly than muscles do. The trainer learns this either the easy way, by reading it in a book or hearing it in a lecture, or the hard way, by pushing an out-of-shape, middle-age client to do too much too soon until the client has to stay home to rest his inflamed shoulder or chronically sore knees.

Most connective tissues are made from collagen fibers, structures that look remarkably like muscle fibers. The key difference between the two types of fibers is that a single collagen fiber does not make up a cell, because it doesn't have its own nucleus. A bundle of collagen fibers has several cells within it, but each individual fiber is not a cell by itself.

This biological technicality is crucial to understanding why collagen fibers don't adapt to exercise the same way muscle fibers do. Bundles of collagen fibers have a direct blood supply (with one exception, explained below), but because they contain relatively few metabolically active cells, they nevertheless take in fewer nutrients and less oxygen than muscles receive. Consequently, they also strengthen and grow more slowly than muscles do, so increases in exercise volume and intensity must be gradual if collagen is to keep up with strengthening muscles.

Here's an interesting paradox: Though muscles are capable of growing more quickly than connective tissues are able to, the former can't get bigger until the latter do. So it's convenient that, as you'll recall from chapter three, muscles get stronger before they get bigger. Stronger muscles pull harder on the connective tissues, which then grow in response to that increased demand, and the bigger connective tissues finally allow the muscles to grow.

Strength training also increases the thickness of the cartilage on joint surfaces (called **HYALINE CARTILAGE**, in case you're interested), which helps with shock absorption. Cartilage, by the way, is that exception we mentioned in reference to blood supply. It's different from tendons, ligaments, and fascia in that it doesn't have its own supply. Instead, it depends on a substance called **SYNOVIAL FLUID** to bring it oxygen and nutrients. Synovial fluid is generated by movement, so immobilizing a joint may kill some parts of the cartilage. Careful post-injury exercise can regenerate dead cartilage. Resurrection is unlikely, however, if you return to exercise too soon or with too much intensity.

YOU'VE GOT SOME NERVES

We've already mentioned that the strength increases you experience at the beginning of a weight-training program are due mostly to your brain's deploying more motor units to perform a given exercise or deploying them more efficiently. The commander of each motor unit is a nerve cell. No matter how many muscle fibers compose a motor unit, there's only one nerve cell, and without the nerve, the unit can't do anything. (In fact, when a nerve is pinched off or otherwise deactivated, its platoon of muscle fibers soon starts dying off.) This is why a new lifter's initial strength gains are called neural, meaning nerve-related, adaptations.

Another type of neural adaptation to strength training is reduced sensitivity of inhibitory mechanisms, including those of **GOLGI TENDON ORGANS (GTOS)**, nerve endings within your tendons that deactivate your muscles when you try to lift an object that's too heavy for your current level of musculoskeletal fitness. GTOs are kind of like an overprotective mother: "Jimmy, don't pick up that weight! You'll hurt yourself!"

In a study published in 1961, researchers tested wrist strength in trained and untrained lifters before and after hypnosis. The untrained guys could wrist-curl 17 percent more weight after hypnosis. In the trained lifters, the difference between pre- and posthypnotic strength wasn't statistically significant. This indicated that strength training, like hypnosis, switches off the inhibitory mechanism of GTOs, convincing that cautious mom to loosen the apron strings a little and allow Jimmy to play with heavier weights.

In the workout programs in this book, you'll make two additional types of neural adjustments. First, the prescribed warmup protocols will ensure that your neural system and your muscles are ready for maximum effort on your most important sets of the most important exercises. Second, in most workouts, you'll work opposing muscle actions: When you do "horizontal pushing" exercises (such as chest presses), you'll also do "horizontal pulling" exercises (rows) in that same workout. Often, you'll perform these two actions in supersets, meaning you'll alternate between one and the other. This will increase your strength in both directions, pushing and pulling, because your neural system, for reasons unknown, relaxes its inhibitions against heavy lifts when you activate the muscles opposite those doing the lifting. So doing a rowing exercise, thereby taxing your upper-back muscles, allows your chest muscles to work harder when you do a press.

Now you know why we're telling you so much about your neuromuscular system: The more you know, the better you lift.

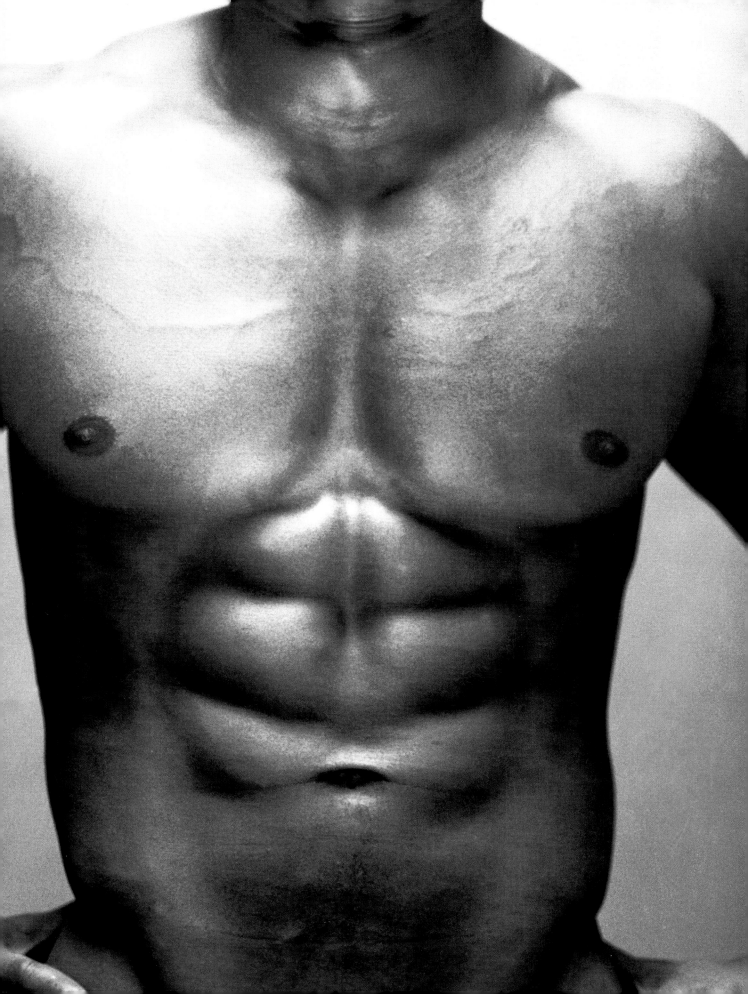

GOOD TO THE BONE

The entire reason muscles exist is to pull bones. We describe many exercises in this book as either "pulling" or "pushing" moves to indicate that they cause your joints to move in one direction or another. In reality, muscles can't push. All physical actions result from muscles and their connective tissues pulling on bones to move your joints.

When bones are pulled by larger, stronger muscles and connective tissues, the bones themselves grow thicker and stronger. Here's how that happens: A strain is applied to a bone, pulling it in a new or more forceful way. The body responds by sending cells called *osteoblasts* to the area that was strained. The osteoblasts spackle the area with new collagen fibers. The collagen then mineralizes, forming new bone tissue. (Here's a fun fact to share at the next PTA meeting: The minimal strain needed to force bone growth is about 10 percent of the force that would break the bone. Of course, as the bone gets bigger, it has more surface area to absorb a strain, so it takes a greater force to break the bone. Now you have yet another reason to use progressively heavier metal as you get more experience in the weight room: to gradually place greater strain on your growing bones and thereby continue that growth.)

Bone growth, technically known as bone remodeling, doesn't begin immediately, as neural adaptations do. It takes 8 to 12 weeks of regular loading for new collagen to form on bones, and then a few more weeks or even months for the collagen to mineralize into complete, functional bone.

It isn't surprising that bone grows most in response to the exercises that use the most muscle mass: squats, deadlifts, and the other usual suspects. Many guys are wary of exercises that put strain on their backs. They shouldn't be. Vertebrae

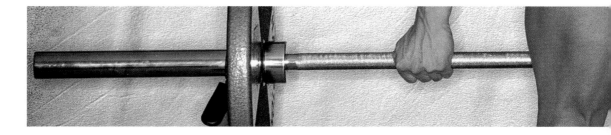

thicken in response to such heavy exercise, and all else being equal, thicker bones are healthier bones.

Like muscles, bones shrink when they're understimulated or immobilized. In fact, they shrink faster with immobility than they grow with activity. So when you return to exercise after a long layoff, you have to remember that your bones have shrunk along with your muscles.

Bones respond to four variables that you can easily manipulate in your workout.

1. LOAD (the amount of weight you lift)

2. SPEED (how quickly you do an exercise)

3. DIRECTION (doing an exercise from a different angle, such as bench-pressing on an incline)

4. VOLUME (number of sets and repetitions)

Of these, the first, load, is the most important. One case study showed that a powerlifter who could squat more than 1,000 pounds had the highest bone density ever recorded in human vertebrae, with no signs of structural damage.

The fourth variable—volume—is almost certainly the least important. That's why our workout programs prescribe fewer sets and repetitions than workouts in other books and magazines recommend.

But we're getting ahead of ourselves. In part two, we'll introduce you to the exercises you'll be doing in the workouts, and then in part three, we'll explain how to implement those exercises.

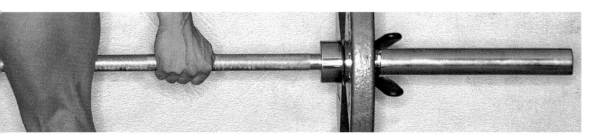

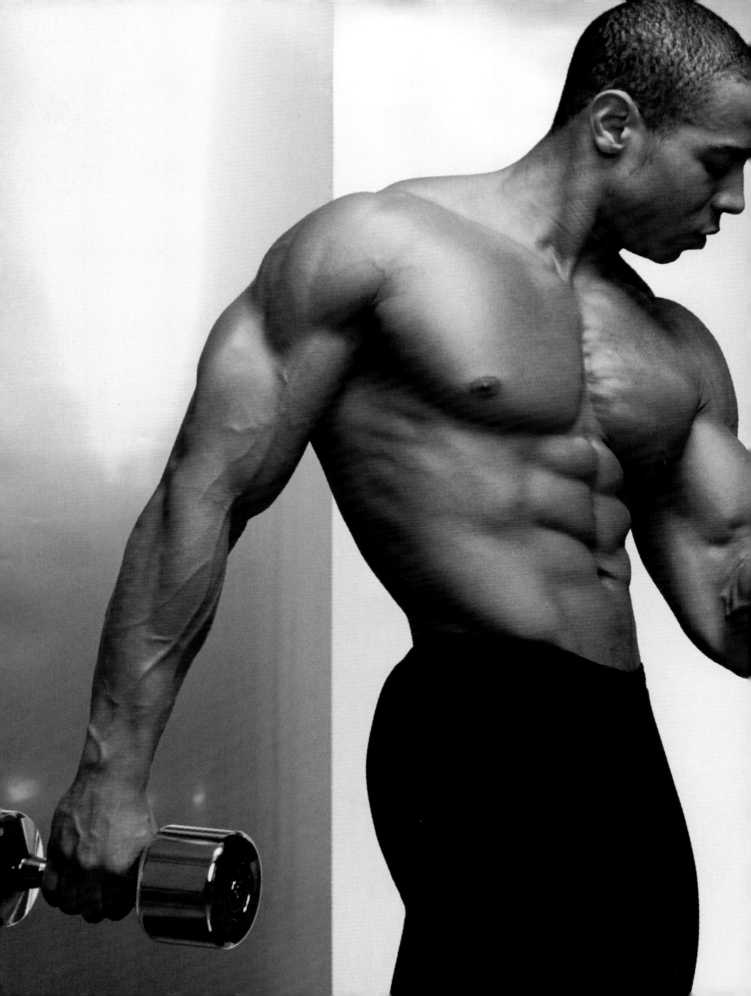

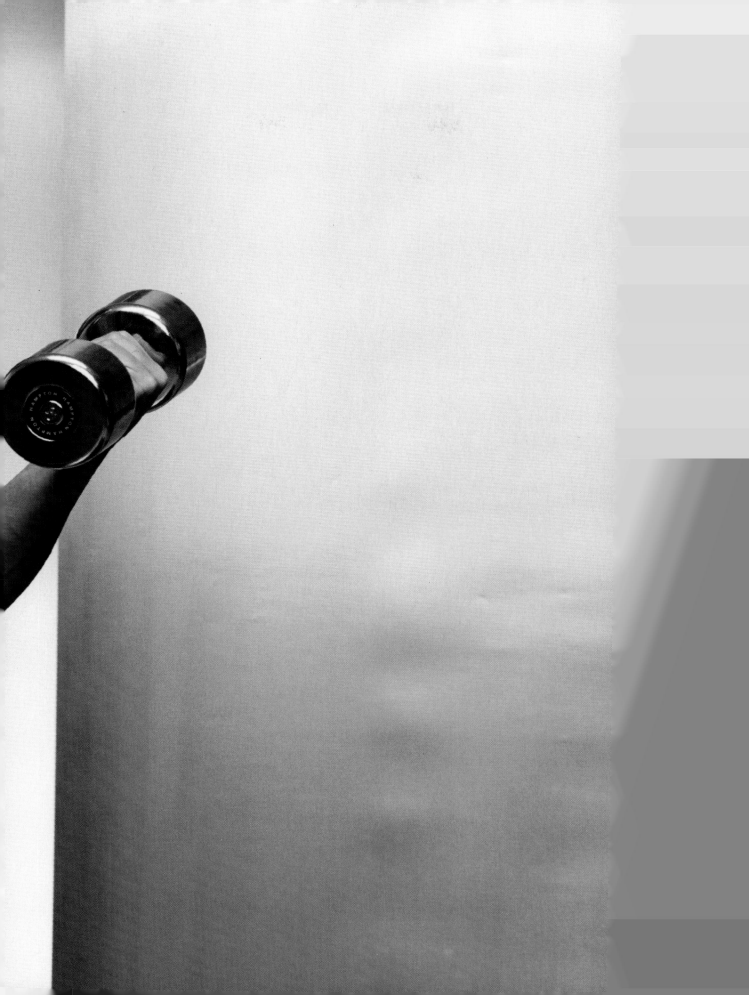

CHAPTER SIX

MUSCLES THAT ACT ON THE SHOULDER

MOST OF US THINK OF THE SHOULDER as a single joint: an arm bone rolling around in a socket. In actuality, the shoulder structure has four joints. Two of them are not generally targeted by strength exercises, but for the record, they are the *acromioclavicular joint*, where the highest ridge of the shoulder blade (acromium) joins the collarbone (clavicle), and the *sternoclavicular joint*, where the breast plate (sternum) and the clavicle meet.

The shoulder joint we all recognize, the ball-and-socket complex, is called the **GLENOHUMERAL JOINT**. (Don't worry; there's no quiz at the end of this book.) This joint has been compared to an egg in a spoon. The egg is the round knob at the top of the upper-arm bone, or humerus. The spoon is the shallow cavity at the edge of the shoulder blade (scapula), in which the knob sits. This structure allows maximum rotation of your upper-arm bone,

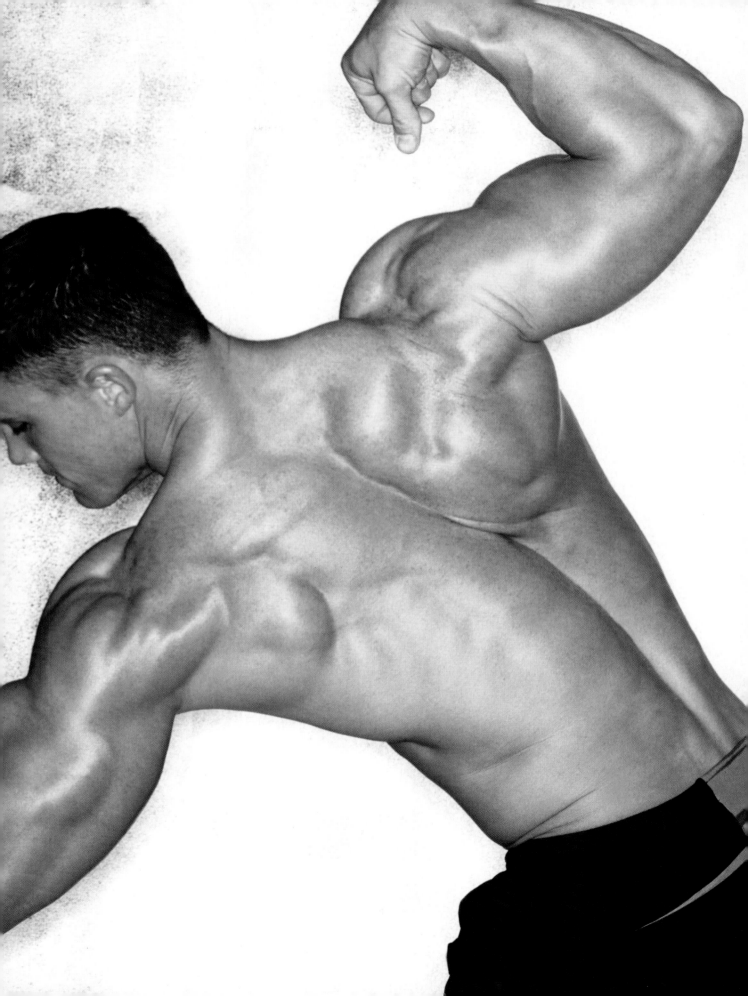

enabling a 98-miles-per-hour fastball. Less than half the knob is in this cavity at any point in the shoulder's rotation, so a complex and sometimes finicky set of 11 muscles and their attendant connective tissues are needed to hold the joint together and put it to full use. This explains why that fastball often necessitates surgery to repair the muscles girding the glenohumeral joint.

The other shoulder joint that comes into play in strength training is the **SCAPULOTHORACIC JOINT**, or the place where each of your two scapulae meets the back of your rib cage. The scapulae are the human equivalent of wings. When you lift your arms out to the sides, the top corners of the scapulae rotate inward, toward your spine, and the bottom corners rotate outward, along your ribs. If you reverse the motion, the tops rotate outward and the bottoms rotate in.

Despite the fact that your scapulae and shoulder joints usually work together in upper-arm motions, they have two different sets of muscles. The trophy muscles—**PECTORALIS MAJOR** (chest), **LATISSIMUS DORSI** (lats), and **DELTOIDS** (delts)—work the shoulder joints. The muscles that work your scapulae—**TRAPEZIUS**, **RHOMBOIDS**, **LEVATOR SCAPULAE**—are much less glamorous. It's not that they don't get bigger and stronger—they do. In fact, the trapezius is probably the strongest upper-body muscle. It's just that though you purposely work your chest, lats, and delts in the gym, you never give much thought to the scapular muscles assisting in such exercises as the bench press, lat pulldown, and shoulder press. You almost never do exercises designed to isolate scapular muscles, with the exception of shrugging exercises (of which you'll do several in our workout programs).

Let's take a closer look at the muscles that make your shoulders go round and round, followed by the exercises that target them. Note that even though we describe the muscles as separate entities in this section, we'll group the exercises according to their functions (horizontal push, vertical pull, et cetera) since they work several muscles together. You'll also observe that the exercise groupings assume that your torso is upright. So a bench press, for which you lie on your back, is still a "horizontal push" exercise because if you were standing, the motion would indeed be horizontal.

PECTORALIS MAJOR

Your pectoral muscle fibers originate in three different places: the collarbone, the breastbone, and the cartilage of several ribs near the breastbone. The fibers all attach to the humerus, but with a twist: The fibers that start at the bottom of the chest attach at a higher point on the humerus than the fibers that start on the top.

Bodybuilders tend to look at their chest muscles as having three distinct portions—upper, middle, lower—that need to be worked separately for maximum development. They're not entirely mistaken, but their isolationist efforts aren't as significant as they think: The twisting of the fibers assures that most chest exercises work most pectoral fibers.

That's why we group most chest exercises as horizontal-push movements. Yes, doing a chest press on an incline bench works the upper fibers more than it does the lower ones, and doing a press on a decline bench hits the lower fibers more than the uppers. Still, most fibers work together most of the time on most chest exercises. So building overall strength with horizontal-push exercises does more to build your chest muscles than would isolating the muscles from every possible angle. (In our workouts, you'll nevertheless work from a variety of angles because your shoulders hate performing the exact same movement over and over with heavy weights.)

The main job of the pectoralis major is to pull your upper arm across the front of your torso, as in a bench press or dumbbell fly. (A small upper-arm muscle, the **CORACOBRACHIALIS**, assists in this motion. It's barely visible even on the best-developed arms, appearing as a small strip of muscle coming out of the armpit between the pecs and lats, beneath the biceps.) The pec major plays a lesser role in pulling your arm down to your side. So if your upper arms are above and in front of your torso and you pull them down, as in a pullup or lat pulldown, your pecs play a small part. If your arms are behind or to the sides of your torso and you push them down, as in a dip or bench dip, your lower pecs handle a substantial part of the load.

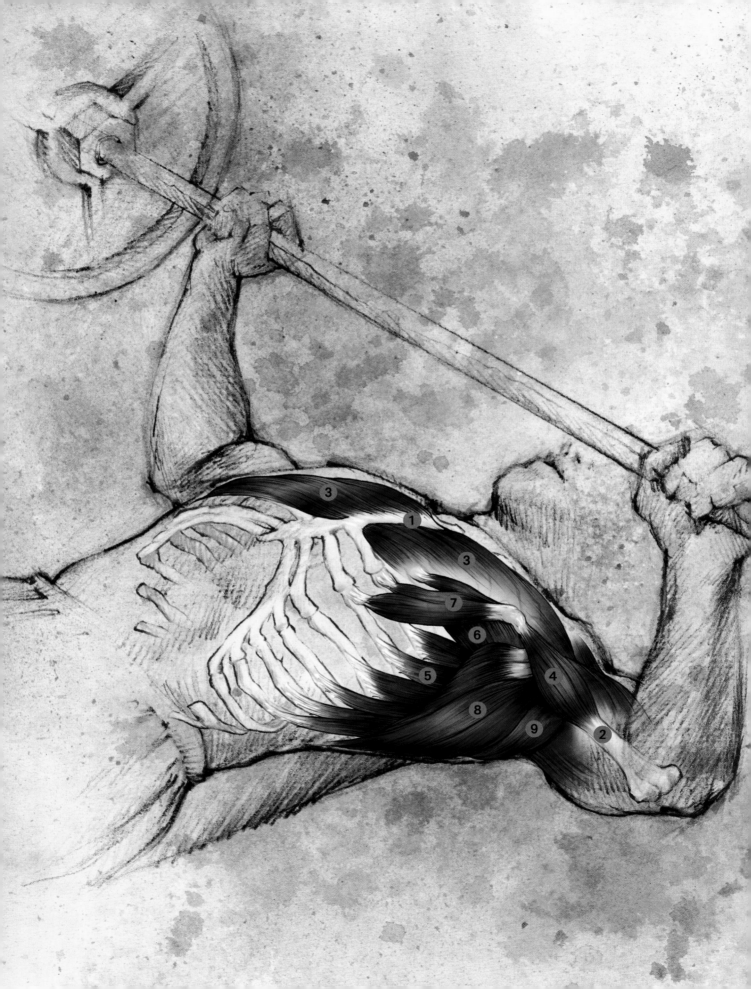

LATISSIMUS DORSI

In terms of square footage, the latissimus dorsi is the body's largest muscle. Its fibers originate along the vertebrae of the lower half of the spine, on the hips, and on the three lowest ribs. They then twist together and attach to your humerus to form the back of your armpit. Everything this muscle does is assisted by the **TERES MAJOR**, a small strip of muscle that originates on the scapula and attaches to the upper arm just above the latissimus.

When your arms are above your shoulders, the lats and teres minor muscles pull your arms to the sides and down, as in pullups and lat pulldowns—the "vertical pull" exercises. These muscles also work in conjunction with your lower pecs when you pull your arms down in front of your body, as when you do pullovers.

DELTOID

This three-part muscle wraps around the cap of the shoulder joint. The front part originates on the outer third of the collarbone. (The other two-thirds of the collarbone serves as the launching point for the uppermost fibers of the pectoralis major.) The rear deltoid starts on the shoulder blade (or, rather, on a diagonal spine that protrudes from and cuts across the top third of the scapula). The middle deltoid springs from the acromion. The three parts come together and attach to the front of the upperarm bone, beneath the biceps.

Because the fibers of the front deltoid originate alongside the fibers of the upper pectoralis major, the two muscles act like conjoined twins on chest presses.

The middle deltoid handles most of the load when you push a weight straight overhead—the "vertical push" exercises, such as

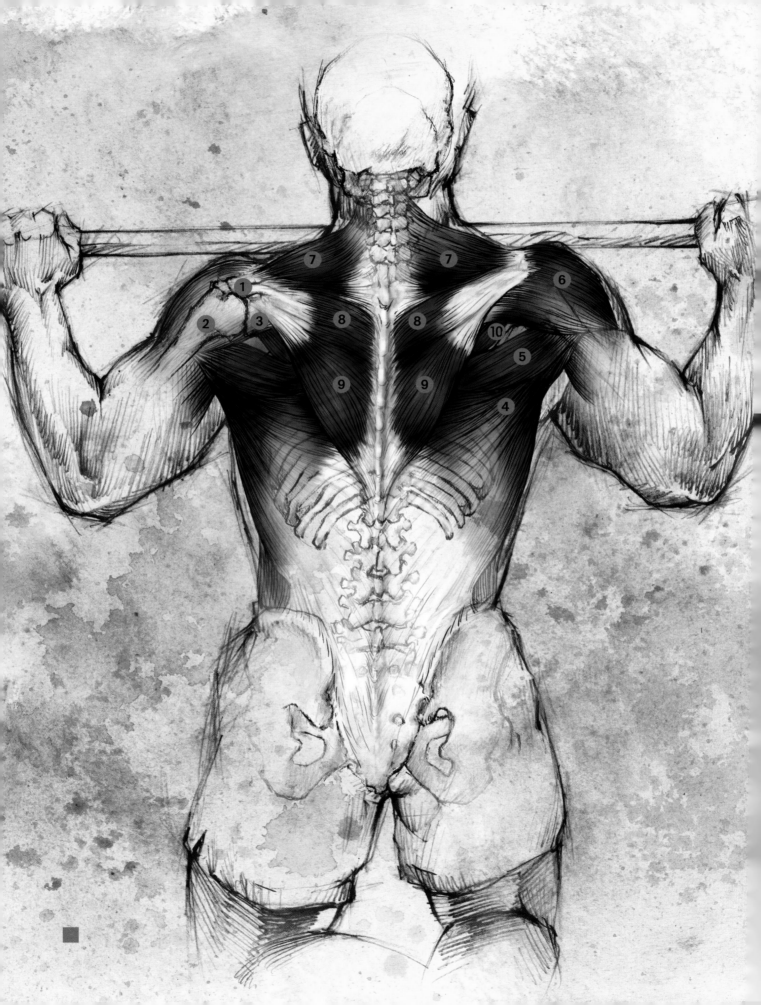

shoulder presses and upright rows. When you lift your arms straight out to your sides, the middle and rear deltoids work hard, along with the **SUPRASPINATUS**, one of the four rotator cuff muscles, which lies beneath the deltoid.

Since the fibers of the rear deltoid begin where the fibers of the upper and middle trapezius end, on the scapula, many of the rear delt's movements are married to those of the trapezius and the other scapular muscles involved in the "horizontal pull" exercises, such as rows.

TRAPEZIUS

The fibers of the trapezius originate at the base of the skull and along the cervical and thoracic vertebrae. (Cervical vertebrae form your neck, and thoracic vertebrae are behind your ribs. Lumbar vertebrae form your lower back.) These trapezius fibers attach along the back of the collarbone and the spiny ridge of the shoulder blade.

Because these fibers run in three different directions, they're responsible for three distinct functions. The uppermost fibers, starting at the skull and running diagonally down to the collar-bone, are most involved in shrugging the shoulders. When they're extremely well developed, as in wrestlers and football linemen, the neck starts to disappear. A smaller muscle, the **LEVATOR SCAPULAE**, assists in the shrugging action. It lies beneath the trapezius, originating on the uppermost cervical vertebrae and ending up on the top edge of the scapula.

The fibers of the middle trapezius pull the scapula in toward the spine, an action called scapular retraction. They're aided by the **RHOMBOID** muscle, which lies beneath the trapezius and de-scends diagonally from the thoracic vertebrae. Scapular retrac-

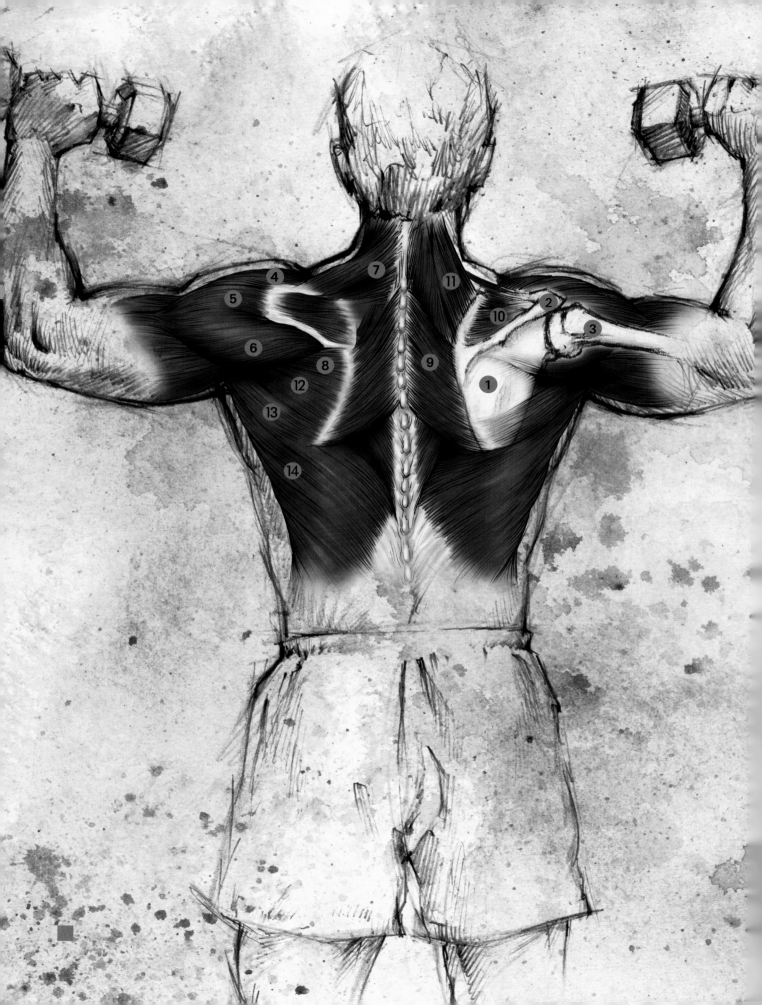

tion, key to horizontal-pulling exercises, is crucial to building balanced strength on the front and back of your upper torso. Many strength coaches and physical therapists now believe that imbalanced upper-body strength leads to shoulder problems that can make your favorite lifts painful and unproductive. This is why you should avoid joining the cult of the pectoralists, guys who do dozens of sets of bench presses a week with only a few minutes spent on the muscles that oppose the chest.

The lower-trap and rhomboid muscles tug your scapula downward, as in the vertical-pull exercises—pullups and lat pulldowns.

PECTORALIS MINOR AND SERRATUS ANTERIOR

You could call these the forgotten scapular muscles, or even the forgotten vanity muscles. The pec minor lies beneath the pec major and isn't externally visible. The serratus, which lies along the ribs, is visible only in the best-developed physiques. They're both worth remembering because a tight pair of pec minor muscles can pull your shoulder joints forward, altering your posture for the worse. And if you're a lean guy, well-developed serratus muscles can make you look like a superhero.

These aren't muscles you have to isolate. The pec minor is involved in such exercises as the pullover, whereas the serratus muscles get involved whenever the scapulae rotate upward and outward, as during an upright row.

ROTATOR CUFF MUSCLES

We've already mentioned one of these: the supraspinatus, which lies beneath the deltoid and assists it in lifting your arms out to

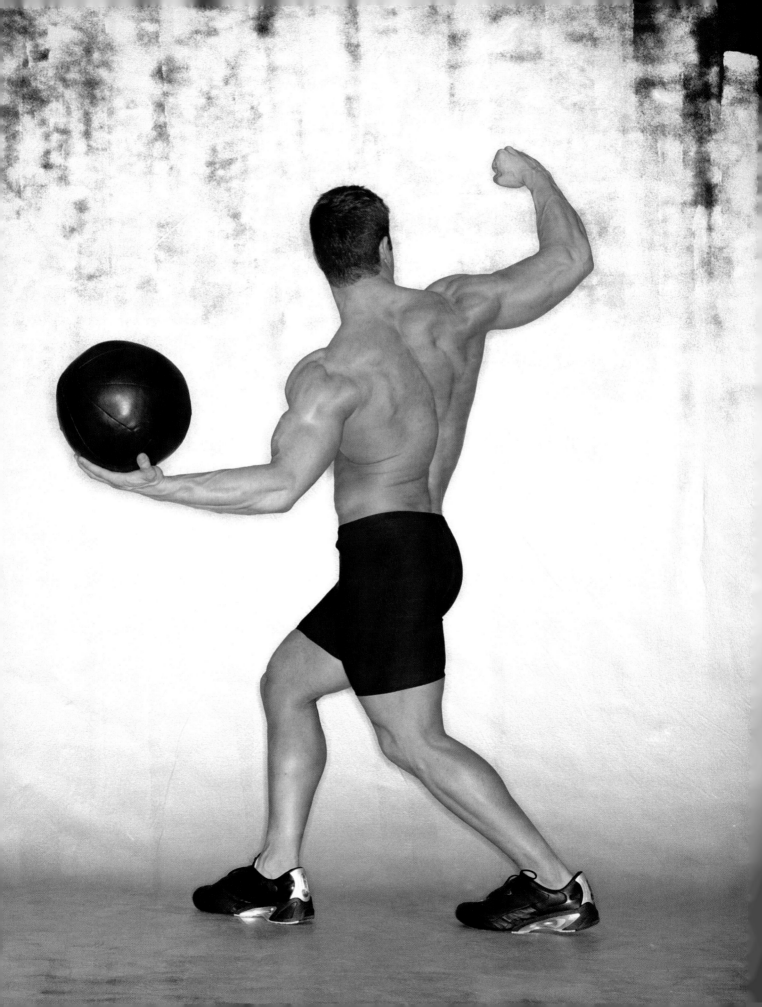

your sides. The other three are the **INFRASPINATUS, TERES MINOR**, and **SUBSCAPULARIS**. Of these, the first two are involved in external rotation, whereas the third helps with internal rotation.

Internal and external rotation are crucial movements. Their role in sports is obvious (throwing involves external rotation on the windup and internal rotation on the pitch). Often overlooked is their role in strength and muscle development.

In serious lifters, internal rotation tends to be maximally developed, if not overdeveloped. This is not because the subscapularis, which lies behind the pec minor, is huge and powerful but because it has a huge and powerful friend: the latissimus dorsi, which, along with the teres major, also works during internal rotation. The pec major is also involved in throwing, so that equals two big, powerful muscles working toward internal rotation along with the small rotator cuff muscle.

Where does that leave the external rotators? When it comes to external rotation—cocking the arm back, as for a throw—for the most part, they're on their own. They do work with the middle and rear deltoids in pulling your arms back when they're perpendicular to your torso, as in some of the horizontal-pulling exercises (particularly the reverse fly and the wide-grip barbell bent-over row).

The infraspinatus is the only rotator cuff muscle that's externally visible. It lies in a triangle between your rear deltoid, teres major, and trapezius. The teres minor lies above the teres major but isn't visually distinct from the infraspinatus—it appears to be all the same muscle.

BARBELL BENCH PRESS

It's easier to ridicule this exercise than to praise it. Among its many sins, it probably contributes to more shoulder injuries than any other strength exercise. And you'd be hard-pressed to discover any specific applications for it, in sports or real life. Sure, professional football linemen do a lot of two-handed shoving. Among the rest of the adult population, literally pushing other people around tends to be frowned upon.

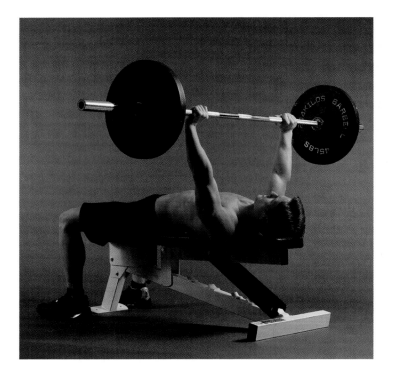

Yet no exercise carries more emotional and hormonal baggage than the barbell bench press. Every man who's spent significant time in a gym measures himself by his maximum bench press. A guy who can't do a single pullup or chinup, who has no idea how to execute a barbell squat or deadlift, who couldn't locate his rotator cuff muscles with a copy of *Gray's Anatomy*, who hasn't seen his abdominal muscles since he was 12 and had no idea abs would one day be really cool—even this guy can tell you his best-ever bench press.

That said, we like the barbell bench press—a lot. We don't care so much about the one-repetition maximum. (Even in the advanced program in chapter sixteen, you'll never do a "true" one-rep max, or the most weight you can lift once.) We simply think the barbell bench press is the best exercise for developing pectoral strength and mass. And it's one of three lifts contested in power-lifting, a legitimate and honorable sport.

SETUP: Lie faceup on a bench, with your feet set on the floor and your hands a bit wider than shoulder-width apart. Most Olympic barbells have a set of rings, or grooves, in the knurling, against which you should place the outsides of your palms, using a standard overhand grip. Extend your arms and move the bar from the uprights to above your chest, keeping your arms straight.

EXECUTION: Slowly lower the bar to your middle chest. Pause, then push the bar straight up to the starting position, over your chest.

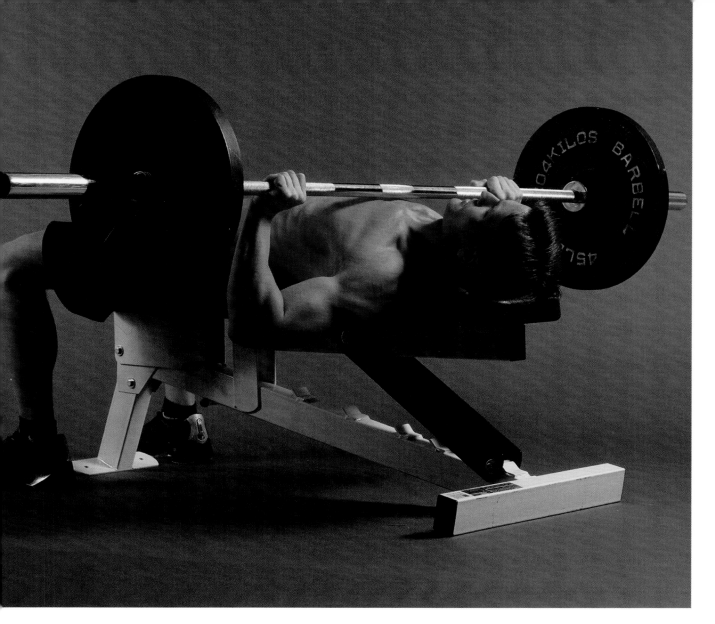

GET STRONGER INSTANTLY: You can most likely improve your bench press by paying attention to your feet and shoulder blades. Feet should be wide apart and flat on the floor, unless the program tells you otherwise (see variation 5 on the next page). Imagine that you're standing up and trying to make this literally a vertical push: You're throwing the bar off your chest for distance. What do you do with your feet? You set them in an athletic position, at least shoulder-width apart, to give your upper-body muscles a solid platform from which they can generate power. Even when you're lying on a bench, your feet contribute to your body's overall strength. So plant them before the lift, and keep them planted. Also, the more acute your knee angle—in other words, the closer your feet are to your head—the more lower-body power you'll generate.

Your shoulder blades will tend to pull away from each other in the top position and then retract again as you're lowering the bar. You'll be stronger, though, if you keep them retracted throughout the exercise. Pull them together before you lower the bar, and keep them together as you lift.

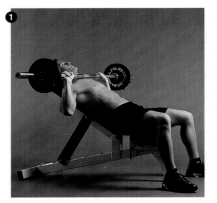

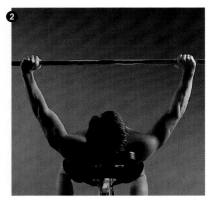

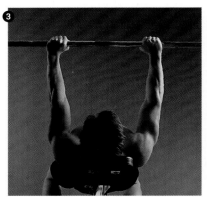

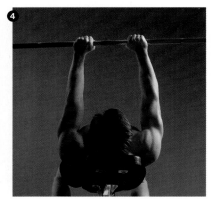

VARIATIONS

❶ INCLINE: Set the incline bench (the one that allows your head to rest higher than your hips) to about a 30-degree angle to the floor. Lower the bar to your upper chest. This variation shifts the emphasis to your upper pectorals and front shoulders.

❷ WIDE GRIP: Place your hands outside the rings on the Olympic barbell. This puts more load on your pectorals and less on your triceps. It can put more strain on your shoulders, so use it carefully, lifting light loads at first and using deliberate movements.

❸ CLOSE GRIP: Position your hands directly above your shoulders, with your thumbs 18 to 24 inches apart. This shifts the load to your triceps and, to a lesser extent, to your lower pectorals. You should be able to use almost as much weight as you would with the conventional bench-press grip—probably 90 to 95 percent of that amount. If you have really strong triceps, you may be able to use equal loads.

❹ VERY CLOSE GRIP: Position your hands 6 to 8 inches apart.

❺ FEET ON BENCH: Place your feet flat on the bench. This gives less stability than you'd have with your feet on the floor.

❻ TO NECK: Lower the bar to your neck or upper chest. Use this variation sparingly to strengthen the shoulders and upper pectorals; it can be very tough on the shoulders if you use too much weight or try to move the bar too fast.

❼ TO LOWER CHEST: This is a powerlifting technique that allows you to move more weight, especially when combined with the back arch described in variation 8. It gives the bar the shortest possible line of

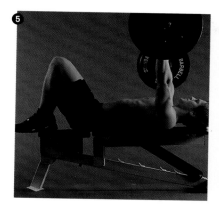

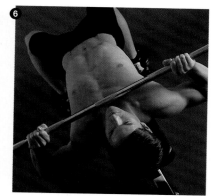

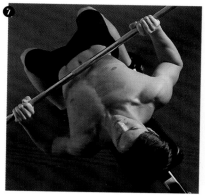

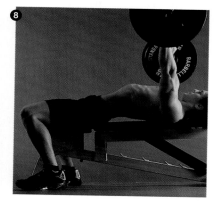

travel from bottom to top. The low-bar technique shifts the emphasis to your lower pectorals, lats, and triceps, which is why it isn't used by bodybuilders, who strive for more upper-chest development.

⑧ ARCHED BACK: Lift your lower back off the bench, shortening the distance between your shoulders and buttocks, and providing a higher platform from which to push the bar off your chest. The higher the platform, the shorter the distance the bar has to travel to complete the lift. This is used only in the max-strength phases of the workout programs, and you shouldn't do it at all if you have lower-back problems.

SAFETY: Anytime you use near-maximal weights and low repetitions (four or fewer), it's a good idea to have a spotter on hand who can help lift the bar off your chest if you unexpectedly fail to complete a repetition. None of our workouts prescribes a maximum bench press. So you shouldn't need to worry about failing to complete a lift until you get to the final stages, when you'll do very low repetition sets. If you need a spotter earlier on, it will probably be because you're using more weight than the workout calls for. Most of the time, you'll be able to tell when you're near failure on a set. So if a workout calls for 10 repetitions, you should know when your muscles are exhausted before you get to the point when someone has to pull the bar off your sternum. However, unspotted bench pressing is the leading cause of death for lifters working out at home, so it never hurts to ask for a spotter if you're going to push your muscles to the limit.

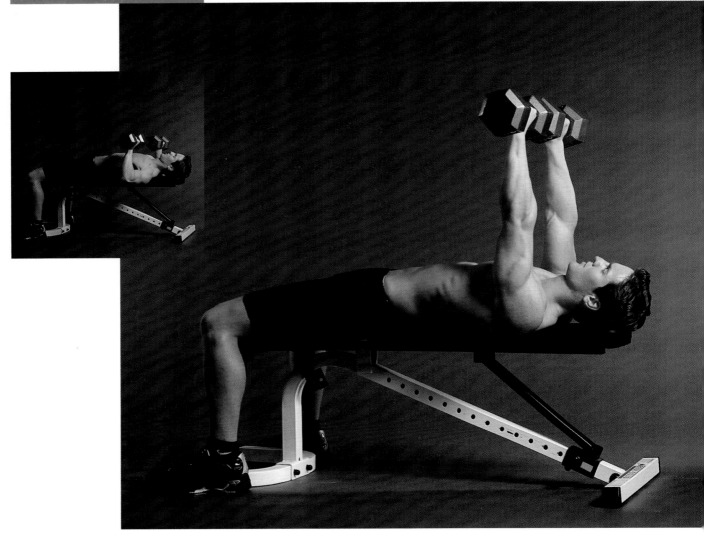

DUMBBELL BENCH PRESS

For pure muscle growth, the dumbbell bench press is probably the best chest exercise. It gives you a slightly deeper range of motion than you get with a barbell, and with your arms working independently, your muscles have to work harder to stabilize themselves. That independent action allows your shoulder joints to choose their own angles of ascent and descent, which means that fewer shoulder injuries are caused by dumbbells than by barbells.

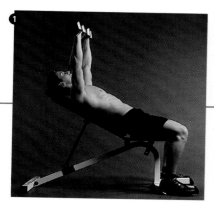

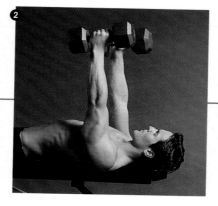

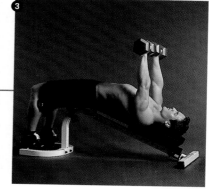

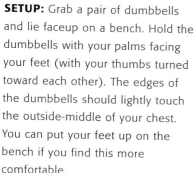

SETUP: Grab a pair of dumbbells and lie faceup on a bench. Hold the dumbbells with your palms facing your feet (with your thumbs turned toward each other). The edges of the dumbbells should lightly touch the outside-middle of your chest. You can put your feet up on the bench if you find this more comfortable.

EXECUTION: Push the dumbbells straight up until your arms are almost fully extended. The dumbbells should come close together in this top position. (They should never clack together at the top of the movement. Hitting the weights together not only takes some tension off your chest muscles but also annoys the hell out of others in the gym. If you must clack, please work out at home.) After a pause, slowly lower the weights back to the starting position.

VARIATIONS

❶ INCLINE: Set the incline bench at about a 30-degree angle to the floor. The rest of the movement is about the same, although the weights will start higher on your chest, near your front deltoids, and the exercise will put more emphasis on your upper chest.

❷ NEUTRAL GRIP: Hold the dumbbells with your palms facing each other.

❸ DECLINE: Set the decline bench (the one that puts your head lower than your hips) about 30 degrees below parallel. The rest of the movement is the same, although as you start using heavier weights, the setup will get increasingly awkward. So you may need a spotter to help you get the weights into position. (On the plus side, you may be able to lift more weight from this angle than in other dumbbell bench press variations.) The decline shifts the emphasis to your lower chest and triceps.

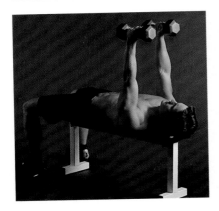

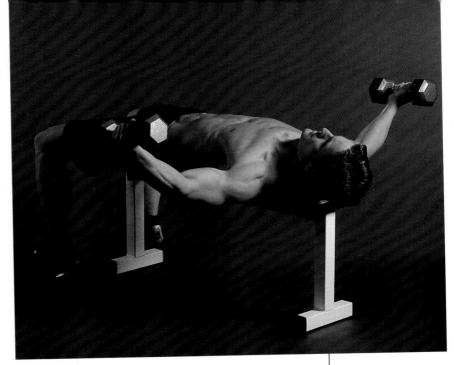

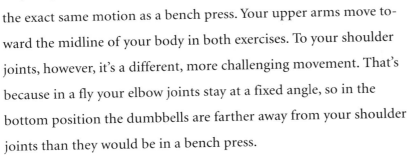

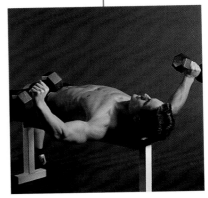

DUMBBELL FLY

To your pectoral muscles, this is the exact same motion as a bench press. Your upper arms move toward the midline of your body in both exercises. To your shoulder joints, however, it's a different, more challenging movement. That's because in a fly your elbow joints stay at a fixed angle, so in the bottom position the dumbbells are farther away from your shoulder joints than they would be in a bench press.

Speaking of the bottom position, on a dumbbell bench press, it's the point at which the weights touch your chest. On a fly, you're limited only by the flexibility of your shoulders and the height of the bench.

All this means two things, fly-wise: (1) You have to use much less weight than you'd use on a bench press, and (2) you have to move the weights slowly and deliberately, taking care not to lower your upper arms past your point of comfort and safety. So start with weights that are light enough to let you figure out your range without risking injury.

SETUP: Lie faceup on a bench, a dumbbell in each hand. Hold the weights directly above your chest, with your elbows slightly bent and your palms facing each other.

EXECUTION: Slowly lower the weights out to your sides, keeping the same angle in your elbow joints. Lower the weights as far as you like (descend to the plane of your torso, at least), but maintain this same range on all repetitions. To return to the starting position, lift the weights back along the same arc, keeping in mind the option of not bringing them up fully. (The higher you raise the weights, the less resistance there is from gravity, so the top of the range of motion—where you could clack the weights together if you wanted to ignore our advice and call attention to yourself in a crowded gym—is functionally useless. A shorter range of motion keeps more tension on the pectoral muscles and increases their fatigue.)

VARIATION

THUMBS IN: Point your thumbs, rather than your palms, toward each other. Maintain the same range of motion.

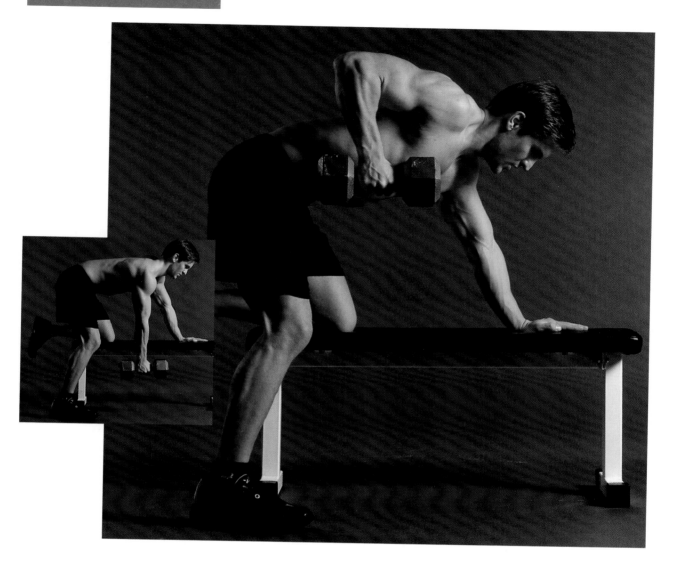

DUMBBELL ONE-ARM BENT-OVER ROW

SETUP: Set a dumbbell on the floor near one end of a bench. Place one knee on the bench near that end, then lean forward and place the corresponding hand on the bench. Reach down, grab the dumbbell, and hold it just off the floor, with your palm turned in toward your torso and your arm straight. Straighten your back and set your torso perpendicular to the bench and the floor, or just above perpendicular (your shoulders can be slightly higher than your hips).

EXECUTION: Pull the dumbbell up to your torso, just below the armpit. Focus on leading with your elbow, initially pulling it straight up toward the ceiling, then angling it back slightly. Your shoulder and elbow joints should be your only moving parts; your lower body and trunk should remain still. Pause, then lower the weight back to the starting position.

VARIATION
REVERSE GRIP: Your palms should face forward.

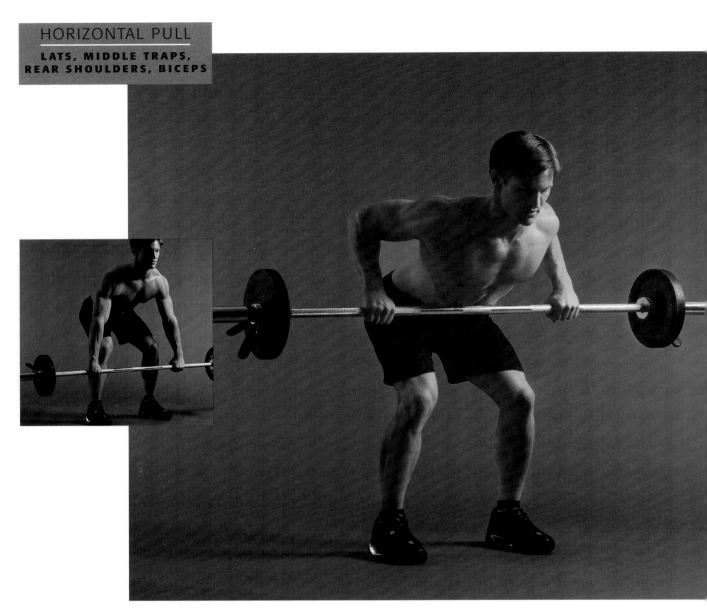

BARBELL BENT-OVER ROW

One of the hallmarks of Ian King–designed training programs is the balance between exercises for the front and back of the upper body. The barbell bent-over row
is this program's most prominent horizontal-pull exercise, the opposite of the barbell bench press.

The exercises aren't precisely equivalent, since on the bench press you have a
platform to support your weight and help with balance, whereas on the row you
have to provide your own platform, using your powerful lower-body muscles. So
the key to the row is to keep your body's center of gravity directly over your legs,
holding your torso in the same plane throughout the exercise.

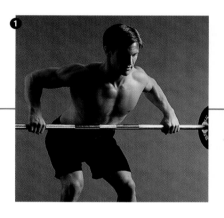

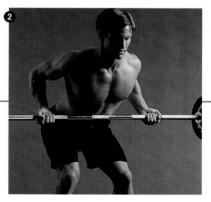

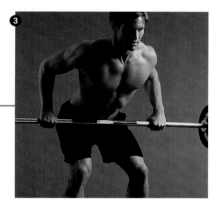

SAFETY: The bent-over row looks as if it would put your lower back in a world of hurt. In fact, it's one of those exercises, like the deadlift, in which the spinal joints actually have little to no range of motion. If you do it right, you should generate enough tension with your midbody muscles to keep your spine protected from any damaging forces.

SETUP: Stand with your feet shoulder width or slightly farther apart. Bend forward at the waist and push your hips back a bit, establishing a center of gravity as close to directly over the legs as possible. Flex your knees slightly—you want them in an athletic posture. Keep your lower back flat or slightly arched, and your torso at an angle slightly above horizontal to the floor. Grasp the barbell with an overhand grip, your hands just inside the lines on the Olympic bar.

EXECUTION: Pull the bar to your upper abdomen, just below your chest, feeling your shoulder blades squeeze together at the top of the movement and keeping your forearms and wrists in a straight line. Pause, then slowly lower the bar until your arms are fully extended.

VARIATIONS

❶ WIDE GRIP: Grab the bar with your hands just outside the rings on the Olympic bar. This shifts emphasis away from your latissimus dorsi and onto your upper-back muscles (rear shoulders, middle trapezius, and rhomboids).

❷ REVERSE GRIP: Grab the bar underhand (palms up), with your hands shoulder-width apart. This gives more work to your biceps, lower lats, and lower traps.

❸ LOW BAR: Pull the bar to your middle abdomen. This shifts emphasis to your lower lats and lower traps.

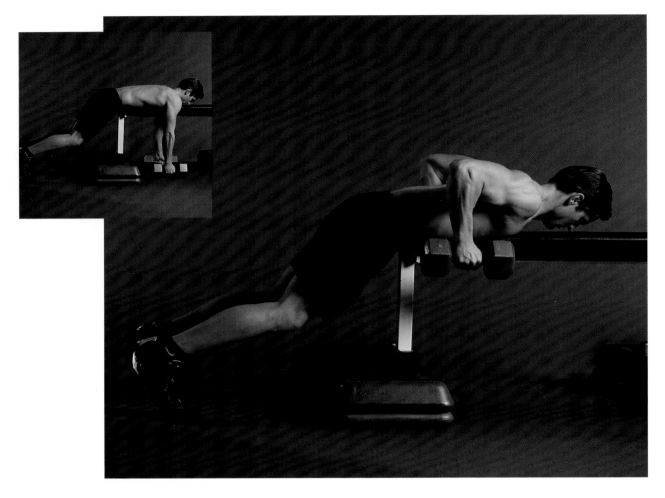

DUMBBELL LYING ROW

SETUP: Grab a pair of dumbbells and lie facedown on a bench. (You'll get a better range of motion if you raise the bench off the floor a few inches, as shown here.) Hold the dumbbells directly below your shoulders, with your palms facing each other.

EXECUTION: Raise the dumbbells as high as you can to the sides of your body, just below your armpits. Focus on squeezing your shoulder blades together at the top, but don't elevate them, because shrugging them calls the upper traps into the movement. Pause, then lower the weights back down toward the floor, but go down only one-third to one-half the way before pausing and starting the next repetition.

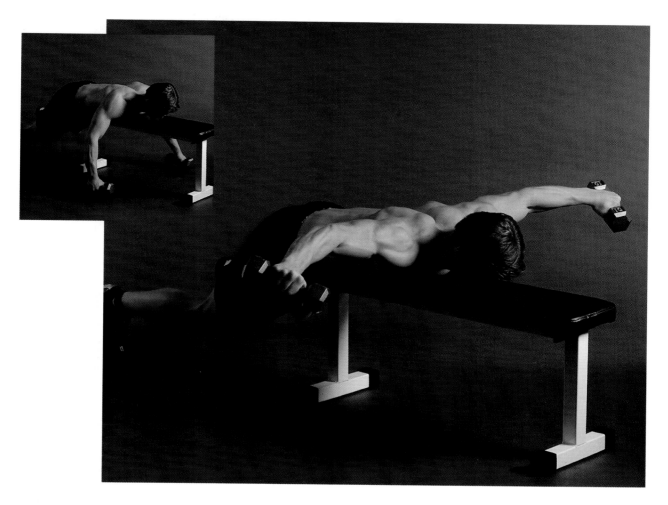

REVERSE DUMBBELL FLY

SETUP: Grab a pair of dumbbells and lie facedown on a bench. Start with your arms nearly straight—you want a slight bend in your elbows—and the dumbbells just off the floor. Your palms should face the floor, and your upper arms should be nearly perpendicular to your torso.

EXECUTION: Raise the dumbbells straight up off the floor, feeling your shoulder blades squeeze together at the top (but not allowing them to elevate). Pause, then slowly lower the weights back down, stopping before they touch the floor.

SEATED
CABLE ROW

This is a deceptively complex exercise, with stiff penalties for poor execution. Novice exercisers often assume it's safe—it does use a machine, after all—so they fail to observe the postural precautions they'd employ if they were working with free weights.

As with any exercise, the first rule is: Don't hurt yourself. We can explain the subtleties of the exercise and offer our opinion on the most effective variations, but all that is moot if you get injured.

If, on the other hand, you learn and consistently observe the proper form for this exercise and its many variations, you can gain strength and muscle mass quickly. And you'll probably find, as many lifters do, that it's among your favorite exercises. Respect is crucial; fear is optional.

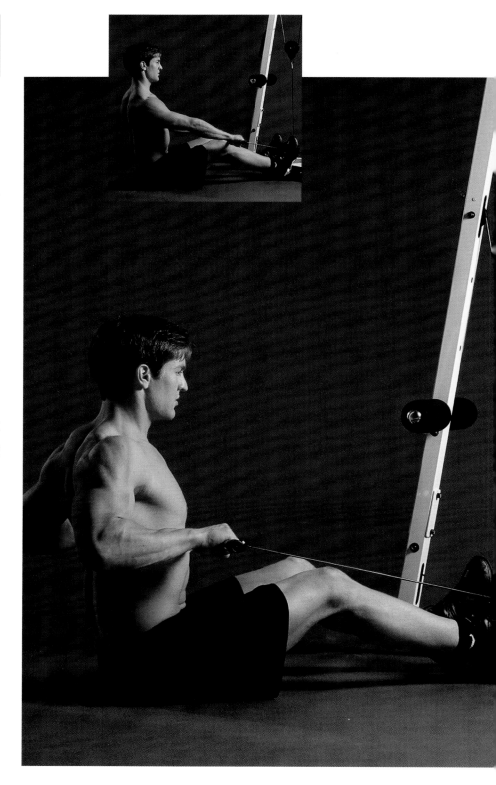

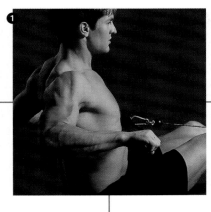

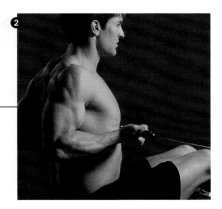

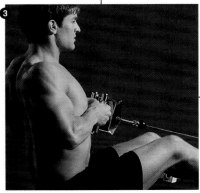

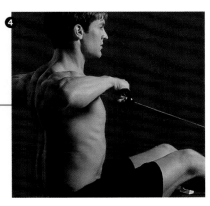

SETUP: Select the appropriate weight on the stack, then attach a straight bar to the cable mechanism. Set your feet on the bracing plates, with your knees close to your chest, and grab the bar with an overhand grip that's the equivalent of the grip you use on the bench press. Push your body back with your feet until your arms are extended and there's tension on the cable. Your knees should be slightly bent. Straighten your back and lean back slightly so your shoulders are just a bit behind your hips.

EXECUTION: Pull the bar to your upper abdomen. Pause, then slowly allow your arms to straighten. Three keys: (1) Your posture must stay fixed throughout the movement—don't lean forward or back. (2) Your shoulder blades must squeeze together in back at the point of full contraction (when the bar touches your torso). (3) Your shoulder blades shouldn't be elevated at any point. If they are, you need to either adjust the range of motion, bringing the bar to a lower point on your abdomen, or decrease the amount of weight you're using.

VARIATIONS

❶ **WIDE GRIP:** Use an overhand grip that's the equivalent of the widest grip you use on the barbell bench press. This shifts the emphasis from your lats to your rear delts, middle traps, and rhomboids.

❷ **REVERSE GRIP:** Use an underhand (palms-up) grip, with your hands about shoulder-width apart. This uses your biceps and lower lats more, and your rear delts and middle traps less.

❸ **NEUTRAL GRIP:** Use the triangle handle, which allows your palms to face each other with your hands a few inches apart. This allows you to use maximum weight and involves many upper-body muscles (including your pectorals, believe it or not).

❹ **HIGH BAR:** Pull the bar to about the middle of your chest, instead of to your upper abdomen. This shifts work to the rear delts and middle and upper traps, and away from the lats.

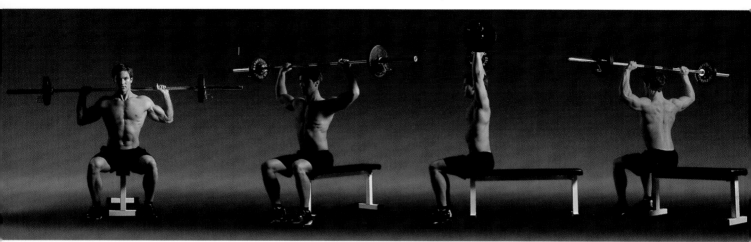

BARBELL SEATED SHOULDER PRESS

The shoulder press, also called the military press, has as checkered a history as any strength exercise. Before the rise of powerlifting in general and the bench press in particular, it was considered the true measure of a man's strength. Now it's used sparingly in most workout programs, because it has the reputation of being a dangerous exercise.

The problem is in the particulars. If you could just lift the weight straight up off your shoulders, there probably wouldn't be much controversy. Of course, you can't do that with a barbell since your head gets in the way. So you have to push the weight up from behind your neck or from the top of your chest. While the behind-the-neck version offers a straight line of movement, it can be tough on your rotator cuffs if your shoulders aren't flexible. And the front version requires that you bend your head backward to get the bar past your chin. Many guys also arch their backs on this movement.

We use the behind-the-neck version as our primary vertical-push exercise, especially in the advanced workouts. We also understand that your shoulders may not allow this movement, particularly if you've had shoulder injuries in the past. If you feel discomfort with the barbell shoulder presses, it's okay to revert to dumbbells. And if even dumbbells are problematic, using a Hammer Strength machine is not the worst thing in the world. Other shoulder-press machines, in our opinion, cause more injuries than they prevent, since they constrict the path your shoulder joints are able to follow.

Ultimately, it pays to learn and get good at the barbell shoulder presses. Proficiency at overhead pressing with a bar makes it easier to learn the most advanced lifts—the cleans, snatches, and push-presses, which are beyond even this book's advanced program. In case you can't master this exercise, there are others that build the same muscles, several of which we describe in this section.

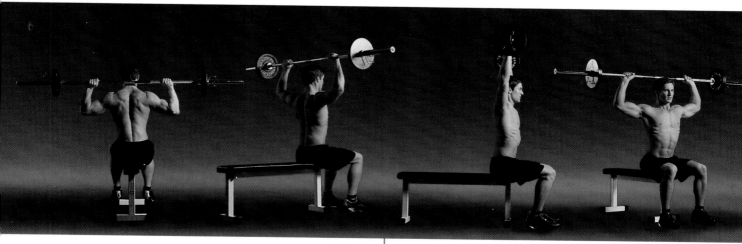

SETUP: Place a bench a couple of paces beyond a squat rack. Set the barbell in the supports of the squat rack, and step under it. Rest it on your upper trapezius, as you would for a squat, and grip it as you would for a bench press, with your hands just inside the rings. Step back to the bench, and sit on the end, with your legs apart and forming a triangle with your hips. Your feet should be flat on the floor.

EXECUTION: Press the bar up in a straight line, without fully locking out your arms. Then lower the bar to the base of your neck or as close to that point as you can get.

SAFETY: As we said, if you can't do this exercise, that's that. If you can do it, you can train more safely and productively if you "groove" one line of ascent and descent and never deviate from it. Deviating from this line of movement is, literally, out of line. You'll pay with neck and shoulder injuries.

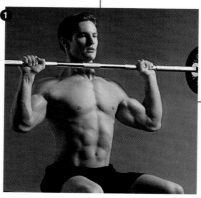

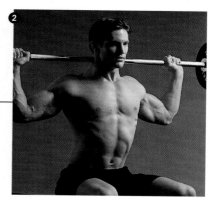

VARIATIONS

❶ TO FRONT: Lower the bar until it's in front of your throat, just above the top of your sternum. This shifts emphasis a bit to your front deltoids, although your middle delts are the prime movers whether you're pressing from the front or the rear.

❷ WIDE GRIP: Grab the bar with your hands just outside the rings on the bar. This version intensifies the work for your deltoids because you get less assistance from your triceps.

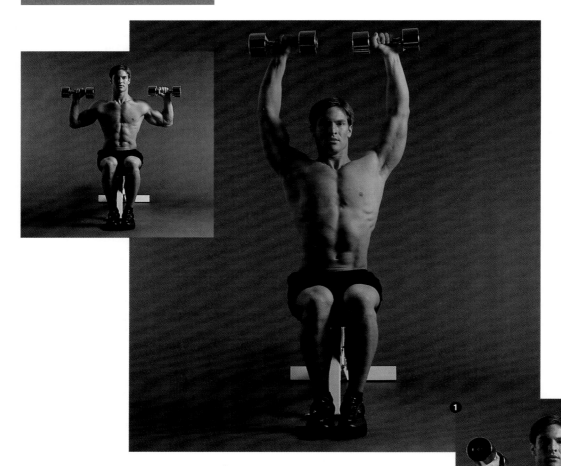

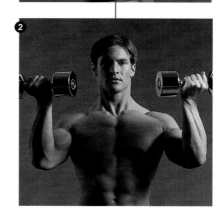

DUMBBELL SEATED SHOULDER PRESS

SETUP: Grab a pair of dumbbells and sit on the end of a bench. Hold the dumbbells at the edges of your shoulders, with your palms facing forward.

EXECUTION: Press the weights up and slightly inward until your arms are almost straight but not locked out. At the top, they should be close to each other without touching. Lower them to your shoulders along the same path.

VARIATIONS

❶ **PALMS IN:** Some find this variation a little easier on the shoulders.

❷ **ARNOLD PRESS:** Start with your palms facing back and the dumbbells next to your ears. As you press the weights overhead, rotate your forearms so your palms face forward. Reverse this path as you lower the weights to the starting position. This variation will have a slightly different effect on your shoulder and forearm muscles, and the twisting action mimics that of punching in martial arts.

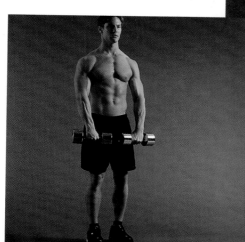

DUMBBELL UPRIGHT ROW

SETUP: Grab a pair of dumbbells and stand holding them at arm's length in front of you, your palms facing your thighs and the weights a few inches apart.

EXECUTION: Raise the weights straight up, keeping your palms close to and facing your body, until they're just under your chin. In the top position, your elbows should be higher than your wrists. Pause, then lower the weights back down until your arms are fully extended, again keeping the action close to your body.

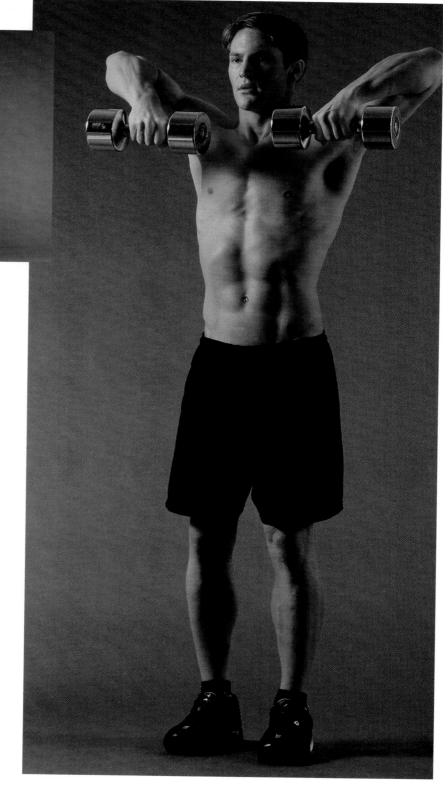

MUSCLES THAT ACT ON THE SHOULDER

BARBELL UPRIGHT ROW

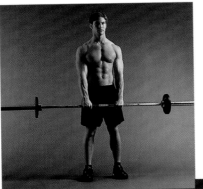

SETUP: Pick up the barbell with an overhand grip, your hands just less than shoulder-width apart. (If you find it more comfortable, you can use a "false" grip, with your thumb on the same side of the bar as your fingers, rather than opposing them.) Hold the bar in front of your body with your arms straight.

EXECUTION: Raise the bar straight up, keeping your palms facing and close to your body, until the bar is just under your chin. In the top position, your elbows should be higher than your wrists. Pause, then lower the bar back down until your arms are fully extended, again keeping the action close to your body.

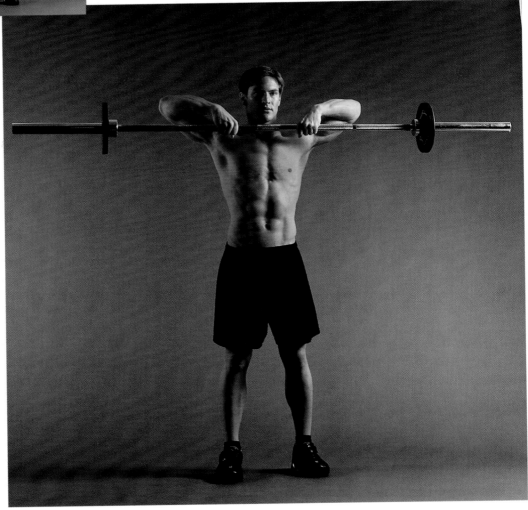

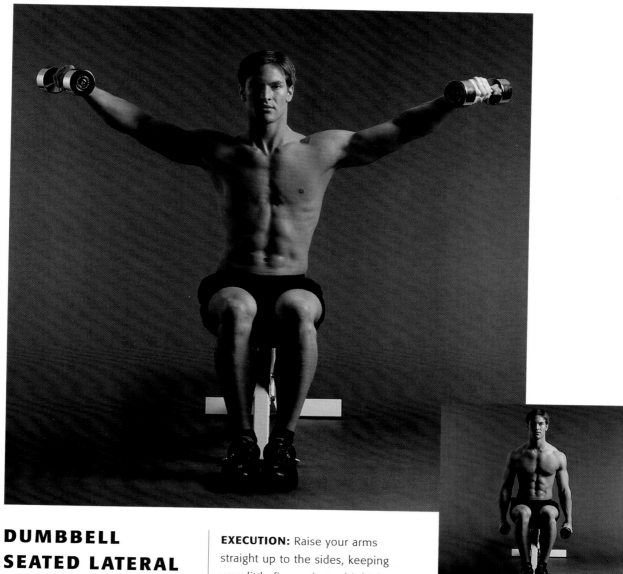

DUMBBELL SEATED LATERAL RAISE

SETUP: Grab a pair of dumbbells and sit on the end of a bench with your feet together. Hold the weights at your sides, with your arms nearly straight (keep a slight bend in your elbow, which you'll maintain throughout the movement) and your palms facing in.

EXECUTION: Raise your arms straight up to the sides, keeping your little fingers just a bit higher than your thumbs. Stop when the weights are even with the top of your head. Pause, then lower them along the same path.

PULLUP/CHINUP

When we say *pullup* we mean an exercise in which your palms are turned away from your body, in an overhand grip; and when we say *chinup*, we mean your palms are turned toward your body, in an underhand grip. The chinup is easier for most guys since it puts the biceps into a stronger position. Also, because of the difference in arm position, the lower-lat and lower-trap muscles work harder in the chinup, while the rear delts, middle traps, and upper lats work harder in the pullup.

Everyone agrees that pulling your body weight over a bar from a dead hang is a great way to develop upper-body strength and muscle mass. Every muscle from your fingers to your gluteals must get involved. The only problem with the pullup/chinup is that so few guys can do it. One survey of members of an American health club found that about 70 percent couldn't do a single one. Presumably, health club members would be among the most fit adults, so you can imagine that the rate of proficiency would be even lower among average, less–exercise-minded Americans.

The rise of the lat pulldown as the most popular vertical-pull exercise may imply that even dedicated exercisers have given up on the pullup and chinup since they have other, easier ways to develop their lat muscles. But the lat pulldown is not the equivalent of the pullup or chinup. It locks your lower body into place so all you have to do is pull with the muscles of your shoulder girdle. (Assisted-pullup machines have the same drawback. The shoulder motion is the same as in a pullup, but since your body isn't hanging in space, it isn't the same overall muscle builder.)

On a pullup or chinup, your abdominals have to contract to keep your body moving along an efficient path. Your shoulder girdle muscles also have to work harder at balancing your body.

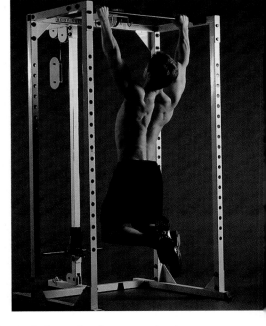

And the gripping muscles in your hands and forearms have to hold on to the bar long enough to give your back muscles a thorough workout.

Our workouts will take you from zero pullups—assuming that's how many you can do now—to multiple reps with your own body weight. You won't stop there. In the intermediate and advanced programs, you'll do multiple sets with weights hanging from a chain attached to a belt around your waist.

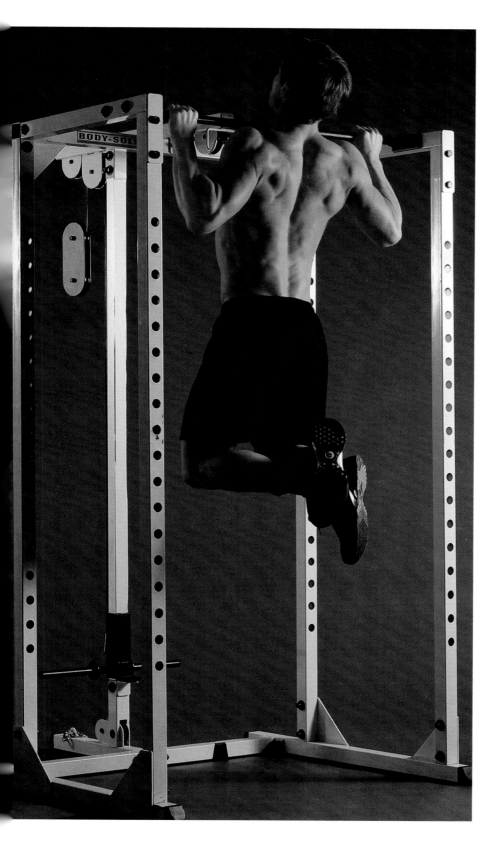

PULLUP SETUP: Grab the chinning bar with an overhand grip that's shoulder width or just a bit wider. Hang at arm's length with your legs bent at the knees and your feet crossed at the ankles.

PULLUP EXECUTION: Pull yourself up until your chin crosses the plane of the bar, then slowly lower yourself without allowing your body to sway.

CHINUP: Grab the bar with an underhand grip that's shoulder width or just a bit narrower, then hang and pull as for a pullup.

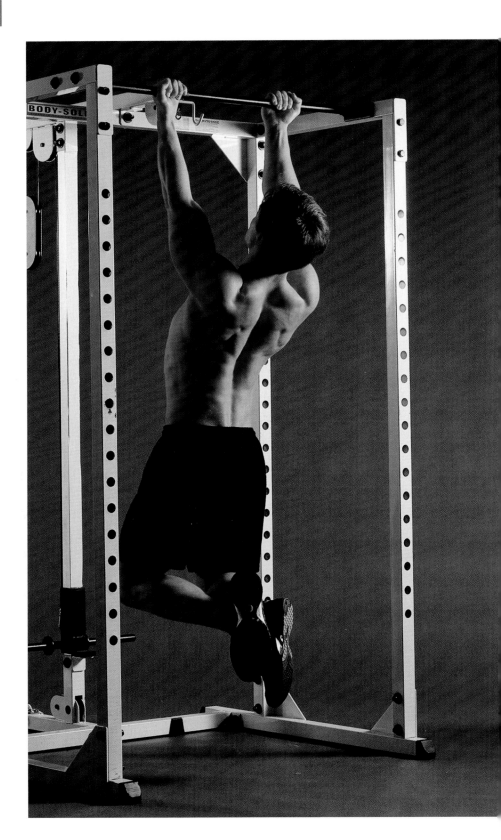

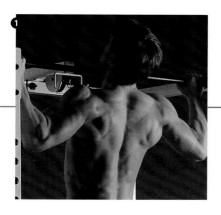

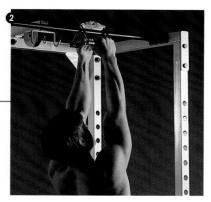

VARIATIONS

❶ WIDE-GRIP PULLUP: Grab the bar overhand with your hands outside shoulder width. This shortens the range of motion for your lats but makes the movement tougher because your arms are in a weakened position.

❷ NEUTRAL-GRIP PULLUP: If your gym has parallel-grip chinning handles, grab those and execute a pullup. If it doesn't, take a triangle handle from the rowing or pulldown station and put it over the chinning bar. Then either pull yourself up and back until your sternum approaches the bar or go straight up, moving your head to either side of the crossbar on alternating repetitions. The benefit of the neutral grip is that your brachialis and brachio-radialis muscles are in their

strongest positions. The risk is that if you use the triangle apparatus, it will fall on your head when you finish your set and let go of the handle.

❸ WEIGHTED PULLUP (NOT PICTURED): When you can complete the required repetitions in a set using your body weight, you need to add weight to make the exercise more challenging. Otherwise, the pullup becomes like the pushup: At a certain point, you shift from building strength to building endurance. The easiest way to add weight is to wear a belt with a chain on the front, allowing you to strap on as much weight as you need. (You haven't lived until you've seen a bodybuilder do pullups with multiple 45-pound plates clanking from his hips.) You can also wear a loaded backpack, filling it with

books, bricks, or weight plates according to your strength. Or you can buy a weighted vest, which is good for pushups but by far the more expensive option for pullups.

WARMUPS AND BACKOFF SETS: Few of us will ever get so good at pullups that we can do multiple warmup sets with body weight, then knock out weighted sets, then do a backoff set (a higher-rep set following heavy, low-rep sets to more thoroughly exhaust the muscles and add more of a muscle-building stimulus) with body weight. It is possible that at some point you may be so strong that you need to do weighted pullups for some of your warmups. Until then, do lat pulldowns for most of your warmups and backoff sets.

LAT PULLDOWN

SETUP: Attach a long, straight bar to the cable apparatus, and select the appropriate weight on the stack. Grab the bar with an overhand grip that's shoulder width or just a bit wider, and lower yourself into position, with your thighs beneath the bracing pads.

EXECUTION: Lean back slightly as you pull the bar down to your upper chest. (A mental trick is to try to push your chest out to meet the bar. That helps you remember to pull your shoulder blades together in back.) In the fully contracted position, your elbows should be slightly behind your torso. Make sure you bring the bar to the exact same point on your chest for each repetition. Control the bar as your arms straighten to return to the starting position.

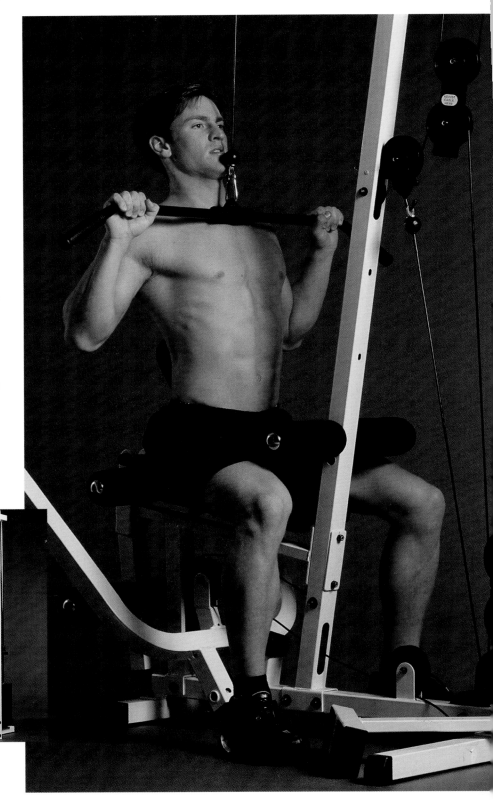

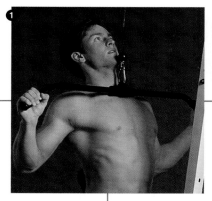

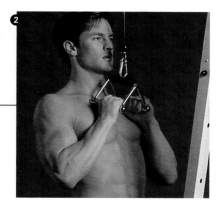

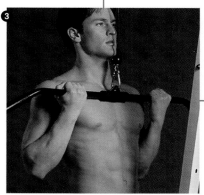

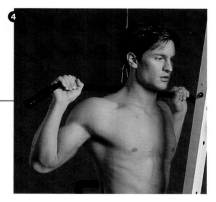

VARIATIONS

❶ **WIDE GRIP:** Grab the bar with your hands outside shoulder width. This is tougher for your lats because your arms can't help as much.

❷ **NEUTRAL GRIP:** When you use the triangle handle to position your hands close together, palms facing each other, your arm and back muscles are in a more powerful position. You can handle maximum loads using this attachment.

❸ **REVERSE GRIP:** Grab the bar with an underhand grip that's shoulder width or just a bit narrower. This is equivalent to the chinup, involving your biceps and lower lats more.

❹ **BEHIND NECK:** When we started lifting, everyone did lat pulldowns behind the neck. Now the front pulldown rules, and the behind-the-neck version is the bogeyman. The front pulldown is a better exercise—studies have shown it produces a more powerful contraction in the lat muscles—but we include the behind-the-neck pulldown in our workouts because it's more clearly the

opposite of the behind-the-neck shoulder press. As with that press, on each repetition you should pull down to the same point on your neck and make the line of pull as straight as possible. Some gym machines simply don't allow a straight pull to the back of the neck, which means you have two options: Either give up on this variation or turn around and face the opposite direction on the apparatus, giving up the bracing pads for your thighs. If you have shoulder problems that make this exercise painful, use the front pulldown instead.

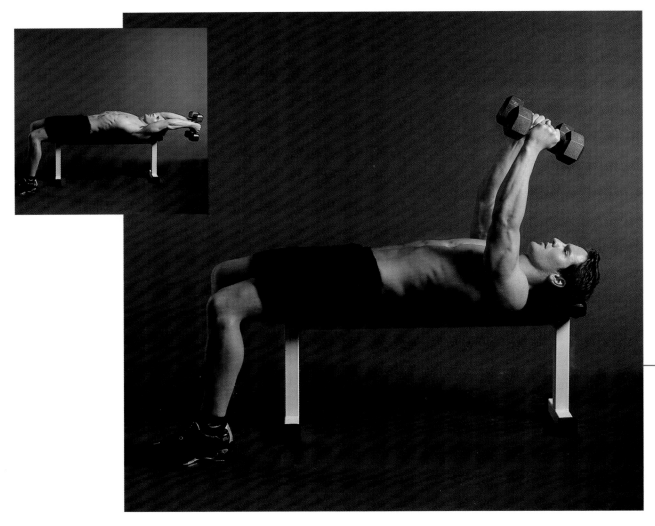

DUMBBELL LYING PULLOVER

SETUP: Pick up a pair of dumbbells, and lie faceup on a bench. Your feet can rest on the floor or the bench. (Placing them on the bench adds an interesting challenge to your balance and also prevents you from arching your back excessively.) Hold the dumbbells over your head with your palms facing each other and your elbows slightly bent.

EXECUTION: Lower the weights behind your head as far as comfort allows while keeping your elbows bent at the same angle. Pull the weights back up over your head. Make sure they stay the same distance apart throughout the movement, and don't pull so far that your arms end up perpendicular to the floor. There's no resistance from gravity at that angle, which means there's no tension on the working muscles—and no tension, no benefit.

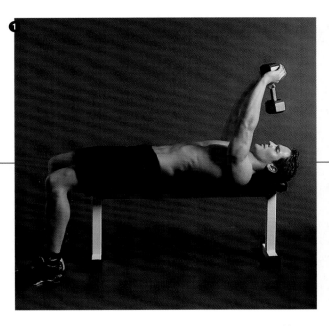

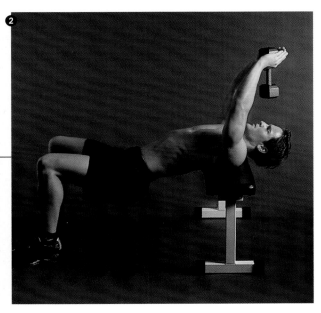

VARIATIONS

❶ ONE DUMBBELL IN TWO HANDS: Cup one hand around the inside end of a dumbbell, then cup the other around that. Using one dumbbell ensures equal strength development on both sides of your torso.

❷ ONE DUMBBELL IN TWO HANDS, ACROSS BENCH: Lie perpendicular to the bench so your shoulders rest on it while your head hangs off one side and your body is supported by your feet on the floor. The movement is the same, except that your hips should be lower than your shoulders, allowing a greater stretch—and thus greater development—in your lats. This variation is a favorite of old-school bodybuilders, who believed it could increase the size of their rib cages. We can't imagine how that could be possible, although you still find the idea advanced in books written by bodybuilding gurus.

BARBELL SHRUG

In our workout programs, the shrug and its many variations are usually performed along with hip-dominant exercises. That's because the trapezius, the muscle targeted by shrugs, is so important in deadlifts, clean pulls, high pulls, and other exercises that involve pulling a weight off the floor.

The shrug helps in your performance of other exercises as well. It allows you to work with heavy weights, improving your grip strength and thereby helping in pullups and rows. This brings up another point: In the gym, you'll see some bodybuilders using wrist straps to help them lift more weight on the shrug and other exercises in which grip strength can dictate the amount of weight you use. While that's fine for them, we want you to go strapless as often as possible—even though sometimes, particularly in the advanced workout program, it makes sense to shrug loads that are too heavy to hold with your bare hands. One of the great benefits of our workout programs is the tremendous improvements you'll see in grip strength, and chronic strap-happiness will limit those gains.

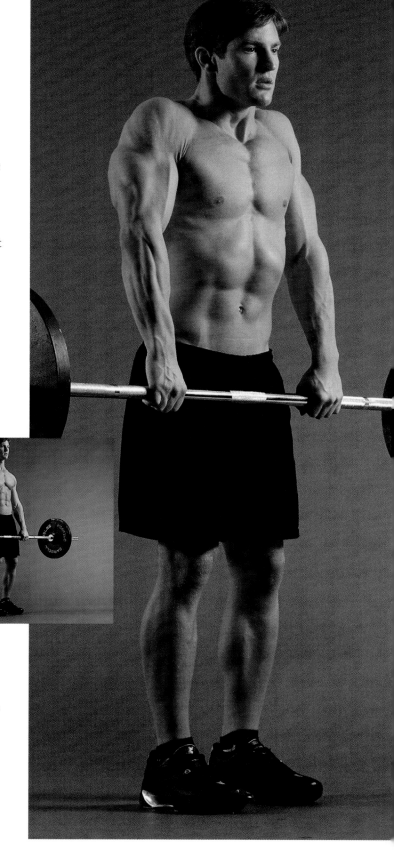

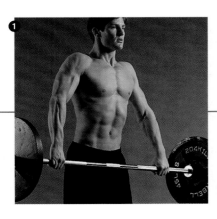

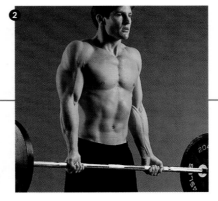

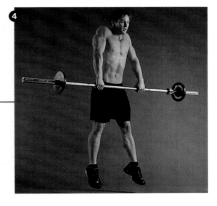

SETUP: Set a barbell above knee height in a rack or on whatever supports you have access to. Grab the bar with an overhand grip that's just beyond shoulder width. Take the bar off the supports and hold it at arm's length.

EXECUTION: Allow your shoulders to sink, then shrug them straight up, as high as you can. Keep your elbows straight and your head vertical (although it's okay to tuck your chin, which may move your head forward a bit). Your chest should rise along with your shoulders. Stop the set when you lose your full range of motion. In other words, we don't want you to use heavy weights that allow you to move the bar only a half-inch; we want you to use your full range of motion throughout every rep in every set.

VARIATIONS

❶ WIDE GRIP: Grab the bar with your hands outside the rings. This changes the action of your traps, since they have to elevate your shoulder blades while the bones are rotated toward each other on top, rather than at their normal distance from each other.

❷ REVERSE GRIP: Grab the bar underhand, with your hands just outside your thighs. This separates your scapulae a bit more, changing the angle from which your traps pull the weight.

❸ EXPLOSIVE, FROM HANG ABOVE KNEES (NOT PICTURED): Start with your torso bent forward, the bar just above your knees, your back flat, and your shoulders over or a bit in front of the bar. Starting the

movement slowly, and building up speed, straighten your torso, then rise up on your toes and shrug your shoulders. At the end of the movement, your body should be aligned in such a way that you could draw a straight line through your shoulders, hips, knees, and ankles.

❹ JUMP, FROM HANG ABOVE KNEES: This variation is the same as the previous except you use a lighter weight and pull so hard that your feet come up off the floor. Bend your knees to absorb the force of landing, then settle and reset your body before the next repetition.

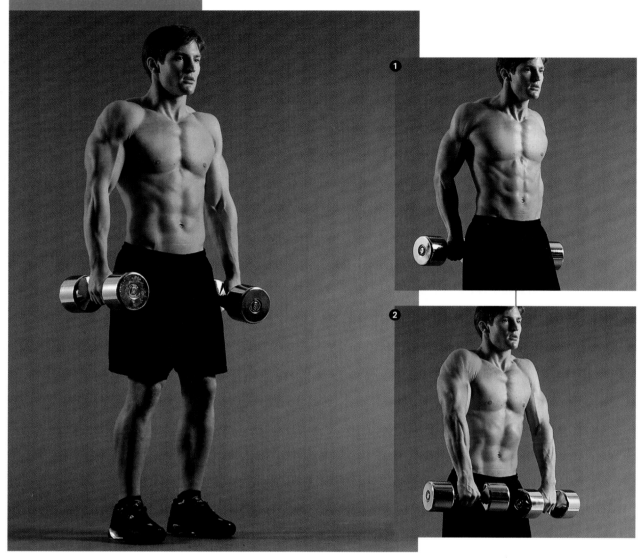

DUMBBELL SHRUG

SETUP: Stand holding a pair of dumbbells at arm's length at your sides, palms facing your body. Plant your feet hip- or shoulder-width apart, with your knees slightly bent. Keep your head straight or just slightly forward, with your chin tucked.

EXECUTION: Allow your shoulders to sink, then shrug them up toward your ears, as high as you can. Keep your arms straight, and don't allow your shoulders to roll forward.

VARIATIONS

❶ BEHIND BODY: Hold the dumbbells behind your butt, palms facing backward. This unusual angle forces your traps to work with the bottoms of your scapulae rotated toward each other.

❷ TO FRONT: Hold the dumbbells in front of your thighs, palms facing your body. At this angle, your scapulae are rotated away from each other, giving your traps another unusual angle of pull.

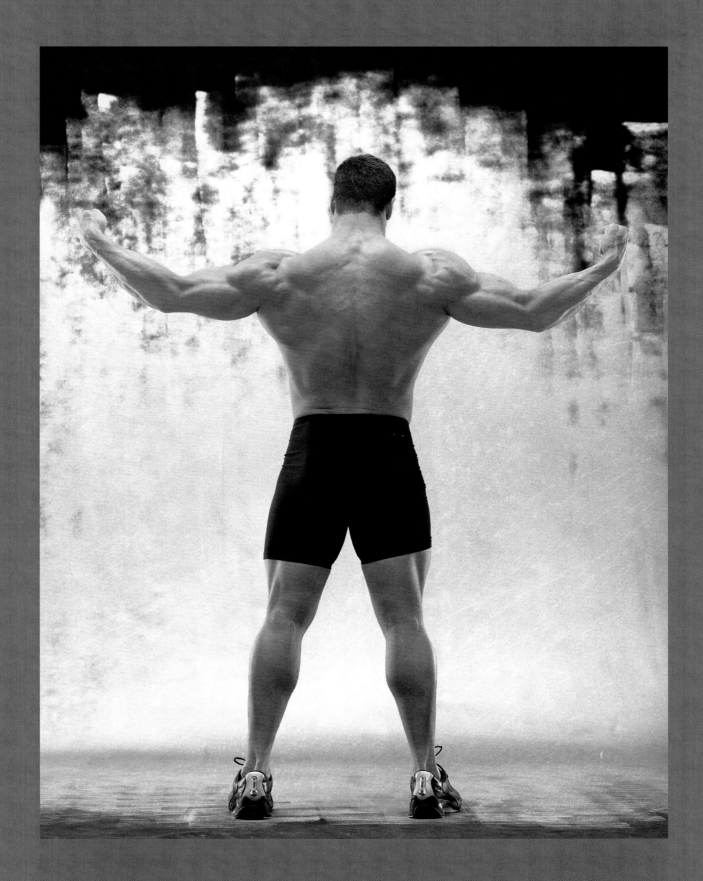

CHAPTER SEVEN

MUSCLES THAT ACT ON THE ELBOW AND WRIST

AT FIRST GLANCE, THE ELBOW JOINT IS PRETTY SIMPLE. It bends, and it straightens. If it were a toy, a toddler would be bored with it in a minute. Once you throw in the movement of the two forearm bones—the radius and ulna, with the former wrapping around the latter—it all gets a little more complicated and interesting. Another complication is the way the muscles that bend and straighten the elbow also play a role in lifting and lowering the upper arm, actions that take place in the shoulder joints.

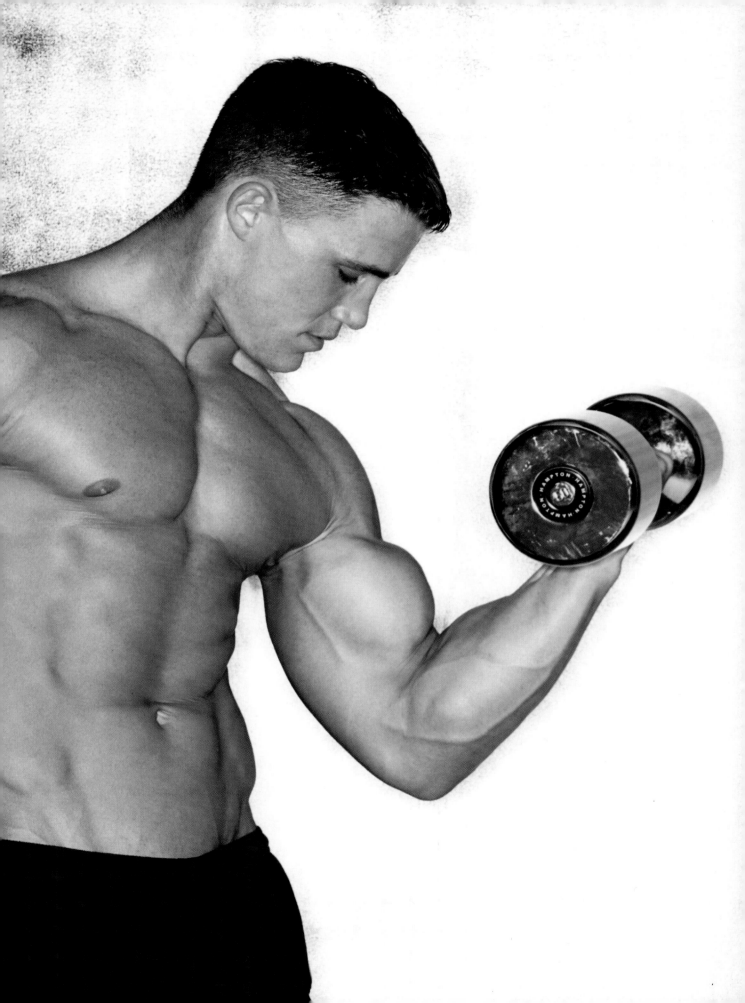

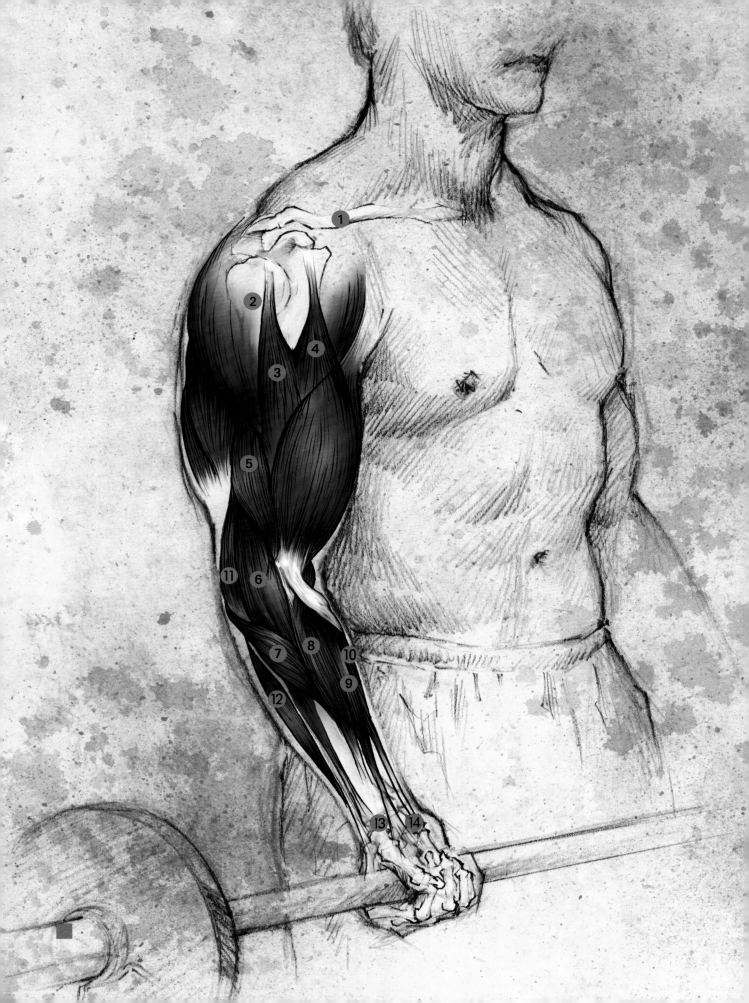

The wrist joint is complex, though its movements are simple: up, down, and side to side. There isn't much need to do special exercises to work the muscles that act on the wrist; they get plenty of work in other strength-training exercises and play a role in virtually everything you do with your hands. (Yes, we thought of that thing. We're just too polite to mention it.) We'll include a pair of simple wrist exercises to build the forearm muscles in the early stages of our workout programs. After that, these muscles are built just by participating in the heavier, more advanced lifts.

BICEPS

That the biceps serves to bend the elbow is painfully obvious. You've been flexing in front of your mirror since before your voice cracked, so you know how this muscle works.

Still, the biceps has a few tricks up your sleeve that you may not know about. It has two heads (hence, the *bi* in its name) that combine to form a tendon that crosses the elbow joint and attaches to the radius. The long head, on the outside of your upper arm, originates on the top of the shoulder blade. It works with the front deltoid and the topmost pectoral fibers to lift your upper arm in front of your body. The short biceps head, on the inside of your upper arm, starts lower on the scapula, so it doesn't get involved in lifting your upper arm.

What the short head does is cooperate with the long head to help perform a motion called *supination*, the act of turning your forearm. (Say your palm is facing back behind you, and you rotate your forearm so your palm faces forward—that's supination.) You have a muscle specifically designed to supinate your wrist (believe it or not, it's called the **SUPINATOR**), located on the outside of your elbow, beneath a forearm muscle. When you have to do this

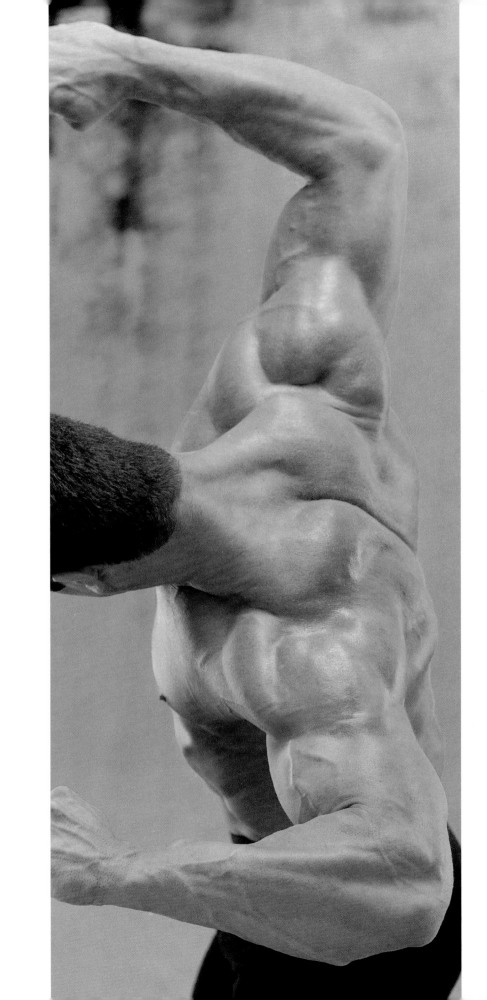

action with a heavy weight involved, your supinator needs help, so the biceps jumps in.

The biceps has a strong but often well-hidden assistant called the **BRACHIALIS**. The brachialis lies between the biceps and the humerus, attaching to the forearm bone called the ulna. It's a thick, strong muscle that takes a leading role when you bend your elbow while your palm is in a neutral position (turned toward the side of your body) or pronated (turned backward, with your thumb pointed toward your thigh). When well-developed, it's visible as a cylinder of muscle popping up between your biceps and triceps.

The brachialis is an assistant that has its own helper, the **BRACHIORADIALIS**. The brachioradialis is viewed mostly as a forearm muscle; it originates near the elbow and attaches near the wrist, so most of its length is along the forearm bones, rather than the upper-arm bone. Nevertheless, its job is elbow flexion. It pulls on the radius while the brachialis yanks on the ulna—all for the glory of the biceps, which gets the credit for elbow flexion no matter how hard other muscles work.

The manner in which these muscles work together is determined by your hand position. With a supinated (palm-up, or underhand) grip, the biceps earn their star billing. With a neutral (palm-in, or hammer) or pronated (palm-down, or overhand) grip, the brachialis and brachioradialis do more to help. And if you start a dumbbell biceps curl with your hand in a neutral position and then supinate your palm (turn it inward, as in the dumbell seated hammer curl, with twist, on page 131), your biceps and supinator make the rotation possible.

In a bilateral exercise (that is, an exercise that works both arms simultaneously), grip width also matters. With a wider grip—your hands farther apart—the short (inner) head of your biceps does more work. With a narrower grip, you get more action from the long (outer) head.

The big question most guys have about their biceps is which exercises and variations will lead to the shape they find most desirable. In chapter five, we reviewed some of the theories about reshaping muscles, so we don't want to repeat ourselves except to say this: Performing a mix of biceps exercises throughout your training program, using progressively heavier weights, remains the best way to bring out whatever shape is possible given your genetics.

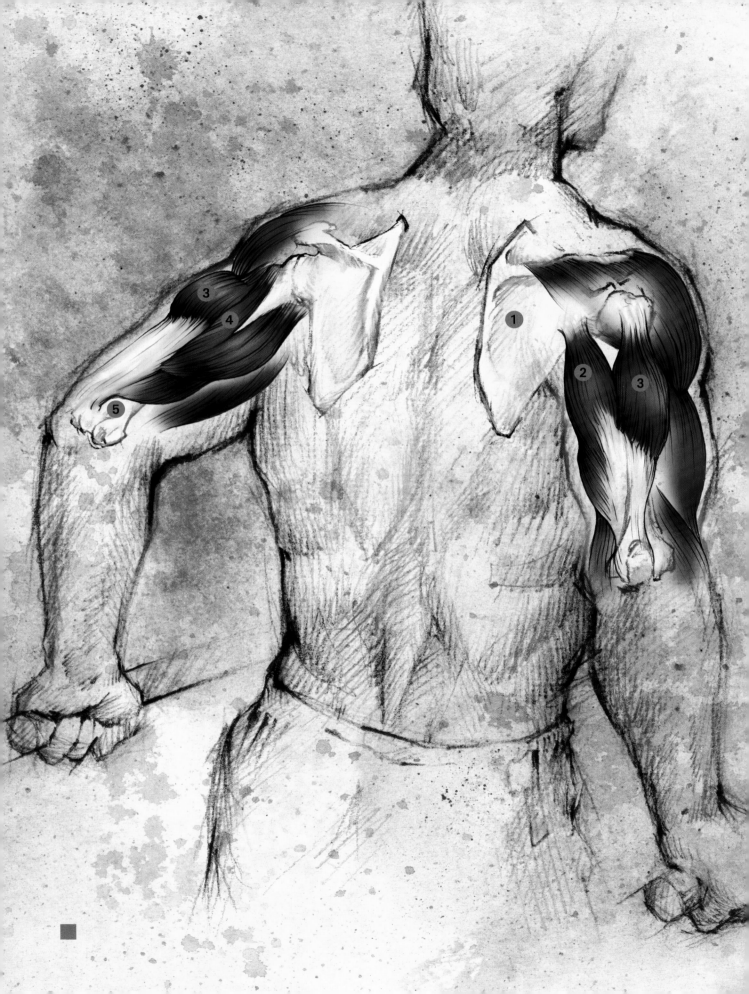

If you want to throw in more exercises in hopes of making the muscle longer or giving it a higher peak, you're on your own.

TRICEPS

Unlike the biceps, the triceps has almost no complexity to its function, hidden or otherwise. It straightens your elbow and plays a supporting role in one shoulder action: lowering your arm to your side when it's extended in front of your body. (Pullovers, shown on pages 112 and 113, are examples of exercises that work your triceps via your shoulders, rather than via your elbows.)

Despite its simplicity, the triceps plays a major role in the weight room, whether you're trying to build strength or muscle mass. If you're a student of the bench press, you know how important triceps strength is to the completion of the lift. Furthermore, the triceps comprises two-thirds of your upper-arm mass, so if you want more eye-catching arms, you have to dedicate at least as much effort to your triceps as to your biceps.

As its name implies, the triceps has three heads. The lateral head is on the outside rear of your upper arm and forms half of the horseshoe shape you see in a well-developed arm. The other half of that curve is formed by the triceps long head, on the inside-rear upper arm. The medial head is the thick part below the lateral head and above the elbow. All three heads come together in a tendon that is attached to the ulna. (If you're keeping track, the triceps and brachialis attach to the ulna, while the biceps and brachioradialis attach to the radius.)

The medial and lateral triceps heads are much like the brachialis in that they're involved in elbow extension—straightening your arm from a bent position—and only elbow extension. The long head has a slightly more interesting life. It originates on

1 SCAPULA

2 TRICEPS LONG HEAD

3 TRICEPS LATERAL HEAD

4 TRICEPS MEDIAL HEAD
(BENEATH LONG HEAD)

5 HUMERUS

the outside edge of the scapula, just below the shoulder joints, so it takes part in some exercises you wouldn't expect, such as the aforementioned pullovers. It even helps a bit in pullups and lat pulldowns, although only to a very limited extent.

Most people in the gym treat the triceps like a fragile, subtle muscle, doing all sorts of elbow-extension exercises on cable apparatuses with various attachments and generally limited ranges of motion. That's fine, especially for beginners.

But the key to triceps development is lifting really, really heavy weights. Since you use the heaviest weights on multi-joint exercises such as bench presses and dips, those are the best triceps exercises, even though they're generally regarded as chest exercises. Positioning your hands close together on the barbell bench press (as shown on page 88) works the triceps even harder.

FOREARM FLEXORS AND EXTENSORS

Hold your arm out in front of you, with your palm facing up. Now bend your wrist so your palm comes closer to you (making a movement called forearm flexion that's mimicked by an exercise called the wrist curl, shown on pages 143 and144). The muscles that jump to attention are the **FLEXOR CARPI RADIALIS** and **FLEXOR CARPI ULNARIS**. (You probably have a weak elbow flexor, called the **PALMARIS LONGUS**, in between these two, unless you're among the 15 percent of people without this muscle. We don't think your career path will be affected if you're palmaris-deficient.)

The two flexors originate on the outside of your humerus and end on your hand, at the knuckles that attach your hand bones (metacarpals) to your finger bones. Because they do cross the elbow joint, they're important stabilizing muscles on biceps and upper-back exercises—any move in which you grip a bar and pull it toward your body or pull your body toward it.

The flexor carpi radialis also has a role in an action called *pronation*, in which your twist your hand from a palm-up or palm-in position to a palm-down position. This makes sense because pronation involves twisting your radius around your ulna. An example would be a cable triceps extension with a rope attachment, in which you rotate your wrists outward at the end of the movement.

Now, hold your arm out in front of you, with your palm facing down. When you bring your knuckles back toward your forearm, you're performing wrist extension, for which you have three muscles: **EXTENSOR CARPI RADIALIS LONGUS**, **EXTENSOR CARPI RADIALIS BREVIS**, and **EXTENSOR CARPI ULNARIS**. (That works out to two extensor muscles for your radius and one for your ulna.) All three muscles originate at the outside edge of the upper-arm bone and play a role in stabilizing the elbow joint during many upper-body exercises. In particular, the ulnaris may help the triceps in elbow-extension exercises.

These forearm muscles also move your wrist laterally, when your thumb or your pinkie moves toward your forearm. The latter action is technically called *ulna flexion*. In sports, it is commonly referred to as the *wrist break*; it's the snap at the end of a baseball or golf swing, or the twist you put on a tennis swing to make the ball spin.

BICEPS EXERCISES

For most muscle groups, it's easy to pick the single best type of exercise: the bench press for your chest, dip for your triceps, pullup for your back, squat for your quadriceps, deadlift for your hamstrings and gluteals. But there is no clear-cut world's-greatest biceps exercise. We're tempted to suggest the chinup since that exercise allows the greatest loads. Unfortunately, during periods when we've relied on it for biceps development we've built plenty of strength but not as much mass as we would have hoped.

Our next choice might be the many dumbbell-curl variations, except for the fact that while those certainly create a great pump and inflict damage on the biceps from every possible angle, they don't seem to improve strength all that much.

So for strength and mass, it seems the barbell curl is the best choice. Curling a straight bar is brutal on the wrists, which is why we finally settle on the EZ-bar biceps curl. The slight variation in hand position allowed by the W-shaped EZ barbell probably activates the brachialis a bit more and the biceps a bit less than does a straight bar. This effect is so subtle that we don't think you'll notice it.

What you will notice is that you'll increase your strength rapidly without developing chronically sore wrists and forearms.

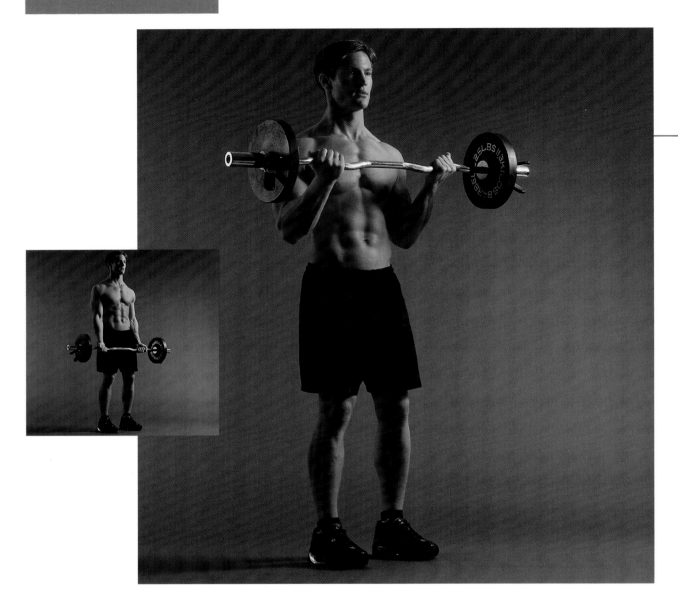

EZ-BAR BICEPS CURL

The EZ-bar curl is an anomaly among exercises in that you can lift more weight while using poor form. So in our advanced program, if you're so inclined, you can add a slight backward lean on your final repetitions in your heaviest sets, provided you do the majority of your repetitions with strict form. Because there may be some injury risk associated with using less-than-perfect form, you have to earn the right to cheat. While you're a beginner or even an intermediate, you need to restrict yourself to strict form until it feels like the only way to do the exercise.

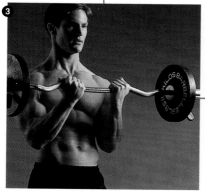

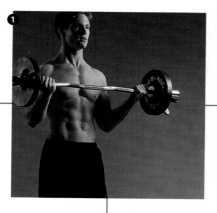

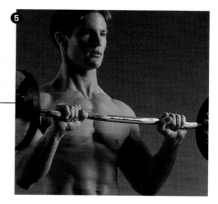

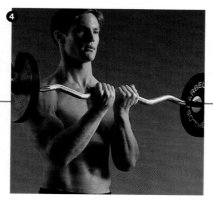

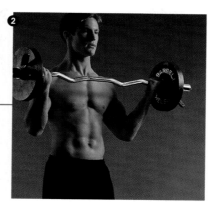

SETUP: Load an EZ-curl bar and grasp it with a shoulder-width, underhand grip. Stand with your feet hip-width apart and your knees slightly bent, or at least unlocked. (This fights the reflex to lean backward as you lift the weight.) Hold the bar at arm's length in front of your thighs.

EXECUTION: Bend your elbows, curling the bar upward. Stop just before the bar hits the "gravity line," the point at which it's moving horizontally and thus meeting no resistance from gravity. This is a subtle shift—it'll take some practice before you regularly stop just short of this point. Pause, then lower the weight to the starting position,

allowing your arms to fully extend. (You'll be tempted to stop short of full extension because it's easier to lift the bar on the next rep when you start with a slight bend in your elbow—your biceps are much stronger in that position than when your arms are straight. And, to tell the truth, it's not much of a problem if you occasionally stop short of full extension in order to lift heavier weights and thus build more mass. If you regularly stop short, your muscles will adapt by shortening themselves, reducing your overall range of motion, and setting you up for injury.)

VARIATIONS

❶ WIDE GRIP: Grasp the bar with a grip that's beyond shoulder width.

This puts more emphasis on the inner (short) head of the biceps.

❷ VERY WIDE GRIP: Grasp the bar with as wide a grip as possible. This puts even more emphasis on the inner head.

❸ CLOSE GRIP: Hold the bar with your hands narrower than shoulder-width apart. This emphasizes the outer (long) head of the biceps.

❹ VERY CLOSE GRIP: Hold the bar with your hands right next to each other. This adds more emphasis to the outer head.

❺ REVERSE GRIP: Take the bar with an overhand, shoulder-width grip. Now you work the brachialis and brachioradialis more than the biceps.

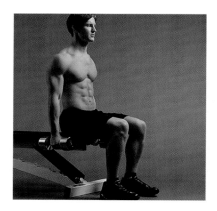

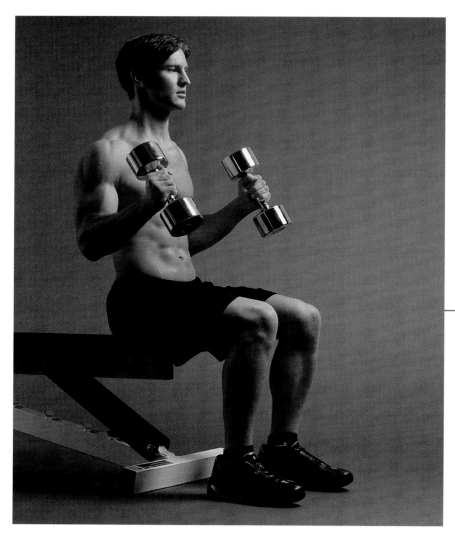

DUMBBELL SEATED HAMMER CURL

SETUP: Grab a pair of dumbbells and sit at the end of a bench with them at arm's length at your sides, palms facing in (hammer grip).

EXECUTION: Keeping your forearms in the neutral position, bend your elbows as high as you can without moving your upper arms. This emphasizes the brachialis, brachioradialis, and long biceps head, and is the strongest position for your elbow flexors. Many bench pressers believe this is the best biceps exercise for improving overall upper-body strength.

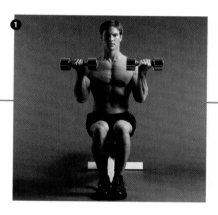

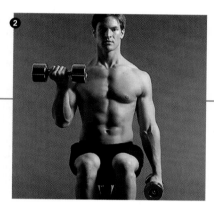

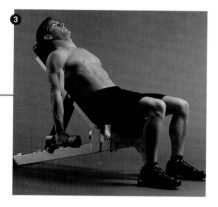

VARIATIONS

❶ WITH TWIST: As you lift the weights, simultaneously rotate your forearms outward, moving your thumbs as far outside as you can by the time you reach the top position (pictured). Lower the weights to the starting position, reversing the twisting motion until your hands are once again in the hammer-grip position when you reach the bottom. Make sure you extend your arms completely at the bottom to get a complete stretch in the biceps.

❷ WITH TWIST, ALTERNATING: Lift one arm at a time. Complete an entire curl with a single arm before you start lifting the other. Resist the temptation to make like the guys in the muscle-magazine photos, who contort to admire their biceps in full flexion. Sit in front of a mirror if you like, but don't change your posture.

❸ INCLINE: This combines the strongest hand position with the weakest arm position, eking a little more muscle development out of the simple hammer curl movement.

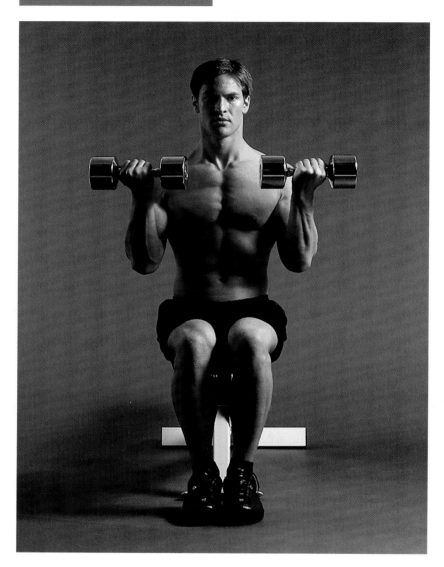

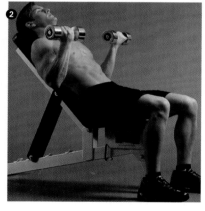

DUMBBELL SEATED BICEPS CURL

SETUP: Grab a pair of dumbbells and sit at the end of a bench with them at arm's length at your sides, palms facing forward.

EXECUTION: Keeping your upper arms in a fixed position perpendicular to the floor, bend your elbows to curl the weights as high as you can.

VARIATION

❶ REVERSE GRIP (NOT PICTURED): Hold the dumbells with an underhand grip. This hits your brachialis harder.

❷ INCLINE: Set an incline bench at a 45-degree angle, or even slightly higher if 45 degrees irritates your shoulders. (The lower you go, the harder it is on your shoulders.) Lie faceup with your arms perpendicular to the floor and behind your torso, with palms forward. Curl the dumbbells as high as you can without moving your upper arms or changing your posture. The angle puts your biceps in a weakened biomechanical position and thus makes them work harder. (Even if your biceps aren't usually sore after an arm workout, they'll ache after this.)

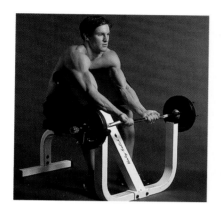

EZ-BAR PREACHER CURL

SETUP: Set the support pad of a preacher bench so you can sit with the top of the pad beneath your armpits and your upper arms at a 45-degree angle to your torso. Load an EZ-curl bar and set it in the supports. Grasp the bar with an underhand, shoulder-width grip, and hold it with your elbows bent slightly.

EXECUTION: Curl the bar up until it's just short of the point at which tension is reduced because the bar is moving horizontally (and thus has no resistance from gravity). Lower the bar to the starting position.

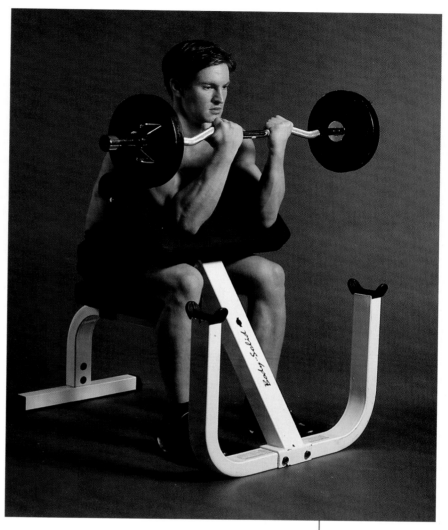

VARIATION

REVERSE GRIP: Use an overhand grip to emphasize the forearm extensors, brachialis, and brachioradialis.

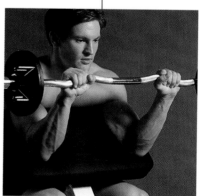

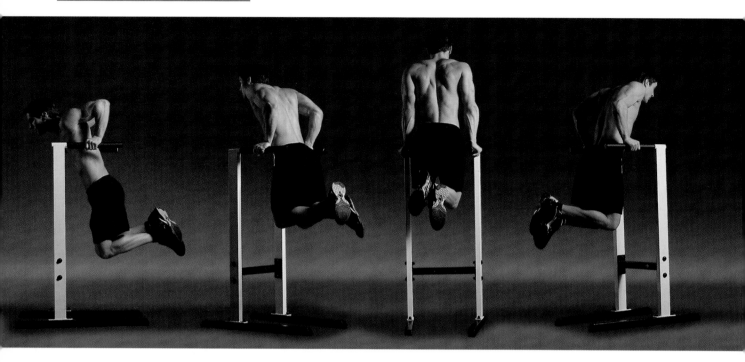

DIP/BENCH DIP

The dip is to the triceps—and thus to the entire upper arm—what the squat is to the quadriceps, and thus to the entire lower body. It's the big, basic movement that works the entire muscle. If you have time for just one triceps exercise, this is the one to do.

It's also a major chest exercise, working the lower and middle pectoral segments, which means that the dip is a two-for-one movement: You get complete triceps development while also working bigger muscles.

The bench dip is the stepping-stone to the parallel-bar dip and is also a good warmup exercise for it. You can add a load beyond your body weight to the bench dip, with a weight plate across your thighs, though that can get a bit awkward. Provided you have access to parallel bars, it's best to learn the dip and use bench dips for warmups and back-off sets.

That said, we should add that the dip is a tough exercise for guys with compromised shoulders. It's a precarious position for your shoulders, with all your weight forward while your upper arms are behind your torso. So if you have existing shoulder problems or find you're developing them after a few attempts at dipping, you may have to skip this exercise. A good substitute exercise (not included in our program) is the decline close-grip bench press, with a barbell or dumbbells. It offers the same pectoral development, although it's probably not as good a triceps exercise.

Even advanced lifters with strong, uninjured

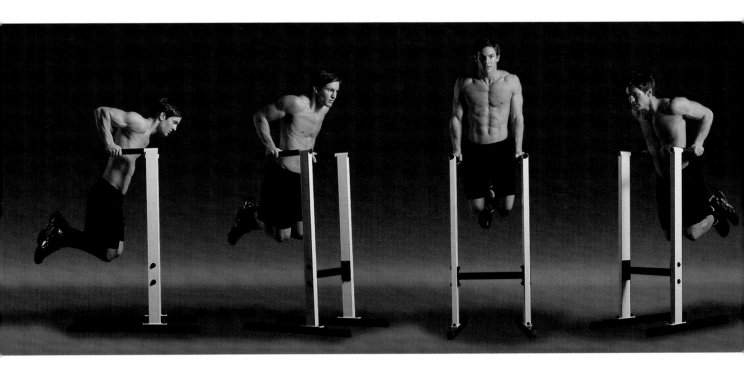

shoulders should show the dip the respect it deserves. Develop your range of motion slowly, over time. Always make your descent deliberate. And increase loads gradually, never adding more than 10 pounds at a time.

Obviously, you have to start with your body weight, and for many guys this will be challenging enough. (You can also use less than your body weight if your gym has a dip machine. While this is okay to start with, we recommend that you wean yourself from the machine sooner rather than later.) When you can do 10 perfect repetitions with your body weight, you need to add some sort of external load. The best solution is to hold a weight plate or dumbbell between your legs using a rope or chain attached to a weight belt. If you do this, make sure you

tightly clamp your legs around the dangling weight. Letting the weight sway could throw off your form. You can also use a backpack with weight plates inside it, if you work out at home.

The more weight you add, and the faster you add it, the more risk you take on. At the lowered position, your pectoral muscles are even more stretched than they are in the bottom position of a bench press, putting you at greater risk for strains and tears.

DIP SETUP: Choose a pair of parallel bars that are truly parallel (not a V-shape that allows you to hold your hands just beyond shoulder width). If you go wider than that, you put more emphasis on your chest muscles—and you also put your shoulders in a more vulnerable position. If possible, use bars that are thicker rather than thinner, minimizing overlap between your thumbs and fingers when you grip the bars. This makes the exercise a little harder, and in this case, harder is more beneficial.

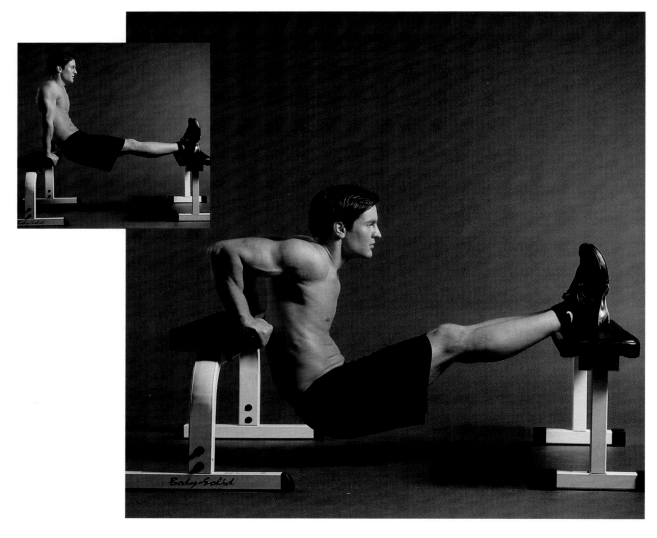

Grasp the bars with an overhand grip and your arms straight. You want your torso to be perpendicular to the floor, a posture you'll maintain throughout the exercise (leaning forward and pushing back will shift emphasis to your chest and shoulders). Bend your knees and cross your ankles.

DIP EXECUTION: Slowly lower your body until your shoulder joints are below your elbows. (Most guys stop short of this position.) Push back up until your elbows are nearly straight but not locked out.

BENCH-DIP SETUP: Place two benches, boxes, or a combination of these about 3 feet apart. Sit on one bench and place your heels on the other. Keeping your palms on the bench beside your body, with fingers forward, lift your body off the bench.

BENCH-DIP EXECUTION: Lower your body down just in front of your sitting bench. How far down you go will be influenced by your strength level and the health of your shoulder joint. Ideally, you want your shoulder joints below your elbows, but this range may not be possible at first. (And, depending on the length of your arms and the height of your benches, you may hit your butt on the floor before you go this far.) If you lack strength or have shoulder-joint issues, use a limited range of movement. If you're unable to do the exercise without pain, skip it altogether.

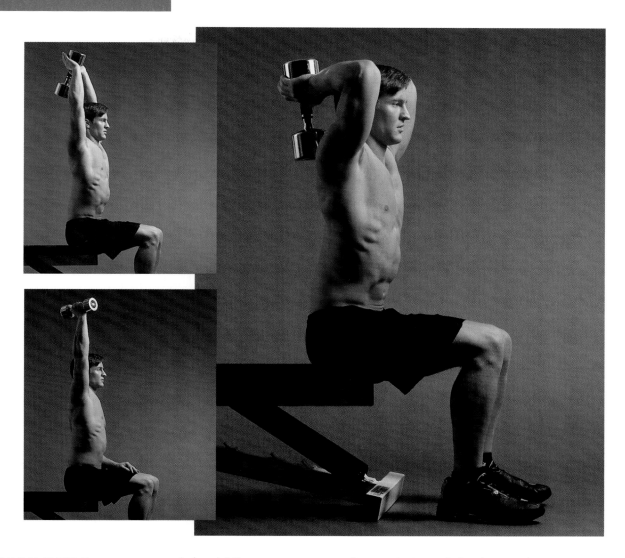

DUMBBELL SEATED OVERHEAD TRICEPS EXTENSION

SETUP (ONE DUMBBELL IN TWO HANDS): To ensure even distribution of load between the two hands, place one palm against the inside end of the dumbbell and the other palm over the back of the first hand. Lift your arms so your elbows are beside your ears.

SETUP (ONE DUMBBELL IN ONE HAND): Sit on the end of a bench, facing a mirror if possible. (Form is everything on this movement.) Grasp a dumbbell in one hand, and raise that hand directly above your head. Place the elbow beside your ear, holding the dumbbell with your palm facing inward. Keep the elbow as high and as far back as possible at all times to maximize the stretch on your triceps.

EXECUTION (ONE DUMBBELL IN TWO HANDS, PICTURED): Lower the dumbbell behind your head as far as you can without changing your posture (arching your back). Ideally, the dumbbell should touch your upper back. Pause, then lift the dumbbell back to the starting position. Keep your elbows stationary and facing forward throughout the movement.

MUSCLES THAT ACT ON THE ELBOW AND WRIST

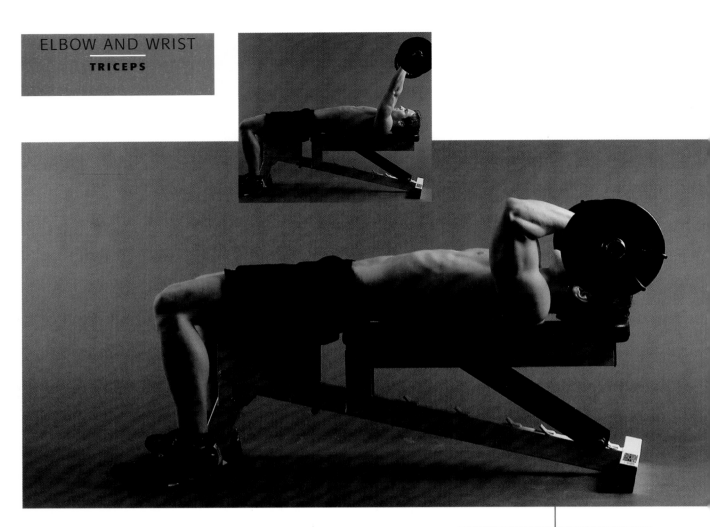

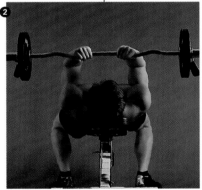

EZ-BAR LYING TRICEPS EXTENSION

SETUP: Load the EZ bar and grasp it with an overhand, shoulder-width grip. Lie faceup on a bench. Hold the bar at arm's length over your face; your arms should be angled slightly back toward your head, rather than vertical.

EXECUTION: Lower the bar to the top of your forehead. Pause, then push the weight back to the starting position, keeping your upper arms in the same position throughout the movement.

AS YOU GAIN EXPERIENCE: Set up so your head hangs off the end of the bench, and your upper arms angle back toward your head. You'll find this more challenging for your triceps.

VARIATIONS

❶ WIDE GRIP (NOT PICTURED): Grasp the bar with a grip that's beyond shoulder width. This shifts the emphasis from the triceps' lateral head to the long and medial heads.

❷ REVERSE GRIP: Grasp the bar with an underhand, shoulder-width grip. This shifts emphasis to the lateral head.

EZ-BAR OVERHEAD TRICEPS EXTENSION

SETUP: Load the EZ bar (make sure you use collars—balance can be tricky), grasp it with an overhand, shoulder-width grip, and stand, holding it overhead with straight arms. If you feel off balance or if you find that you arch your back too much on the movement, you can rest your butt against a sturdy, stable support, such as a preacher bench.

EXECUTION: Lower the bar behind your head as far as you can without changing your elbow position. Pause, then push back up to the starting position. Keeping your elbows high, still, and ideally, the same distance apart throughout the lift, use the fullest range of motion available without any elbow movement.

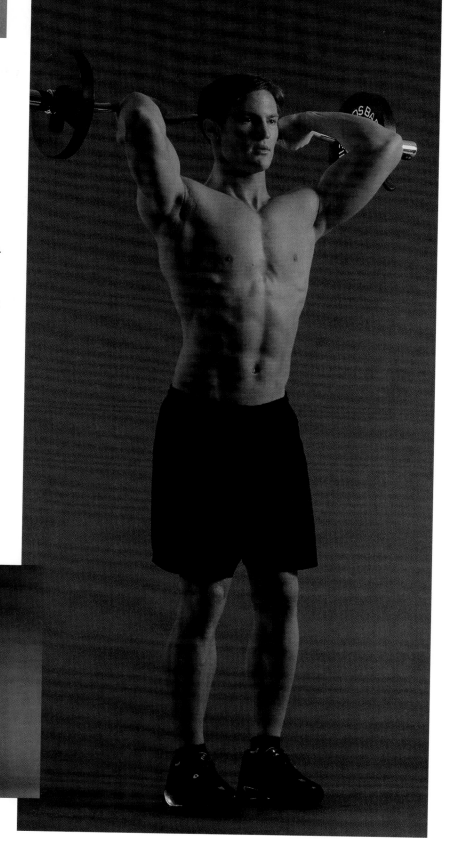

MUSCLES THAT ACT ON THE ELBOW AND WRIST

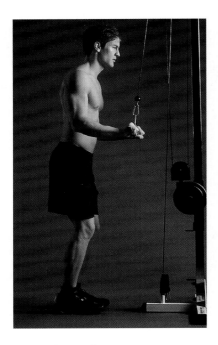

TRICEPS PUSHDOWN

SETUP: Attach a straight bar to the cable apparatus, and select the appropriate weight. Stand facing the bar, with the cable even with the midline of your body, then grasp the bar with an overhand, shoulder-width grip. Pull it down so your elbows are bent 90 degrees and tucked against the sides of your torso. Tilt your hips forward slightly, and bend your knees.

EXECUTION: Push the bar down until your arms are fully extended. Pause, then return to the starting position. The trick to this exercise—which may be the first triceps exercise you learned when you

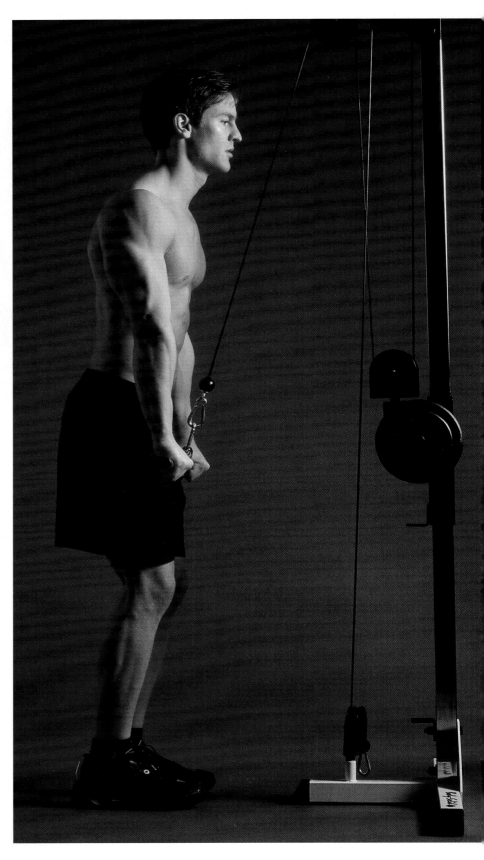

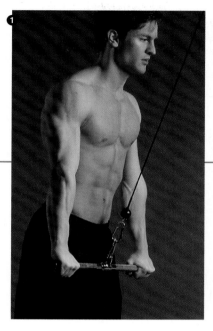

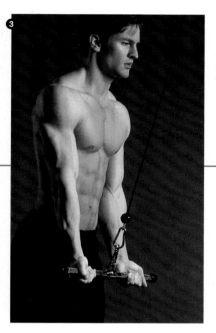

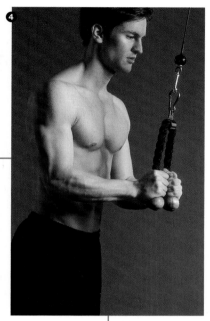

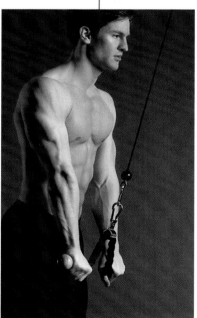

joined your gym—is to keep your elbows against your torso throughout the movement, ensuring that the only motion occurs in your elbow joints. Typical health-club execution of this exercise involves shoulder and hip movement, turning a simple triceps exercise into a standing version of the close-grip bench press by involving upper-body muscles that are better worked with other exercises.

VARIATIONS

❶ WIDE GRIP: Grasp the bar with your hands beyond shoulder-width to emphasize the long and medial heads more and the lateral head less.

❷ CLOSE GRIP (NOT PICTURED): Grasp the bar with a grip that's narrower than shoulder width.

❸ REVERSE GRIP: Hold the bar with an underhand, shoulder-width grip, which puts more emphasis on the lateral triceps head.

❹ NEUTRAL GRIP: Use the rope attachment so you can start with your hands facing each other. If you rotate your hands outward at the end of the movement, you'll involve all three triceps heads and several forearm muscles.

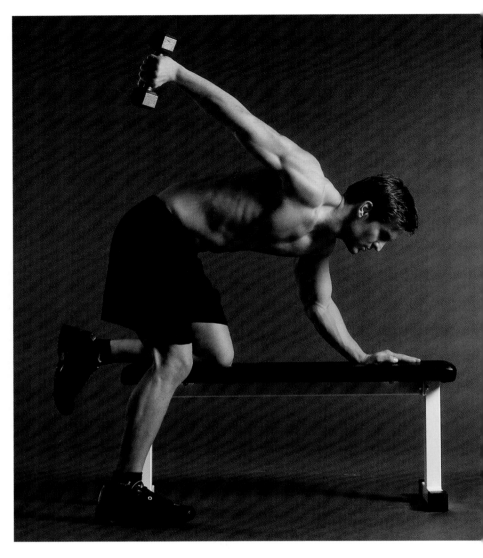

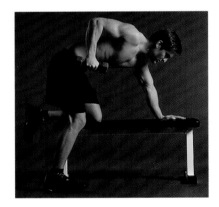

DUMBBELL TRICEPS KICKBACK

Get past the girly reputation of this exercise and you'll find it surprisingly challenging and effective. You don't need heavy weights to get good results. Just use the strict form we describe and you'll discover the benefits of a complete triceps contraction with your upper arm behind, rather than in front of, your torso.

SETUP: Pick up a dumbbell and rest your free hand and the corresponding knee on a bench. Hold your working arm so your upper arm is against your torso but slightly above horizontal. In other words, your elbow should be just above your torso, and it absolutely must be higher than your shoulder. (Doing this sideways next to a mirror helps—you should be able to see your arm from the side to ensure strict form.) Your elbow should be bent about 90 degrees so there's some tension in your triceps.

EXECUTION: Straighten your arm without moving your upper arm from its position. Pause—this hesitation here, in the fully contracted position, is probably more important than the pause in any other exercise—and then lower the dumbbell to the starting position. Don't go past the starting position, to the point at which the weight hangs effortlessly and there's no resistance from gravity. You don't want to give your triceps a running start on the next repetition.

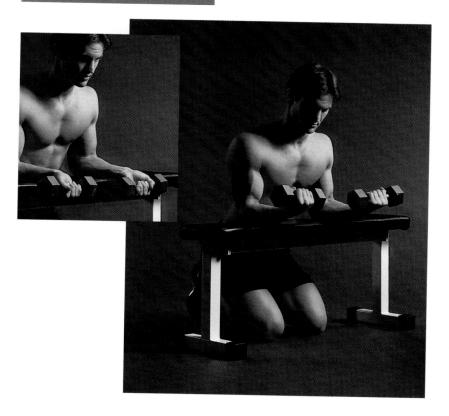

DUMBBELL WRIST CURL

SETUP: Grab a pair of dumbbells and kneel alongside a bench, laying your forearms on the bench, palms up, with your hands just off the edge.

EXECUTION: Curl the dumbbells as high as you can without moving your forearms or anything else in any way. Pause, and then lower the weights, allowing them to roll to your fingertips. Use this full range of motion on every repetition; when you can't do the entire movement, the set is over.

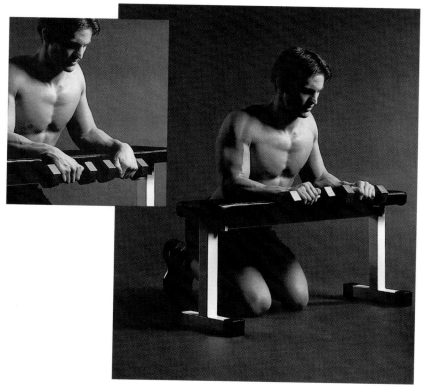

DUMBBELL WRIST EXTENSION

SETUP: Grab a pair of dumbbells and kneel alongside a bench, laying your forearms on the bench, palms down, with your hands just off the edge.

EXECUTION: Raise the dumbbells as high as you can without moving your forearms. Pause, then lower the weights as far as you can. There's no need to allow the weights to roll down your fingers.

MUSCLES THAT ACT ON THE ELBOW AND WRIST

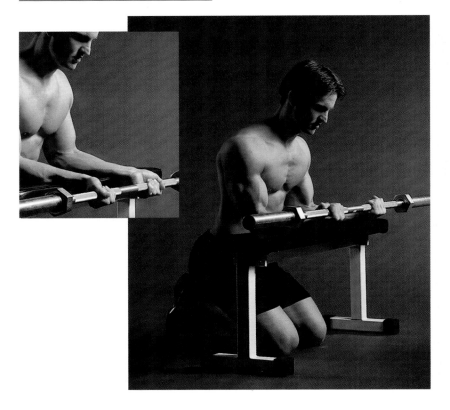

BARBELL WRIST CURL

SETUP: Grasp a light barbell with an underhand, shoulder-width grip, and kneel alongside a bench, laying your forearms on the bench with your hands just off the edge.

EXECUTION: Curl the bar as high as you can without moving your forearms. Pause, then lower the bar, allowing it to roll to your fingertips. Use this full range of motion on every repetition; when you can't do the entire movement, the set is over.
  If the barbell causes wrist strain, use an EZ-curl bar. And if you attempt a warmup set but find you can't complete all the reps, even using the lightest barbell in the gym, consider that warmup your work set. Move on to the next exercise in your routine.

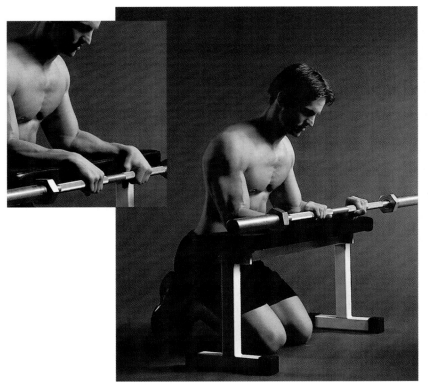

BARBELL WRIST EXTENSION

SETUP: Grasp a light barbell with an overhand, shoulder-width grip, and kneel alongside a bench, laying your forearms on the bench with your hands just off the edge.

EXECUTION: Curl the bar as high as you can without moving your forearms. Pause, then lower the bar as far as you can. You may prefer to use an EZ-curl bar. And if you can't complete all the reps on a warmup set with the lightest barbell in the gym, that's your work set, and you should move on.

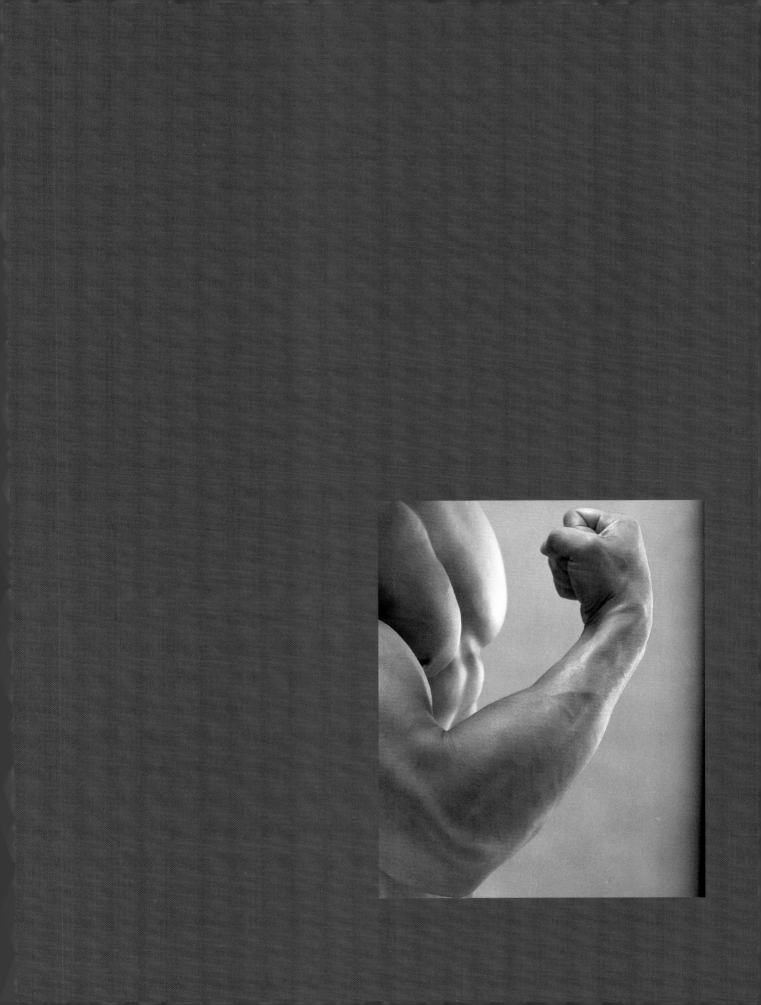

CHAPTER EIGHT

MUSCLES THAT ACT ON THE SPINE

IF YOU'RE A FATHER, you may have noticed that your baby was born with a somewhat flat spine. Soon after a child starts walking, the spine develops the S-shape it will retain in adulthood. If your child is naturally thin, another thing you may have noted is that once the baby fat burns off, a kid has visible and well-defined abs. The 6-year-old son of one of our authors is active without having any interest whatsoever in formal exercise or athletics. Nevertheless, because he's a skinny boy who climbs everything that doesn't move (and a few things that don't move fast enough), he has a perfect little abdominal six-pack.

What's the connection between spinal curvature and effortless pediatric six-packs? Just this: The posture and muscular definition that come naturally to children can get pretty damned complicated for adults.

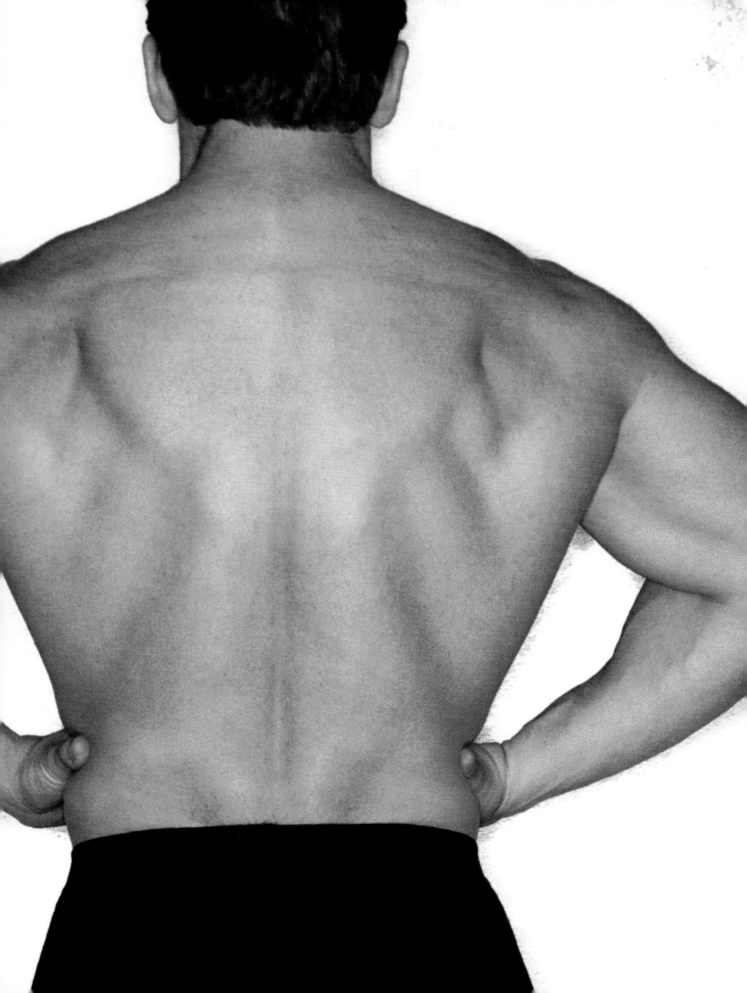

Most adults—up to 80 percent, experts say—will suffer lower-back pain at some point. Most of the U.S. population is overweight and sedentary, and this is intimately related to the previous statistic. All is made worse if the excess weight is in the form of visceral fat, the stuff that accumulates around your internal organs and creates a protruding belly (or, as our friends in the malted-beverage industry would prefer you didn't call it, a beer gut).

Two fundamental strategies for avoiding back pain are regular exercise and weight management. We suspect that those are a given for anyone who has purchased this book.

We also suspect you didn't buy this book for information on back pain. However, given the prevalence of back problems, it's difficult to separate the topic from our discussion of midsection muscle building. So in composing the following sections on developing the muscles of the abdomen and lower back, we had three goals:

1. To help you develop the midbody muscles with the most aesthetic appeal

2. To help you develop the muscles that will improve the structural integrity of your spine as well as your athletic performance

3. To help you increase endurance and control in the midbody muscles that will help you avoid back pain or alleviate pain you currently have

Now that we've delivered our mission statement, let's look at the most coveted muscles in the history of Western civilization.

ABDOMINALS

Biologists describe the muscles closest to the skin—and farthest from the center of the body—as the most superficial. This is a perfect description of your **RECTUS ABDOMINIS**, your six-pack muscle. It matters most for appearance and plays an important role in athletic performance. But it may be the least important abdominal muscle when it comes to lower-back stability and integrity.

The rectus originates on the crest of the pubic bone and attaches to the sternum and to the cartilage of the fifth, sixth, and seventh ribs. The six upper-abdominal segments are separated like ice cubes in a tray by tough connective tissue called **FASCIA**. The strip of fascia down the middle is called the **LINEA ALBA**. (If you can see your linea alba right now, congratulations; you're leaner than we are.) The lower rectus actually has two segments beneath the belly button, but it's nearly impossible to get so lean and muscular that this muscle separation is visible.

The rectus has a fairly simple function, called spinal flexion, or bending the trunk forward at the waist. Where it gets complicated is in the details of how best to develop the muscle. Trainers may tell you that there's no such thing as an "upper" or "lower" rectus. Technically, they're right, but the segments of the muscle are so clearly divided that they're governed by distinct motor units. And laboratory studies using electromyographic (EMG) analysis have shown that the upper and lower rectus respond differently to trunk-flexion exercises that start with the legs (as in toes to sky, shown on page 155) than to exercises that begin with the upper body moving toward the pelvis (as in the curlup on page 156).

The **EXTERNAL OBLIQUES**, located on the sides of the rectus abdominis, are more interesting and versatile muscles, as well as the widest muscles on your body. The fibers originate on the lower eight ribs and run diagonally to attach along the top of the pelvis. They work with your **INTERNAL OBLIQUES**, which lie beneath them. The internal oblique fibers run diagonally upward from the lumbar fascia (in the lower back) and pelvis and attach to the cartilage of the eighth, ninth, and tenth ribs. Put another way, the external oblique fibers run diagonally downward from the middle of the rib cage, while the internal oblique fibers run diagonally upward from the pelvis. (The bottommost internal oblique fibers, however, are more horizontal.)

The obliques are astoundingly versatile muscles. They work with the rectus abdominis in spinal flexion—and work damned hard at it. In fact, the fibers of the external obliques attach to the linea alba at the bottom, and the fibers of the internal obliques attach to the linea alba at the top. So whether you're doing a curlup or a leg raise, the fibers of your obliques are working at both ends.

They also control twisting at the waist, one of the most important sports-related muscle actions. Think about this for a moment: When you twist at the waist

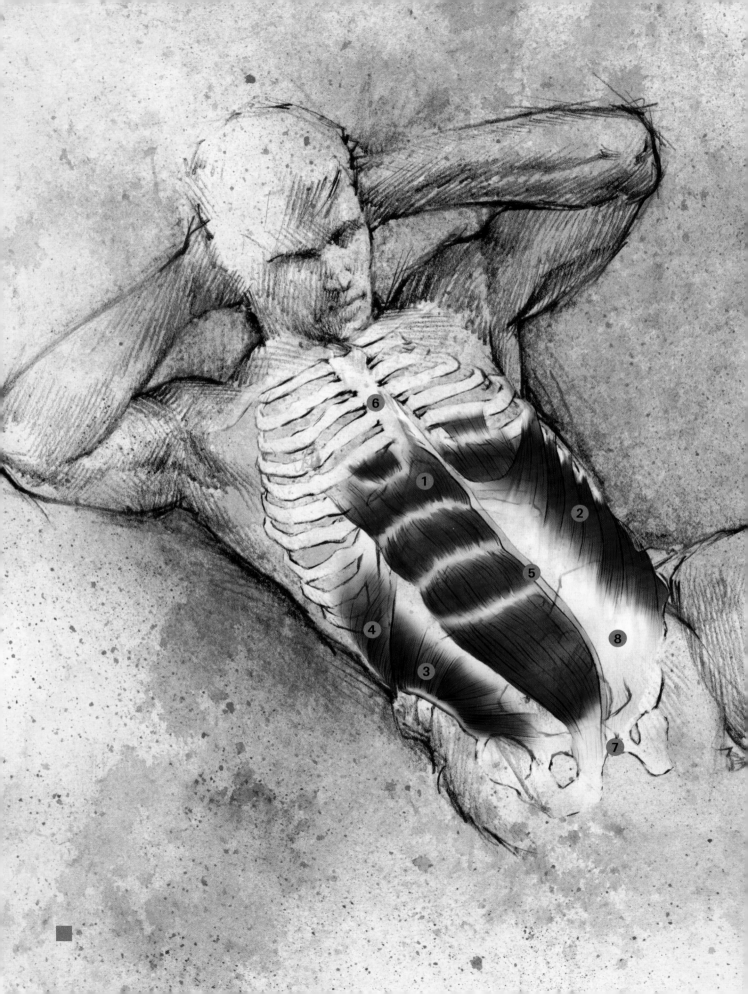

1. **RECTUS ABDOMINIS**
2. **EXTERNAL OBLIQUES**
3. **INTERNAL OBLIQUES (BENEATH EXTERNAL OBLIQUES)**
4. **TRANSVERSUS ABDOMINIS (BENEATH INTERNAL OBLIQUES)**
5. **LINEA ALBA**
6. **STERNUM**
7. **PUBIC BONE**
8. **FASCIA**

to hit a golf ball, tennis ball, baseball, or oddball (hey, fisticuffs happen), when you turn to kick a soccer ball, and when you throw a football or baseball, you use your obliques to generate force by rotating your torso.

Because the fibers run perpendicular to each other, the external and internal obliques alternate duties when you twist. For instance, when you twist to the left, you use the external obliques on your left side and the internal obliques on the right side.

The obliques also help you bend and straighten your body to the sides. This time, the internal and external obliques work together on the same side of your body. Thus, when you crunch your torso to the left, the internal and external obliques on the left side pull your ribs closer to your hip. When you straighten your body after it's bent to one side, the obliques on the pulling side work together, along with your lower-back muscles.

Because the internal obliques originate in the rear of your midsection, they're also considered postural muscles. That is, they have to contract throughout the day to keep you upright. You can work them anytime you're sitting or standing by pulling in your waist and straightening your back.

One more abdominal muscle worth discussing is the ***TRANS-VERSUS ABDOMINIS***. This thin patch of muscle lies beneath the internal obliques, with fibers that run horizontally from the pelvis, the cartilage of the lower ribs, and the lumbar fascia to the midline of the torso. It has two jobs: (1) preventing the internal organs from pushing your belly outward and (2) forcing air out of your body. In other words, it matters for appearance (keeping your belly flat) and for performance (helping you exhale air forcefully at the end of a movement, as in a martial arts punch). It doesn't have any direct role in flexing, twisting, or straightening your spine.

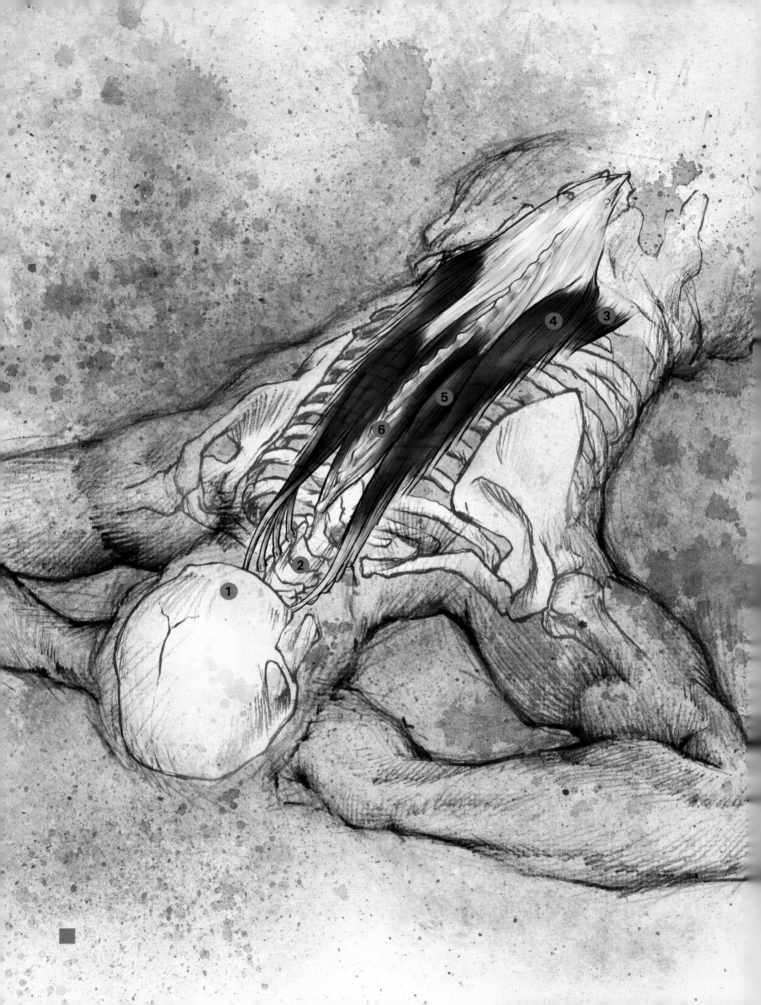

LOWER BACK

Your lower back has two sets of muscles: one for the heavy lifting and one for the less glamorous job of stabilizing the part of your spine that carries all your weight.

The heavy-lifting set is called the **ERECTOR SPINAE**, or spinal erectors. You have two spinal erectors, one on each side of your spine, and three sets of muscles in each spinal-erector set: **ILIOCOSTALIS (OUTERMOST)**, **LONGISSIMUS (MIDDLE)**, and **SPINALIS (INNERMOST)**. Each set of erectors has three individual muscles with such designations as *lumborum*, *thoracis*, *cervicus*, and *capitis*. If you're Latin-challenged, the easy way to make sense of all these terms is to remember that lumborum muscles are nearest the butt (the lumbar area), the thoracis muscles are near the mid-body (or thorax), the cervicus designation means near the neck (the cervical area), and the capitis is nearest the skull (just think of what's chopped off when one is decapitated). The spinal erectors spread up your back, like vines climbing a brick wall. They comprise the longest muscle group on your body.

When you're bent forward at the waist, these muscles straighten you up. They also take your back into hyperextension, an action that sounds dangerous. Indeed it can be devastating—or at least damned painful—to hyperextend a knee or elbow. Your back, however, hyperextends often, with no negative consequences. When you're standing upright your back is fully extended. If you could draw a straight line from your ear through your shoulder and hip, you're standing with good posture in a fully extended position. Hyperextension is nothing more than arching your back to lean backward.

In experienced lifters, the spinal erectors are well-developed, like twin ridges flanking the groove of the spine. That's because these muscles have to work hard to support the lower back during heavy-duty exercises—deadlifts, squats, good mornings, bent-over rows.

The spinal erectors are also involved in side-bending and backward-twisting exercises, along with the **QUADRATUS LUMBORUM**, a set of muscles that lie beneath each set of erectors. Each set of these underlying muscles originates on the top of the pelvis and the lower lumbar vertebrae and attaches to the bottom rib. These muscles look like less ambitious versions of the spinal erectors, and they share the same duties.

Beneath the quadratus lumborum and the spinal erectors are several small muscles that act like struts supporting a bridge—the bridge being your lower and middle back. These have a small role in spinal movement, but mostly they shore up your spine. (The **MULTIFIDUS** in the lower back is an important example.) New research on lower-back injury and rehabilitation shows that it's most important to develop endurance in these muscles. Strength is fine, but endurance can make the difference between injuring and not injuring your lower back. The pushup hold, shown on page 172, is designed to build endurance and structural integrity in these tiny but crucial muscles.

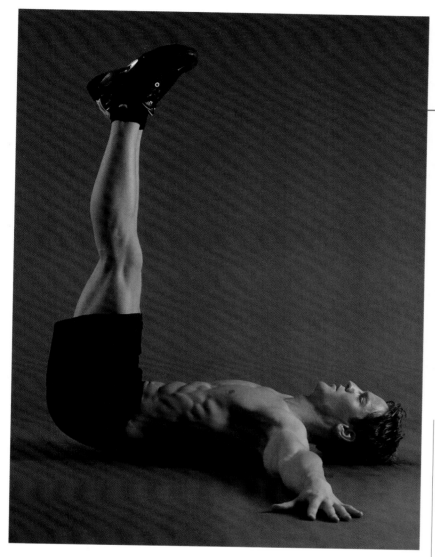

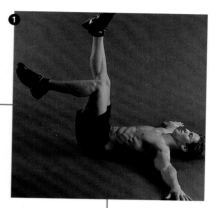

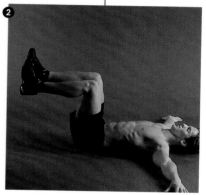

TOES TO SKY

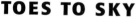

SETUP: Lie faceup on the floor, arms outstretched at 90-degree angles to your torso. Lift your legs straight up so they're together and vertical.

EXECUTION: Lift your pelvis as far as you can off the floor while keeping your legs vertical, and hold for the duration specified in your particular workout. Lower your hips.

PERFORMANCE TIPS:

The range of motion will be small—even the most accomplished exerciser won't be able to lift his pelvis more than a few inches off the floor. So don't compromise the described form to get more lift.

Keep your head still. You may be inclined to lift it, but resist.

Initiate the movement smoothly, in a controlled fashion. Avoid any sudden movements.

VARIATIONS

❶ ONE KNEE BENT: Same setup, but bend one knee 90 degrees before the first repetition. At the end of this rep, after you've lowered your hips back to the floor, straighten that leg and bend the other knee to 90 degrees. Now perform your second rep. Keep alternating until you've finished the set.

Again, your legs shouldn't move in any direction except up, and initially you may not experience very much vertical displacement of the hips.

❷ KNEES TO SKY: Same as above, except you perform all reps with both knees bent at 90 degrees so your lower legs are parallel to the floor.

MUSCLES THAT ACT ON THE SPINE

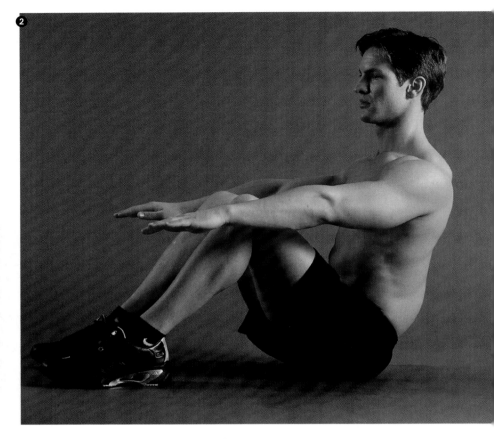

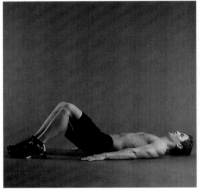

CURLUP

SETUP: Lie faceup on the floor with your knees bent about 90 degrees and your feet flat on the floor. Don't anchor your feet under anything. Your arm position will vary depending on which of the variations you do (variation 2 is shown above).

EXECUTION: Slowly raise your torso at a constant speed—whichever is specified in your particular workout—without jerking or accelerating through any part of the movement (with one exception, described below). Lower yourself just as smoothly and deliberately.

VARIATIONS
❶ CHEAT UP + SLOW LOWER: Raise yourself any way you can, at any speed (for example, throw your hands over your head to generate momentum). Whatever you choose to do, don't aggravate your neck or back. Then lower yourself at the tempo specified in your particular workout, making sure your speed stays the same throughout the descent (your natural inclination is to go faster at the bottom, since that's harder). Your goal is to perform ever-slower repetitions as you improve at the exercise.

❷ ARMS STRAIGHT AND PARALLEL TO FLOOR: Extend your arms straight out in front of you as you curl up.

❸ ARMS STRAIGHT AND PARALLEL TO FLOOR + TWIST: Same as above, with a twist to one side or the other on each repetition.

❹ HANDS ON OPPOSITE ELBOWS: Set up with your arms resting on your chest, and as you curl up, raise your arms so they're parallel to the floor in the top position. Reverse this on the way down so your arms are back on your chest at the end of the repetition.

❺ HANDS ON OPPOSITE SHOULDERS: This is the same as above, except that you start with your hands on your shoulders.

❻ HANDS ON OPPOSITE ELBOWS + TWIST: As you come up, twist so your right elbow touches your left knee. Go down, then come up so your left elbow touches your right knee. That's 2 reps.

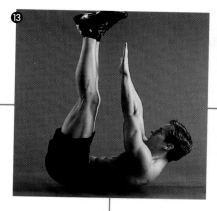

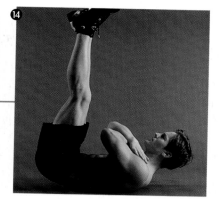

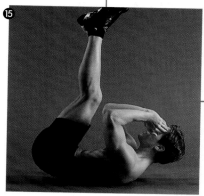

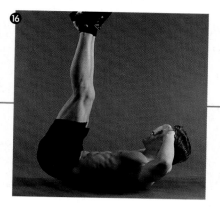

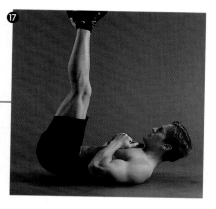

❼ HANDS ON OPPOSITE SHOULDERS + TWIST: With this different hand position, twist an elbow to the opposite knee. This variation forces you to use an even greater range of motion because you have to come up higher to touch elbow to knee.

❽ HANDS ON FOREHEAD, ELBOWS IN: Set your fingers on the same sides of your forehead (right fingers on right temple, left on left). Point your elbows straight ahead on the way up and the way down.

❾ HANDS ON FOREHEAD, ELBOWS IN + TWIST: Twist as you come up, so your right elbow touches your left knee. Go down, then come up so your left elbow touches your right knee. That's 2

reps. Maintain the same elbow angle throughout the set; in other words, don't move your elbow forward to cut the distance to your knee.

❿ HANDS ON FOREHEAD, ELBOWS OUT: Hold your hands to your forehead and point your elbows out 45 degrees. Keep your elbows out to the sides throughout the movement.

⓫ HANDS ON FOREHEAD, ELBOWS OUT + TWIST

⓬ WEIGHTED: Hold a weight plate on your chest.

⓭ LEGS IN AIR, ARMS VERTICAL TOWARD TOES: Raise your legs so they're vertical. Start with your arms extended straight up from your shoulders. As you curl your head and

shoulders up, reach toward your toes. (Don't try to touch your toes; just reach toward them as far as your natural range of motion allows.)

⓮ LEGS IN AIR, HANDS ON OPPOSITE SHOULDERS, ARMS ACROSS CHEST: Without raising your arms, curl your head and shoulders up toward your legs. Then slowly lower.

⓯ LEGS IN AIR, HANDS ON FOREHEAD, ELBOWS IN: On this variation and the next two, the range of motion is short but the muscle contraction is intense.

⓰ LEGS IN AIR, HANDS ON FOREHEAD, ELBOWS OUT

⓱ LEGS IN AIR, WEIGHT ON CHEST

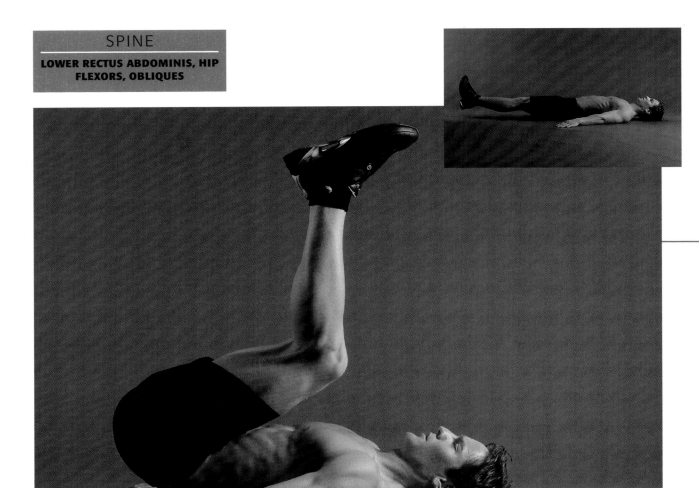

KNEE-UP

SETUP: Lie faceup on the floor. Bend your hips and knees 90 degrees so your lower legs are parallel to the floor. Suck in your tummy and push your lower back as flat against the floor as you can. You must maintain this lower-back-to-the-floor position throughout.

EXECUTION: Lift your knees to your chest, maintaining their 90-degree angle. Your lower back will round as you do this. Once your knees are on your chest, reverse the action, this time straightening your legs as you lower them (see inset photo). Lower them as far as you can without compromising your lower-back position. (Ideally, you want them almost parallel to the floor.) Then bend your knees before starting the next rep. Don't let your legs touch the floor between reps.

VARIATIONS

❶ **INCLINE:** Lie faceup on a slant board (head above hips), and perform the exercise as described above. Keep your lower back on the board throughout the movement; you want it either flat (at the beginning and end of each rep) or rounded—never arched.

❷ **VERTICAL:** This exercise is commonly known as a *hanging knee raise*, but we refer to it differently to establish the progression from the knee-up through the incline knee-up to the vertical knee-up. You can do it one of three ways: (1) on a captain's chair, which you'll find in most gyms; (2) using special elbow straps designed to hang from a chinning bar and allow your upper arms to remain parallel to the floor;

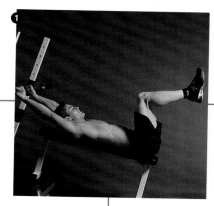

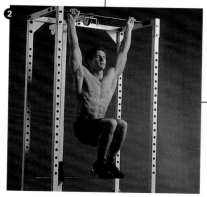

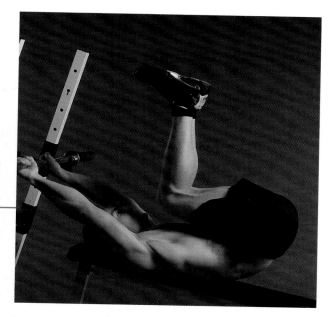

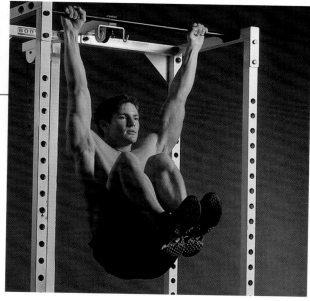

(3) the old-school way, hanging from a chinup bar.

Start with your hips and knees bent 90 degrees. Pull your knees to your chest, rounding your back. Then slowly lower them until your thighs are once again parallel to the floor. When you're hanging from a bar, with or without elbow straps, your biggest battle is keeping your body from swaying. (This won't be a problem on the captain's chair, which has a back rest to prevent swaying.) Combat this by pausing at the top position, then slowly lowering your thighs to a count of three. Though you won't be able to do as many reps this way, the quality will more than make up for the lack of quantity.

If you need to make the exercise more difficult (trust us, very few people do), you can start it with your legs fully extended, then bend your knees as you round your back and bring your knees to your chest. An even more difficult option is the hanging leg raise, in which you start with straight legs, bring them up straight until your feet are above your head as you round your back, then lower them without bending your knees.

SAFETY: The vertical knee-up is an advanced exercise involving the hip flexors, muscles that pull hard on the lumbar spine. If you experience lower-back discomfort, switch back to the incline knee-up.

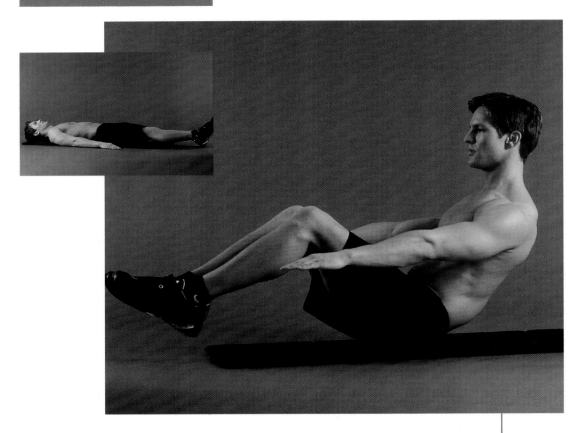

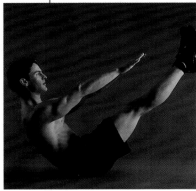

MODIFIED V-SIT

SETUP: Lie faceup on the floor, with your legs straight and together and your arms at your sides.

EXECUTION: Your goal is to come up so your trunk and thighs form a V shape. The trick is lifting your trunk and legs at the same speed so they reach their end range of motion at the same moment. Bend your knees as you come up, and then straighten them as you lower yourself to the start position. Keep your arms parallel to the floor at all times. To make the exercise more challenging, keep your heels, upper back, or arms off the floor between repetitions.

VARIATION

FULL V-SIT: Start with your arms back over your head. Come up with your arms, legs, and trunk simultaneously so your trunk forms a V with your legs, which remain straight. You are an absolute stud if you can fold up your body so your arms and feet meet at a point straight up over the floor.

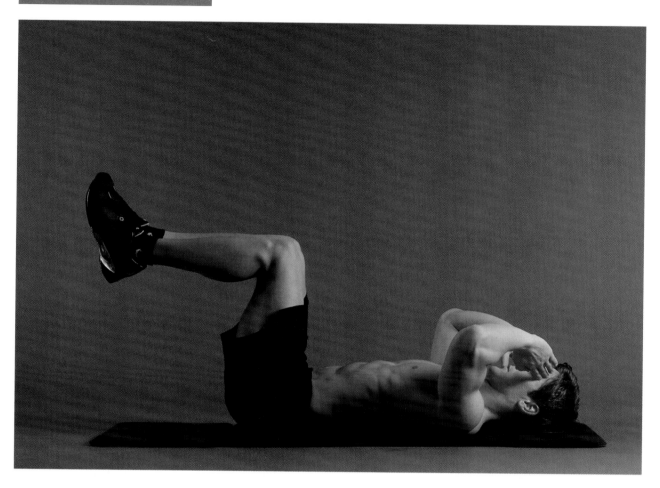

WRIST-TO-KNEE CURLUP

SETUP: Lie faceup on the floor, with your hands on your forehead and your elbows pointing out at 45 degrees. Don't change your elbow angle during the exercise. Raise your legs until your hips and knees are at 90-degrees angles, which means that your lower legs should be parallel to the floor.

EXECUTION (NOT PICTURED): Simultaneously raise your shoulders and hips off the floor. Then rotate at the waist so one knee and the opposite wrist meet. At the same time, cycle your other leg outward. Then "unrotate" as you lower back down to the start position, but don't let your hips and shoulders come to a full rest on the floor. That's 1 rep. Repeat with the other wrist and its opposite knee rotating together. Continue alternating to finish the set.

VARIATION
FULL LYING POSITION (NOT PICTURED): Start with straight legs. As you rise, bend your knee to touch it with the opposite wrist (or, if you can't manage that range of motion, with your elbow). Straighten your leg again at the end of the repetition.

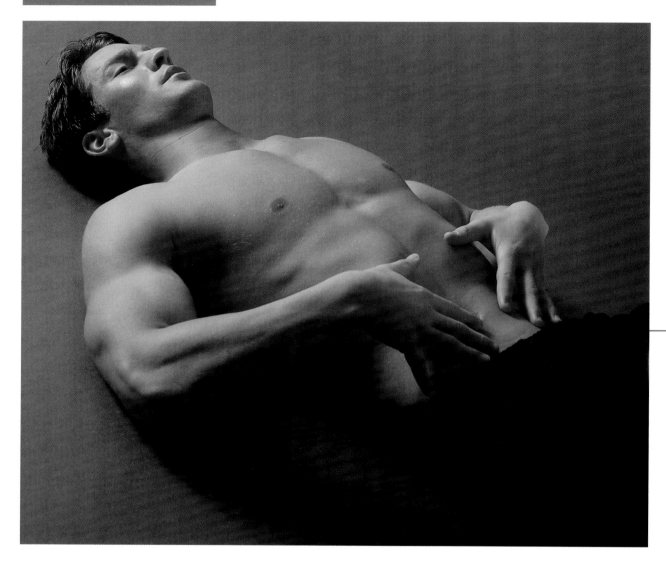

THIN TUMMY

SETUP: Lie faceup on the floor, with your knees bent and your feet flat. Place both hands under your belt line, with your fingers heading down into the pubic area and the thumbs placed higher up on the rectus abdominis (upper-abdominal region).

EXECUTION: Contract your lower-abdominal muscles, "thinning" your tummy between the belly button and groin. Your upper-abdominal muscles should be hollowed (not contracted and pushed out). Hold this position for 5 seconds. Then relax and reset the muscles before repeating.

PERFORMANCE TIPS: Use your fingers to provide feedback. Initially, you may struggle to even find the muscles you want to contract. With practice, you'll not only find them but also learn to control their contraction, which is key to developing these muscles, improving your posture, and performing all the exercises in our workout programs. Yes, learning to control your midsection muscles is a key to biceps curls, deadlifts, and the rest. In other words, it all begins right here.

At first you may find yourself holding your breath, which is natural. It's important to learn to breathe normally during these

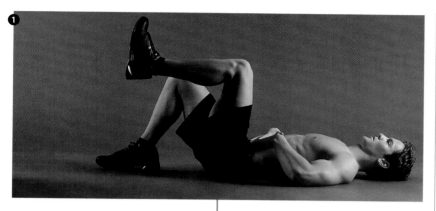

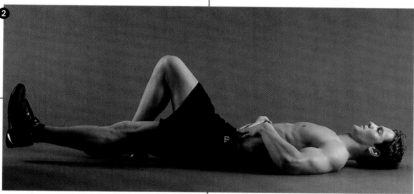

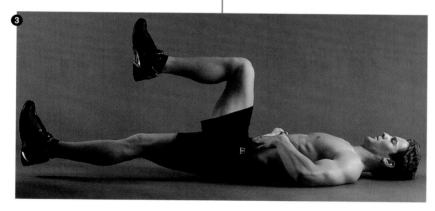

② LIFT AND CYCLE OUT ONE LEG: Create the thin-tummy position (using your hands for feedback), lift up one leg until the lower leg is parallel to the floor, and then extend that leg until it's parallel to and almost touching the floor (as pictured). Then reverse the movement—bend the knee 90 degrees, and place your foot back on the floor. That's one repetition. Repeat with the other leg.

Throughout this movement, it's critical to maintain the thinness of the tummy and keep the hips in place. If you feel you're losing the desired abdominal or hip position, terminate the repetition or even the whole set. Develop the full range of motion gradually; focus most on the quality of the movement, rather than the range, at first.

③ BOTH LEGS UP, CYCLE OUT ONE LEG: Lie faceup on the floor and lift up both legs until your hips and knees are at 90-degree angles, with your lower legs parallel to the floor. Create the thin-tummy position (using your hands for feedback). Extend one leg until it's parallel to and almost touching the floor (as pictured). Then reverse the movement, lifting it back up. That's 1 rep. Repeat with the other leg.

As with the previous variation, you must maintain the abdominal and hip positions throughout, even at the expense of range of motion. Quality is everything.

isometric contractions. Try it, and feel the increased tension in the muscles as you do so.

VARIATIONS

① LIFT ONE LEG: Create the thin-tummy position (using your hands for feedback), and then lift up one leg until the lower leg is parallel to the floor (as pictured). Then lower it back down. That's 1 repetition. Repeat with the other leg.

During this movement, aim to keep your tummy thin and tight, and your hips flat. You need to initiate this movement slowly and keep it smooth and slow throughout.

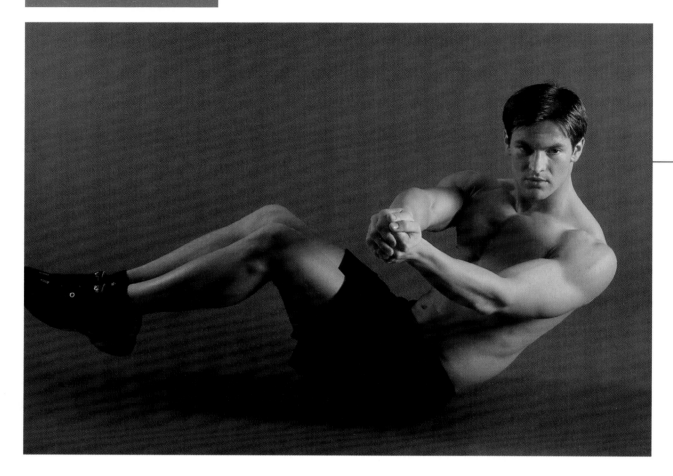

RUSSIAN TWIST

SETUP: Sit on the floor, with your knees bent 90 degrees and your feet just off the floor. Lean your trunk back to a 45-degree angle (or farther, if you can). Keep your spine flat. Clasp your hands together and extend your arms straight out from your trunk, putting them at a 45-degree angle to the floor, more or less.

EXECUTION: Rotate your trunk from side to side, keeping your legs still. Make sure you rotate from your waist, not your shoulders. Each twist to one side is a repetition, so a set of 10 reps is five twists to each side.

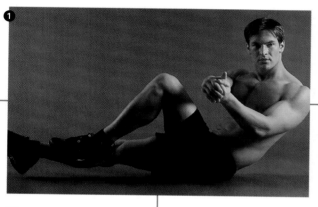

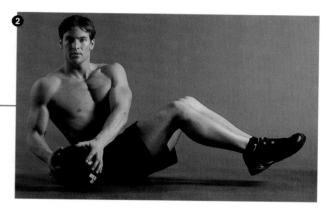

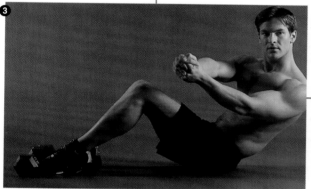

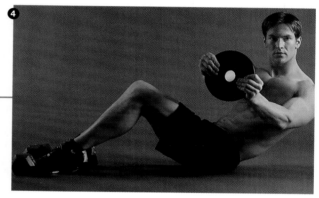

VARIATIONS

❶ LEG CYCLE: Start with one knee up toward your chest and the other leg extended, as if you were cycling. "Pedal" as you twist, retracting the leg on the side to which you're twisting (that is, as you twist to the left, bring up your left knee and extend your right leg to complete one rep; then as you twist right, retract your right knee and extend your left for a second rep).

❷ MEDICINE BALL IN HANDS: Hold a medicine ball (or, the first time you try it, perhaps something lighter, such as a basketball), and get into the standard Russian-twist position, with your feet lifted slightly off the floor. Then twist, extending the range of motion so you touch the ball to the floor on each repetition.

❸ FEET ANCHORED: Anchor your feet with a pair of heavy dumbbells, an abdominal board, two sleeping dogs—anything that won't move. This allows you to use heavier weights and establish more muscle isolation, since your legs won't move as you twist.

❹ FEET ANCHORED, WEIGHT IN HANDS: Same as the previous variation, but holding a weight plate in your hands.

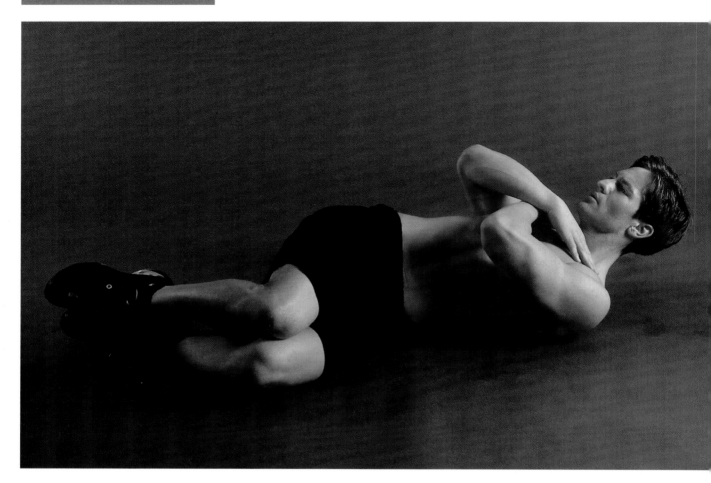

SIDE RAISE

SETUP: Lie faceup on the floor, with your knees together and bent to about 90 degrees. Roll your knees to one side so they're on the floor, keeping your shoulders and upper back flat on the floor. Cross your hands over your chest, touching opposite shoulders.

EXECUTION: Flex your trunk toward the ceiling. Pause, then lower back down at the speed indicated in your particular workout.

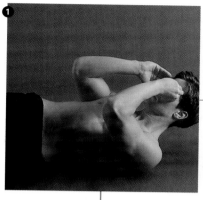

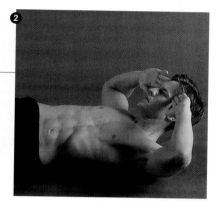

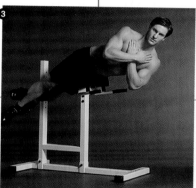

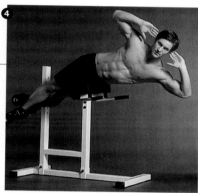

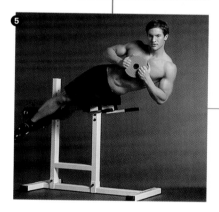

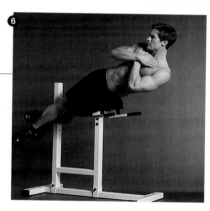

VARIATIONS

❶ HANDS ON FOREHEAD, ELBOWS IN: A change in hand position increases the difficulty.

❷ HANDS ON FOREHEAD, ELBOWS OUT: Here's another hand position.

❸ ON ROMAN CHAIR: The Roman chair is an apparatus found in most gyms and usually used for back extensions. It allows you to support your hips and legs against pads and braces, with your trunk free to move. (You can use a regular bench if you have a spotter to hold your feet.) Position yourself sideways, with one leg crossed over the other and both feet braced. Cross your hands over your chest, lower yourself as far as possible and comfortable, then pull yourself back up.

❹ ON ROMAN CHAIR, HANDS ON FOREHEAD, ELBOWS OUT: This is the same as above, with the different hand position.

❺ ON ROMAN CHAIR, WEIGHT ON CHEST: Hold a weight plate against your chest.

❻ ON ROMAN CHAIR + TWIST TO CEILING: Once you raise yourself, twist at the waist so your chest points toward the ceiling.

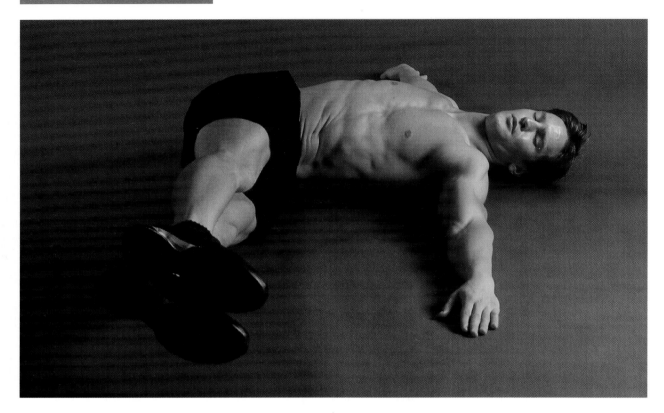

LATERAL
LEG LOWERING

SETUP: Lie faceup on the floor, with your legs together in the air and your arms out at 90 degrees to your body. Keep your head down on the floor.

EXECUTION: Lower your legs to one side, going all the way down to but not resting on the floor and keeping them at a 90-degree angle to your upper body. Keep your head and upper body still. Lift your legs back up to the vertical to complete the rep, then lower them over to the other side in the same way.

SEATED THIN TUMMY + CHEEK SQUEEZE

SETUP: Sit on the end of a bench or on a Swiss ball (the big inflatable exercise ball you find in all gyms nowadays), with your knees and feet together, your feet on the floor, your chest up, and your back straight. Place your hands on your abdomen, as in the thin tummy on page 162.

EXECUTION: Contract your lower abs, creating a thin tummy. Simultaneously contract your gluteals, raising you up an inch or so on the bench or ball. The co-contraction of the glutes should intensify the contraction of the abs.

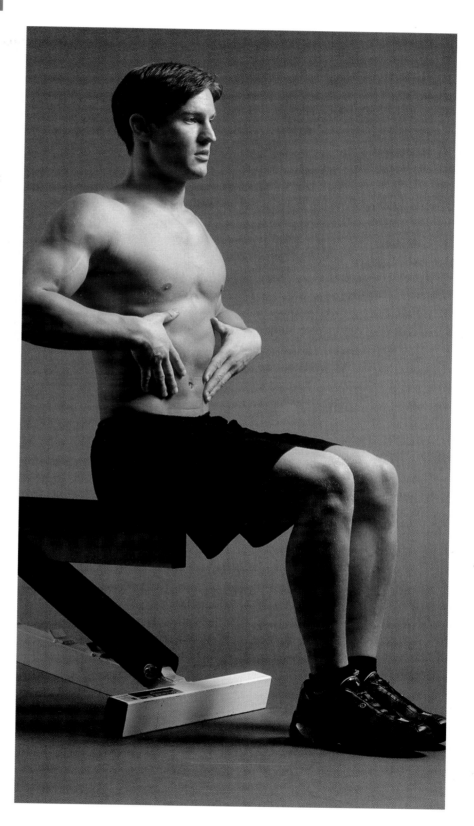

MUSCLES THAT ACT ON THE SPINE

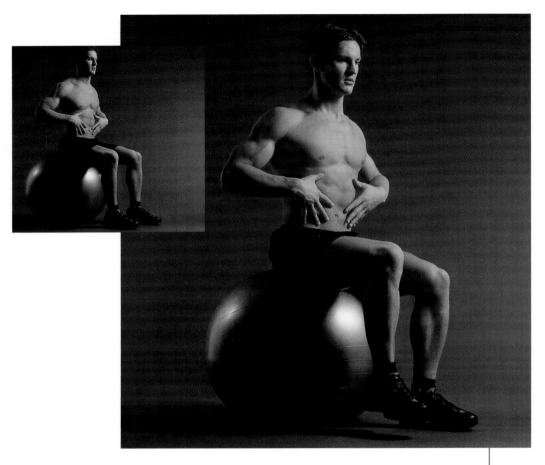

SWISS-BALL ALTERNATE LEG LIFT

SETUP: Sit on a Swiss ball and start in the thin tummy + cheek squeeze co-contraction described on the previous page.

EXECUTION: Raise one leg a few inches off the floor, maintaining the co-contraction of abs and gluteals. Slowly lower at the speed prescribed in your particular workout. Repeat with the opposite leg without releasing the co-contraction. That's two repetitions. The key is to keep your back flat as you do this. If your hips move forward and your back arches, the emphasis of the exercise switches from your abdominals to your hip flexors.

VARIATION

LYING: Set your upper back and shoulders on the Swiss ball, and set your feet shoulder-width apart and flat on the floor. Your knees should be bent at 90-degree angles. Lift your hips so there's a straight line between your knees and shoulders. Co-contract your lower abs and gluteals, and lift one leg at the prescribed speed, then lift the other. Each leg lift is 1 repetition.

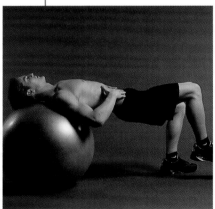

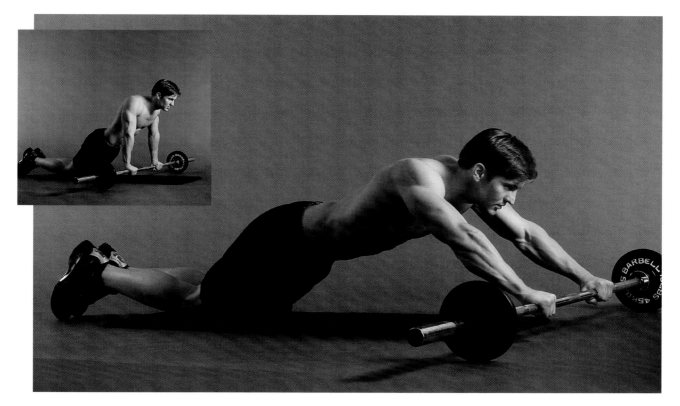

BARBELL ROLLOUT

SETUP: Load a barbell with the smallest weight plates that allow the bar to roll. Kneel in front of the barbell, and grab it with an overhand, shoulder-width grip.

EXECUTION: Keeping your arms relatively straight, roll the bar out in front of you and lower your trunk down toward the floor. Then pull the bar back to the starting position.

PERFORMANCE TIPS: Keep your thighs, hips, and trunk in line; your body should form a straight line between your knees and shoulders throughout the movement—you don't want any arching or sagging in your lower back, nor do you want your hips to go up in the air during the return phase.

If you can, go all the way down till your body is nearly touching but not resting on the floor. It could take months, if not years, to build up to this range of motion. The key is that you maintain perfect form through every inch of the motion.

As you try to increase your range of motion, you can also increase the weight you put on the bar. While you should start as light as possible, as mentioned, increasing the load you have to pull back to the starting position adds a different, extremely beneficial challenge.

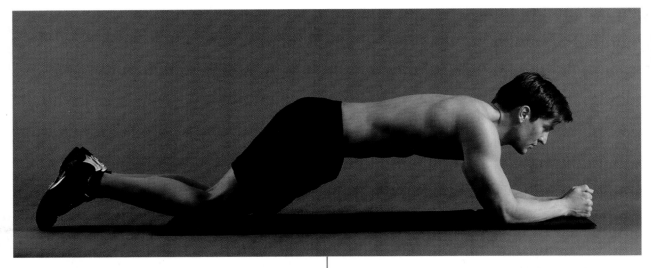

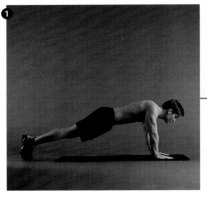 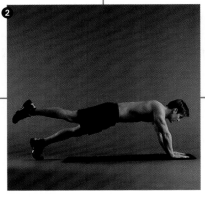 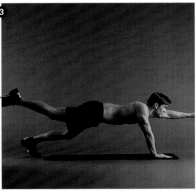

PUSHUP HOLD

SETUP: Lie facedown on the floor, with your legs straight and together. Set your hands beneath your chest, with your forearms parallel to each other and your hands a few inches apart.

EXECUTION: Raise your body onto your elbows and knees (or elbows and feet, if you're up for a bigger challenge), with your body forming a straight line from ankles to shoulders. (The line won't necessarily be parallel to the floor.) Hold for the prescribed duration, lower to the start position, and repeat.

VARIATIONS

❶ **HANDS AND FEET:** Execute the same movement from a standard pushup position.

❷ **LIFT LEG, THEN ARM:** From a standard, feet-and-knees pushup position, lift a leg until it's in line with your trunk. Hold for the prescribed duration, then lower it and raise the opposite arm. After you lower that, raise the other leg, then the other arm. That's 4 repetitions. Focus on achieving balance without compromising posture—the straight line between ankles and shoulders.

❸ **LIFT LEG WITH OPPOSITE ARM:** One repetition is when you successfully balance with an arm and its opposite leg lifted at the same time.

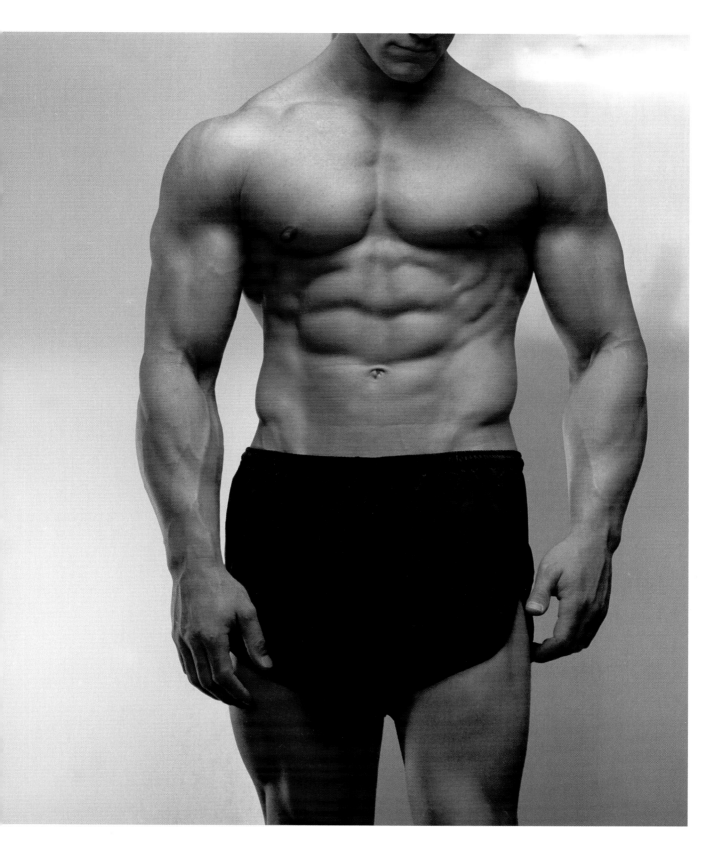

MUSCLES THAT ACT ON THE

HIP

YOU'VE PROBABLY HEARD of the muscle group known as **HIP FLEXORS**, Most likely in the context of advice such as "Don't do full situps—you'll just end up using your hip flexors!" These muscles are involved in a simple and important movement called, appropriately, **HIP FLEXION**. Right now, lift one of your leg out in front of you. (Just do it, even if you're sitting down or lying on your bed.) There, you just performed hip flexion.

Why should you care whether hip flexor muscles get involved in your abdominal exercises? The short answer is: You shouldn't, unless you have serious lower-back problems. Before we give you the long answer, we need to introduce you to the opposite movement: **HIP EXTENSION**. Bend forward at your hips, keeping your back flat and your legs straight. Now straighten back up. That's hip extension—moving your torso away from your thighs. When you lift your leg out behind you, that's also hip extension.

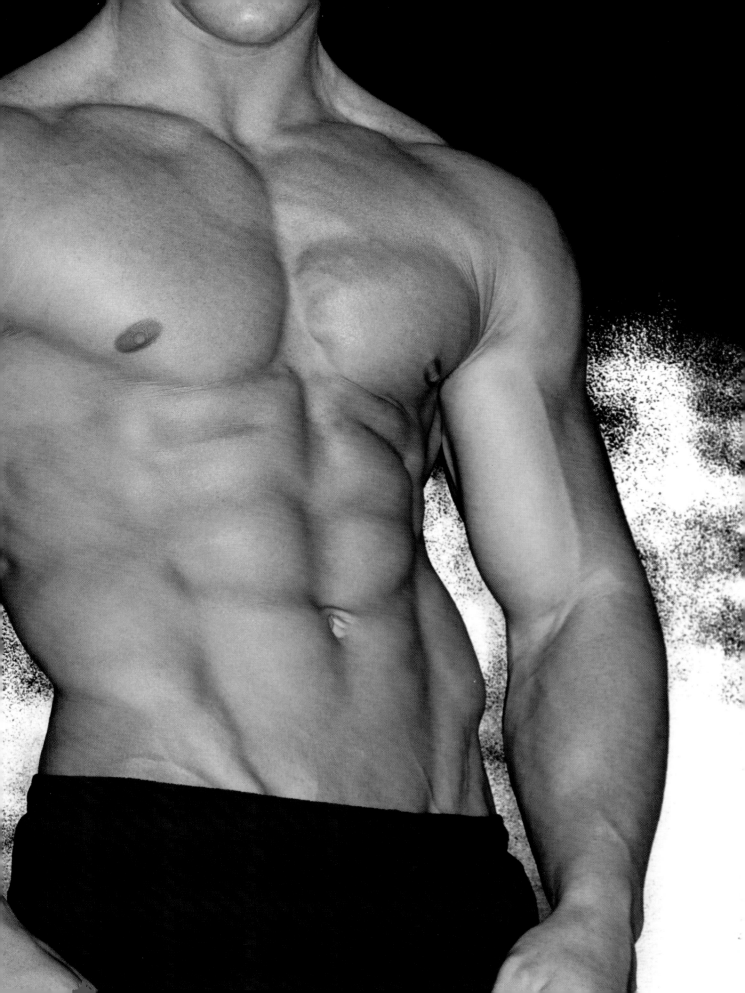

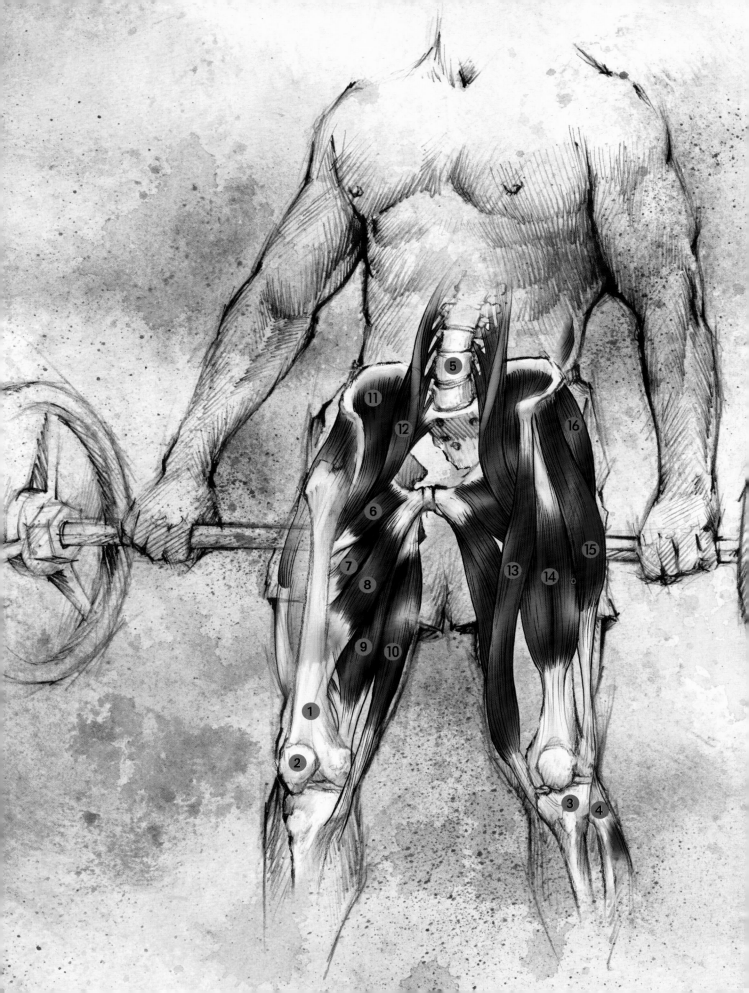

HIP FLEXORS

Sometime during the past couple of decades, physical therapists and trainers began warning that the hip flexor muscles must be kept out of all abdominal movements. The reasoning behind this advice has to do with the functioning of a deep pelvic muscle called the **PSOAS MAJOR** that originates on the vertebrae of the lower back and attaches to the inside top of the thigh bone (femur). When it flexes (shortens), it pulls the lower back into a more pronounced arch. Strong abdominal muscles are necessary to resist that pull and keep the lower back flat or in its natural arch when you're exercising. So you have to take precautions to build abdominal strength before performing movements—such as hanging leg raises—that force the psoas to tug hard on your lumbar vertebrae. And if you already have back pain, you may not be able to risk those advanced movements at all.

However, we think it's a terrible idea to try to take all hip flexion out of your exercise routine. The functions of the hip flexors, as we'll soon explain, are simply too important for you to leave the muscles untrained.

Though you can't see the psoas, you can feel it in many contexts. If it's too tight, you'll have trouble doing squats with a good range of motion, and you may suffer some back pain. If it's loose and weak, the top of your pelvis will tend to rotate backward, giving you a "buttless" look and a slovenly posture. So your goal is to keep this muscle strong with aggressive ab exercises through a full range of motion, as well as to keep it limber with stretches. It's also helpful to perform hip-extension exercises, thereby keeping the flexors and extensors in balance.

The psoas works in conjunction with the **ILIACUS**, a muscle that originates on the inside of your pelvis and joins up with the psoas on the front of the pelvis. The two muscles share a tendon and are so closely linked that they're usually referred to as the **ILIOPSOAS**.

The biggest hip flexor visible to the naked eye is the **RECTUS FEMORIS**, part of the quadriceps group and the only part of the quadriceps that crosses the hip joint. It originates on the outside front of the pelvis and ends in the tendon it shares with the three other quadriceps muscles. (We'll discuss the other quads in the next chapter because they act on the knee joint.) That tendon crosses the knee joint, which is why the rectus femoris works in the leg extension (shown on page 215) as well as in hip flexion.

Another visible hip flexor, if you're really lean, is the **SARTORIUS**, the body's longest muscle. No exercises isolate the sartorius, but it's interesting to note all those in which the "tailor's muscle" participates. (It's called that because tailors used to sit cross-legged on the floor, engaging the sartorius along with the gluteals to externally rotate the hip joint.) The sartorius starts on the outside of the pelvis, crosses the femur diagonally, and attaches to the tibia, just below the inside of the knee. In crossing both the hip and knee joints, it not only acts as a hip flexor to lift your leg in front of your body but also works with the gluteals and other hip extensors to lift your leg to the side. In addition, it plays a minor role in bending your knee out of a straight position.

The final hip flexor is called the **TENSOR FASCIA LATAE**, which is situated toward the front of the thigh and isn't interesting enough to mention again.

ADDUCTORS

The process of pulling your leg in toward the midline of your body is called **ADDUCTION**. It's one of those terms that's easiest to remember if you think of its opposite, **ABDUCTION**. Since you already know that abduction involves forcefully carrying something away from something else, it's easy to figure out that *hip-joint abduction* means pulling your leg away from your torso. (The major muscle involved in this action is the gluteus medius, which we'll describe shortly.) It goes to follow that *hip-joint adduction*, the opposite movement, means pulling the leg in closer toward your torso.

The muscles involved in adduction, arrayed along the inner thigh, are surprisingly big—among the largest in the body. At first glance, it's hard to figure out why so much muscle tissue is devoted to an action like adduction. About the only sports movement that's adductor-centric is soccer-style kicking, in which you swing your leg diagonally, rather than straight ahead. Of course, the fact that you can kick a ball farther soccer-style than you can straight on demonstrates how strong these muscles are.

On second glance, the adductors' size and strength make sense since the muscles play big roles in stabilizing your body during lateral movement. This function is important in soccer, hockey, basketball, racket sports, and baseball (where the first step in the field or off the bases is almost always lateral). In the gym, women tend to work the adductors directly, whereas men rarely do. These muscles grow even without direct stimulation, however, as you'll notice when you do heavy squats in our workout programs. Your adductors will grow along with all your other lower-body muscles.

So what exactly are they? The largest is the **ADDUCTOR MAGNUS**, which originates on the pubic bone at the bottom of the pelvis and attaches to the thigh bone at the inside top of the knee. The others—**ADDUCTOR LONGUS, ADDUCTOR BREVIS,** and **PECTINEUS**—are progressively shorter and closer to the hip joint. The **GRACILIS** is the only adductor that crosses the knee joint. It attaches to the tibia just below the knee on the inside of your shin, right next to the sartorius's attachment point.

GLUTEALS

The **GLUTEUS MAXIMUS** is your body's strongest muscle. Fully developed, it looks like a construction helmet atop the back of your thigh. It originates along the pelvis and lumbar fascia, attaching along the outside of the thigh bone and along a thick strip of connective tissue called the **FASCIA LATA**.

In addition to executing hip extension, the maximus controls the outward rotation of your thigh. The top part helps lift your leg out to the side, and the bottom part helps pull your thigh back toward your body once it's out to the side.

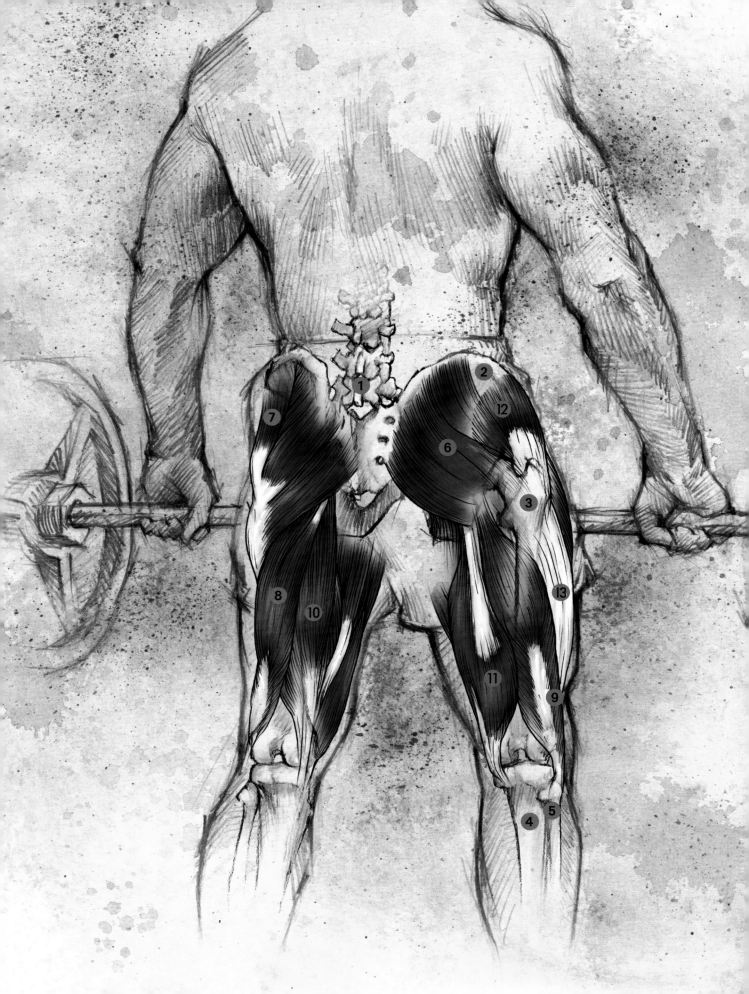

The prime mover when you lift your leg sideways is the *GLUTEUS MEDIUS*, on the outside of the hip. Aesthetically, this muscle helps create a dimple effect when your gluteals are viewed in profile. No one can see this unless you're naked or wearing really tight shorts, so unless you're an exotic dancer, you develop the gluteus medius solely for the enjoyment of the special person(s) in your life.

The front fibers of the medius are active in hip flexion and inward rotation of the thigh, along with the *GLUTEUS MINIMUS*, which lies beneath the medius. The rear fibers of the medius assist in hip extension and outward rotation of the thigh. Both the medius and minimus tend to be especially well developed in soccer players and martial artists, since these muscles are important in kicking.

HAMSTRINGS

When you look at someone with well-developed hamstrings, you see two really big muscles that split more or less down the middle of the leg, and some more separations toward the inside of the leg. The outermost of the two big masses is the *BICEPS FEMORIS*, or, more accurately, the long head of the biceps femoris. (Like the biceps in your upper arm the largest of the hamstring muscles has two heads.) The long head is the one toward the outside of the thigh. It starts at the bottom of the pelvic bone. The short head originates on the femur, and thus is the only part of the hamstring group that doesn't cross the hip joint. Put another way, the short head is the only part of the hamstrings that's involved exclusively in knee flexion (or bending), with no role in hip extension. The heads of the biceps femoris attach to both lower-leg bones (tibia and fibula), on the outside of the knee.

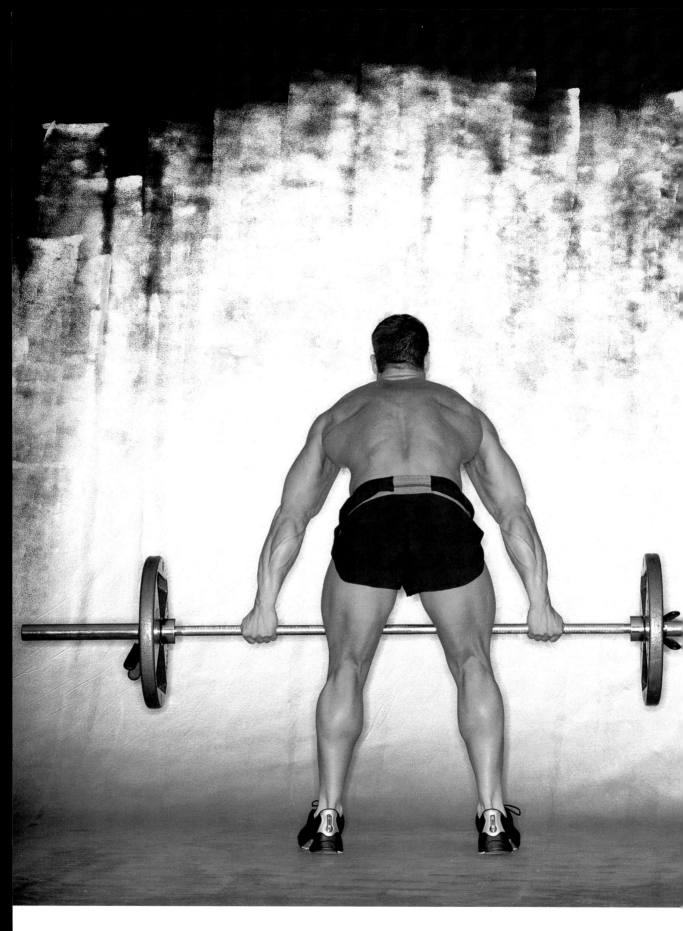

The other big hunk o' hamstring is actually two muscles. The **SEMITENDINO-SUS** is a smaller muscle that starts on the lower pelvis (sharing a tendon with the biceps femoris) and runs alongside the biceps femoris before attaching to the tibia, on the inside of the knee. The **SEMIMEMBRANOSUS** lies alongside the semitendinosus on the inside rear of the thigh, beginning and ending in the same places. It has a longer tendon at the top and a shorter one at the bottom.

These muscles have tremendous growth potential and respond to heavy weights and fast movements, which is why you never see a powerlifter or Olympic weight lifter with skinny legs. Interestingly, they don't respond well when you try to work them at both ends at once. They move powerfully during hip extension or knee flexion only if you perform the two actions separately.

Now that you know that most of the hamstring muscles cross both the hip and knee joints, you have an advantage over most other guys in the gym, who have the hamstring muscles figured all wrong. They treat the hams as if they acted exclusively on the knee joint, working them solely on the leg curl machine.

We aren't knocking the leg curl as a decent exercise to help build hamstring size. It's just that the movement is nearly useless in real life. After all, how important is it to bend your knee up behind you? You use that movement in . . . what? Checking the bottom of your shoe to see what you just stepped in? (The knee bend that occurs during walking and running is more a function of lack of quadriceps tension than of deliberate contraction of the hamstrings.)

That's why our workout programs build size, strength, and power in your hamstrings through hip extension, the thrusting movement that propels you in running and jumping. Hip extension is the primary action in the deadlift, the gym exercise in which you'll probably be able to lift the most weight. And along with knee extension, or straightening, it's also important in the squat. You'll thank us when you see the results: bigger, stronger legs with more power for sprinting, spiking, rebounding, blocking, or whatever else you do in your favorite sport.

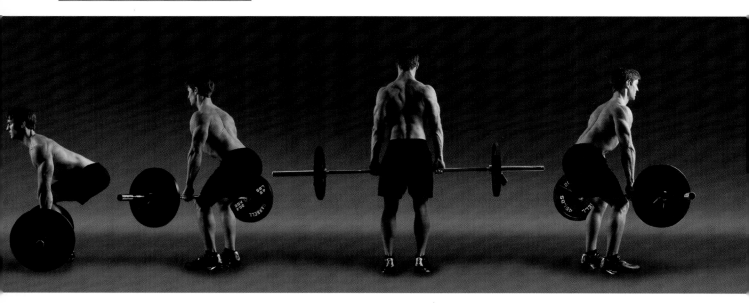

DEADLIFT

Have you ever watched a strongman competition on television? Most of the events start with picking something up off the ground. That's a deadlift—the most basic and practical of all strength-building movements. Need to help a friend move his sofa? Deadlift. Need to hoist bags of fertilizer off the ground while you're working in the yard? Deadlift. Need to pick up a sleeping child off the floor and carry her up to bed? Deadlift.

So one of the most important goals of our workout programs is to make you a good deadlifter, not only by increasing strength in your thighs and gluteals but also by improving your midsection strength and stability, and by building trapezius strength, since your traps have to keep your scapulae together and down throughout the movement. We showed midsection and trapezius exercises in previous chapters. Now let's get into the biggest of the big movements.

Because of the complexity of the lift, we'll take a slightly different approach to the description.

SETUP
- Load a barbell and roll it up to your shins.
- Set your feet shoulder-width apart.
- Set your shoulders over the bar as you grab it with an overhand grip, just outside your knees.
- Keep your back flat, in a straight line from your pelvis to your head.
- Keep your shoulder blades pulled together and down in back.

JUST BEFORE THE LIFT
- Straighten your legs a bit to take up slack—you want tension on the bar at the start.
- Pull in your lower abs (thin tummy) to ensure a neutral pelvis, neither arched nor rounded.
- Squeeze your glutes together— this is where you want the power to come from.
- Tighten your shoulder blades.

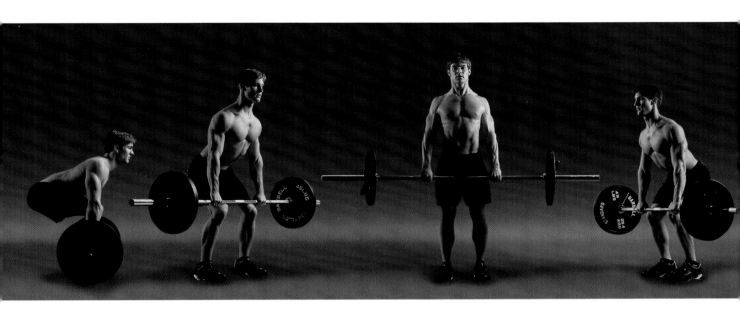

FIRST PULL, FROM FLOOR TO JUST ABOVE KNEES

■ Straighten your legs—imagine pushing your feet through the floor, with your glutes as the prime movers.

■ As your legs extend, your trunk and hips should remain at or near the same angle. This is critical—lack of compliance causes more injuries in this exercise than any other technical error. You may want to have a spotter watch you to make sure you maintain a similar angle.

■ The bar should stay in contact with your skin at all times.

SECOND PULL, FROM JUST ABOVE KNEES TO MID-THIGHS

■ Stand up, forcing your hips forward with the driving force of your glutes.

■ Finish in an upright posture, with your shoulders back and down, and your lower back still flat.

■ The bar should have stayed in contact with your skin throughout both parts of the lift.

LOWERING

■ Slide the bar down your thighs and shins to the floor. The lowering doesn't have to be exactly the reverse of the technique you used to raise the bar. You aren't trying to develop muscle here; you just want to get the bar back on the floor without hurting your back or annoying everyone in the gym by simply letting the bar fall.

■ Start every repetition with the bar resting on the floor. Keep the "dead" in deadlift.

YOUR LOWER BACK: If you notice a strain on your lower back, you're using a different technique than the one just described. The back is a stabilizer between the shoulder girdle and the glutes, so you shouldn't feel any particular strain there.

However, if you have preexisting lower-back problems, you may not be able to lift with the form we've described. Your lower back and gluteal muscles could have an abnormal firing pattern, so even if you get into the proper positions, the wrong muscles could contract and relax. In that case, try the **SUMO DEADLIFT**, in which you set your feet wide apart, toes pointed slightly outward, and grip the bar with your hands inside your knees. In this position, you'll start the lift with your torso more upright, taking away some of the potential for back strain.

VARIATIONS

❶ WIDE GRIP: Grab the bar with your hands outside the lines. The major difference you'll feel is in your trapezius—the contraction as you lift the bar off the floor will seem much more intense.

❷ ALTERNATING/MIXED GRIP: This is a medium grip—just outside your knees—in which one hand goes over the bar and one goes under. Experiment to find which of the two possible over-under combinations is most comfortable for you. You don't have to alternate which hand goes over and which goes under; you'll use this grip only for the heaviest sets, so there's no danger your body will grow lopsided in response to this technique.

❸ OFF BLOCKS: Rest the weight plates on blocks or on other plates stacked on the floor so the bar starts off higher than the floor. You use this extra height to train with weights that are heavier than those you could lift off the floor. The extra few inches should allow you to work toward lifting 10 to 20 percent more weight.

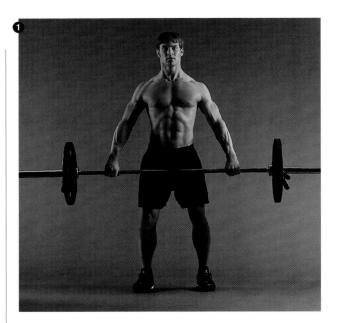

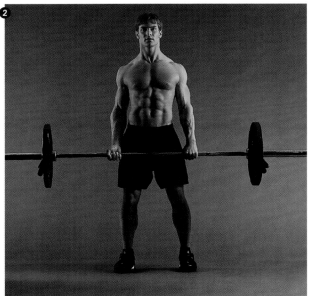

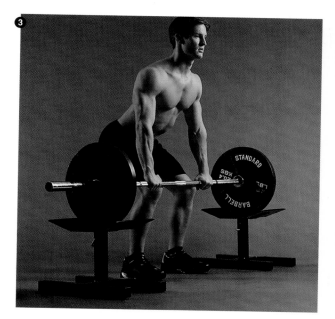

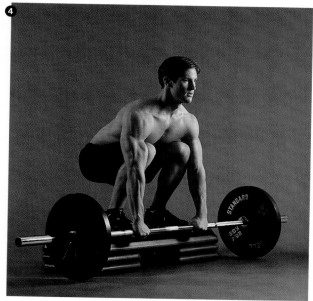

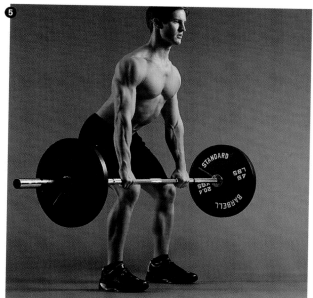

❹ STANDING ON BLOCKS: Keep the barbell on the floor while you stand on low blocks or weight plates. This exaggerates the range of motion and makes you stronger pulling the weight off the floor. If you have lower-back problems, you should use less weight, and perhaps skip this variation.

❺ HANG START: Load the bar on the supports of a power rack (not pictured), then lift it off, step back, and start with the bar just above your knees.

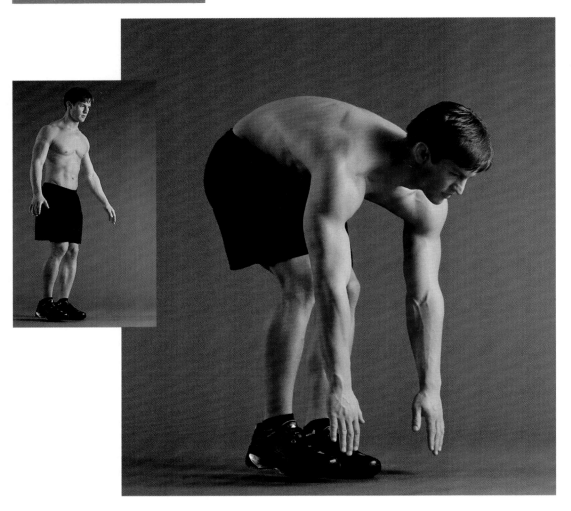

SINGLE-LEG STIFF-LEGGED DEADLIFT

SETUP: Stand on one foot, with the other foot just slightly off the floor. Keep your legs parallel, as if you were standing on both feet instead of one.

EXECUTION: Bend at the waist and reach slowly toward the floor, rounding your back to extend your range of motion. Touch the floor with the fingers of both hands if you can, and then straighten up to the starting position. Your goal is to develop enough balance to do an entire set without once touching the floor with your nonworking foot. You may be able to do only a few repetitions your first time, but persist. You'll develop the muscles in your ankle and the sole of your foot, and those will help you in most of the exercises in this chapter.

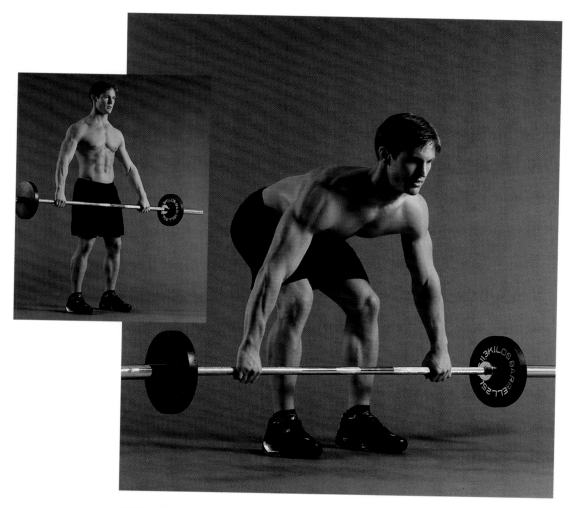

STIFF-LEGGED DEADLIFT, CHEST UP, WIDE GRIP

SETUP: Stand holding a barbell with a wide grip, your hands outside the rings. Plant your feet shoulder-width apart, and bend your knees slightly (maintain this angle throughout the lift).

EXECUTION: Bend forward at the waist, keeping your chest up and your back flat, as you push your hips backward. When you can't go any farther without rounding your back, stop and feel the stretch in your hamstrings. Contract your glutes and push forward with your hips to straighten your body back to the starting position. The key to this exercise is hamstring isolation; if you allow your lower-back posture to change, you take work away from the hamstrings and put it on your spinal extensors, which is not the goal.

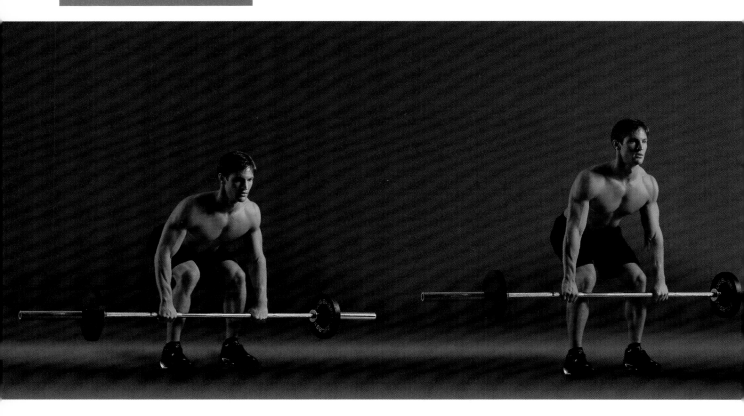

CLEAN PULL

The clean pull and the variation listed as a high pull are high-speed deadlifts, with lighter weights and more action from your calves, trapezius, and (in the high pull) shoulders. They develop power for sports that involve leaping and sprinting, and they also help improve your performance in lifts performed at slower speeds. Even if your only goal is to get bigger—not stronger or better in sports—these lifts still help. You won't necessarily see improvements in muscle size when you incorporate clean pulls and high pulls into your routines, but the strength you'll gain as a result of improved performance in other exercises eventually brings muscle gains. (For what it's worth, many guys report size gains, particularly in the upper back and shoulders, after trying these lifts for the first time. This goes to show that the best workout for you is the one you haven't tried yet.)

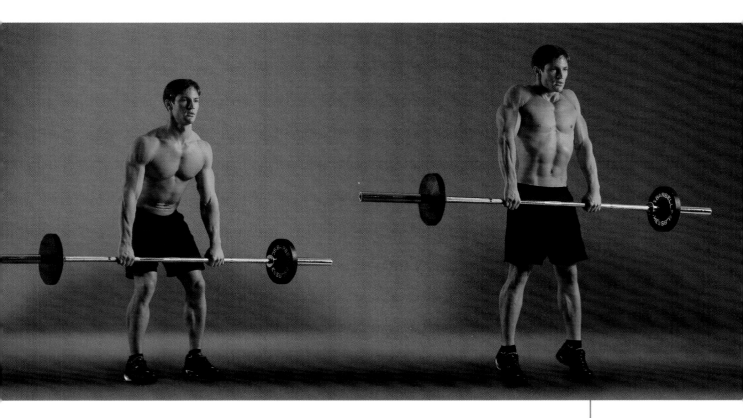

SETUP: Load a bar with one-quarter to one-third of the weight you'd use in the deadlift. Set up as you would for a deadlift, using an overhand grip that's just outside your knees (see page 184).

EXECUTION: The first pull, to just above your knees, is exactly the same as in the deadlift, except that you'll move faster because you're using a lighter weight. On the second pull, in which you straighten your hips, accelerate so powerfully that you come up on your toes and shrug your shoulders. In other words, perform the second pull as if you were going to fling the bar up over your head, but keep your arms straight. Then lower the bar to the floor with control; don't worry about making this lowering action the exact reverse of the lift.

VARIATION

HIGH PULL: This is the same exercise except you bend your elbows and pull the bar up to your chest, keeping your elbows over the bar. If you were doing it slower, it would look like a deadlift combined with an upright row. Once again, it helps to think of flipping the bar up over your head. This is the first half of that motion.

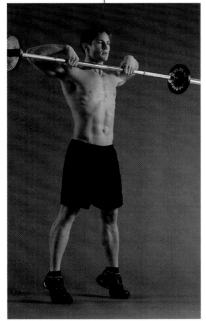

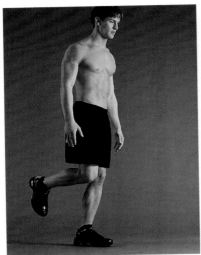

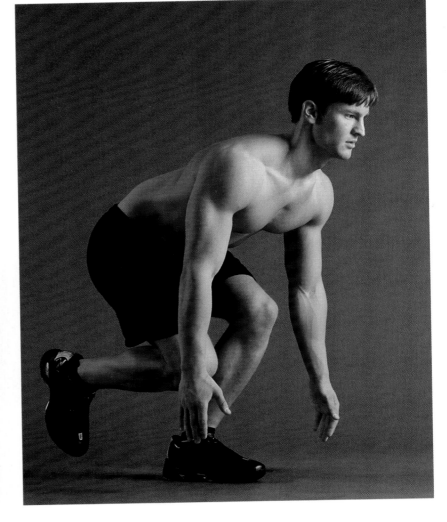

KING DEADLIFT

SETUP: Stand on one foot, with the other leg bent at the knee so its shin is behind you and parallel to the floor. Your thighs should be parallel, as if you were standing on two legs. Your hands can be at your sides or on your hips.

EXECUTION: Lower your body until the knee of your nonworking leg is as close to the floor as you can get it. You can bend forward at the waist as much as you want. Pause, then straighten up to the starting position. This is a surprisingly difficult and humbling exercise; your goal is to increase your range of motion from one workout to the next.

PROGRESSION: When you can do 15 to 20 repetitions with the full range of motion—nonworking knee brushing the floor on each rep—you can try the exercise while holding dumbbells in your hands. Few ever get to that point.

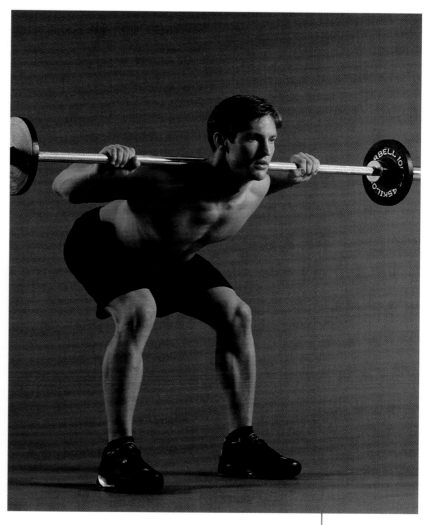

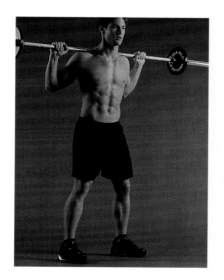

GOOD MORNING

SETUP: Stand with a bar on your shoulders, your feet shoulder-width apart, and your knees bent slightly. Maintain this knee angle throughout the movement.

EXECUTION: Bend forward at the hips as far as you can without losing the flat or slightly arched posture in your lower back. (With good flexibility, you'll end up with your torso parallel to the floor.) Contract your glutes and push your hips

forward to return to the starting position.

VARIATION

ROUNDED BACK: Using a very light load, round your back as you bend forward. With superior flexibility, you can get your head down near your knees. If you have lower-back problems or if you are extremely overweight, lower your torso only as far as you can without rounding your back.

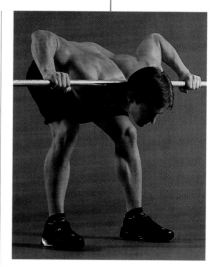

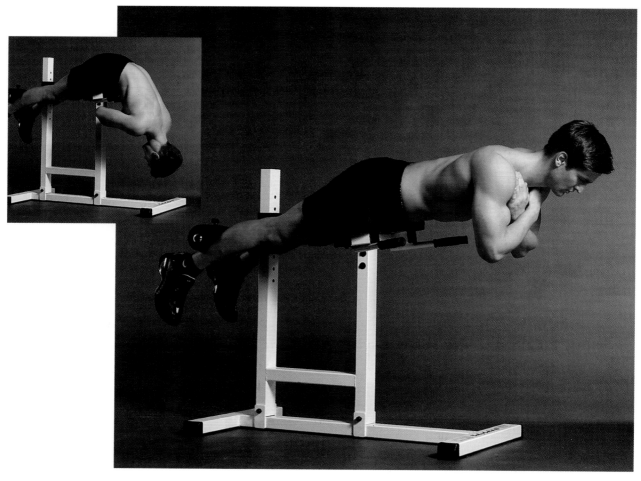

BACK EXTENSION

SETUP: Lie facedown in a back-extension apparatus—also called a Roman chair—or, if you have someone to hold your legs, on a regular flat bench. Your hips and legs should be supported, but your trunk should hang off the end. Your hands can be crossed on your chest (easiest), behind your ears, or straight out in front of you (hardest).

EXECUTION: Lower your upper body until your head is nearly on the floor. Then raise your torso back up until it forms a straight line with your legs.

LOWER BACK: This is one of the few exercises in which we want you to round your lower back. If you have lower-back problems, you may not want to do this exercise as described. Instead, lower your torso as far as you can without rounding your back, then straighten to the starting position.

EXTENSION VERSUS HYPER-EXTENSION: This exercise is often called a *hyperextension*, implying a movement in which you raise your torso past the point at which it forms a straight line with your legs. We don't want you to

hyperextend; doing so would put unnecessary pressure on your spinal disks. We do, however, want you to exercise your spinal extensor muscles through a range of motion, from flexion through extension—a movement they're designed to perform safely. Your extensor muscles are probably up to the challenge of moving the initial load, which is your body weight. If, however, you're extremely overweight, you may want to start by observing the earlier lower-back caution.

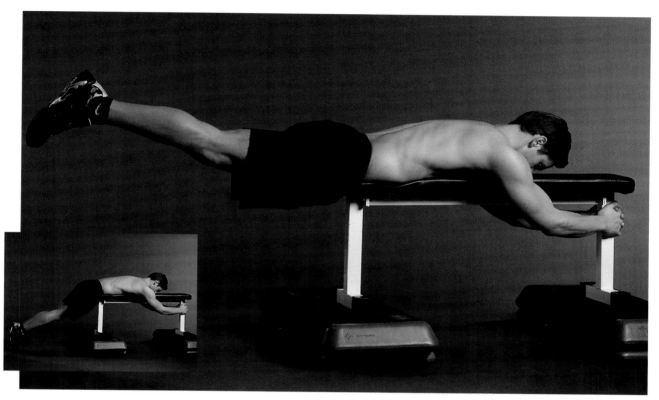

PRONE HIP-THIGH EXTENSION

SETUP: Lie facedown on a bench with your hips and legs hanging off the end. (If you can, prop up the bench to get a greater range of motion. Some gyms have taller benches that are better suited to this exercise than the standard flat benches used primarily for chest presses.) Grab the legs on the front of the bench for balance.

EXECUTION: Contract your gluteals to raise your legs until your thighs are in line with your torso. (Your feet will be slightly higher because you'll naturally have a small bend in your knees as you lift your legs.) Pause, then lower your legs, but don't allow your feet to touch the floor.

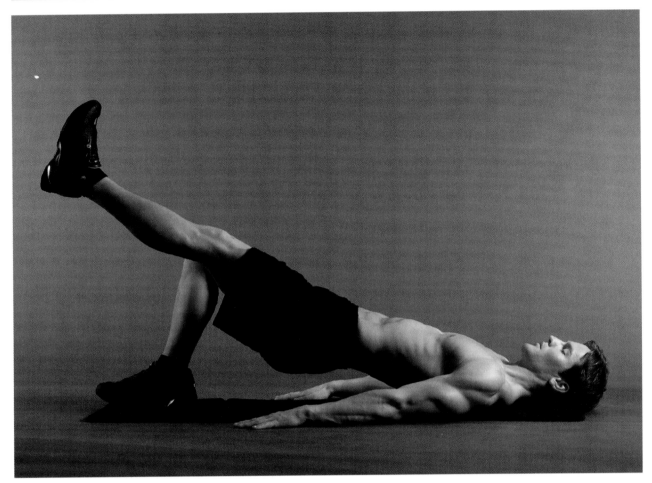

SUPINE HIP-THIGH EXTENSION

SETUP: Lie faceup on the floor. Bend one leg 90 degrees, with your foot flat on the floor. Extend the other leg straight out.

EXECUTION: Push down with the foot on the floor and raise your extended leg until its thigh is parallel to the thigh of your bent leg. Your glutes will come off the floor as you do this. Pause, feeling the contraction in your glutes and hamstrings, then slowly lower yourself, stopping just before your glutes and your straight leg touch the floor. Finish all your reps with one leg before repeating the set with the other.

LOWER BACK: You shouldn't feel any lower-back strain, but if you do, tighten your lower abdominals (thin tummy) to help flatten your back.

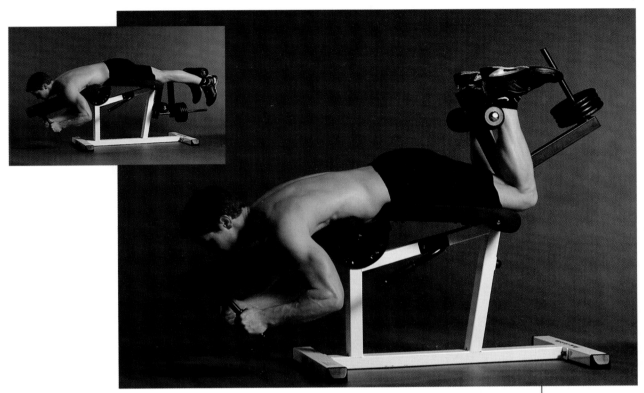

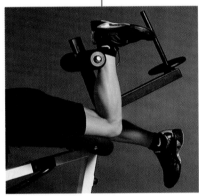

LEG CURL

This is technically a knee-dominant exercise; it works only your knee joint. And earlier in this chapter, we did spend a few sentences disparaging it. Despite all that, it's a nice exercise for building hamstring muscle mass, thereby making your body better able to do the more challenging and beneficial hip-extension exercises—the deadlifts, good mornings, and others.

SETUP: Lie on the leg curl machine and put one or both ankles beneath the pads. You can also use a standing or seated leg curl machine, if you prefer. Just use the same one for each workout in any particular stage of our programs. In other words, don't do the seated machine one week, the standing one the next week, and the lying one the week after, because you won't have any useful way to monitor your progress.

EXECUTION: Curl up the weight without lifting your hips off the pad (or changing your posture in either of the other leg curl machines). Pause when your hamstrings are fully contracted, slowly lower the weight with control, then when your hamstrings are fully stretched, pause again before starting the next repetition. Don't let the weight plates rest against each other at the end of a rep; you want to keep tension on your muscles.

VARIATION

SINGLE LEG: Curl just one leg at a time. Finish all your reps with one leg before working the other.

MUSCLES THAT ACT ON THE KNEE AND ANKLE

ONE OF THE OLDEST MAXIMS IN THE WEIGHT ROOM is that if you aren't doing squats, you aren't really lifting. Of all the strength exercises, the squat uses the most muscles—over 250. It also uses the biggest and strongest muscles: gluteals, hamstrings, and the main focus of this chapter, quadriceps.

The leg extension and leg press also work the quadriceps, and the leg extension does so more directly than the squat. Still, you never hear anyone say, "If you ain't leg-extendin', you ain't really liftin'." That's because the mighty quadriceps muscles do their best work when they're teamed up with the hip extensors. Isolate

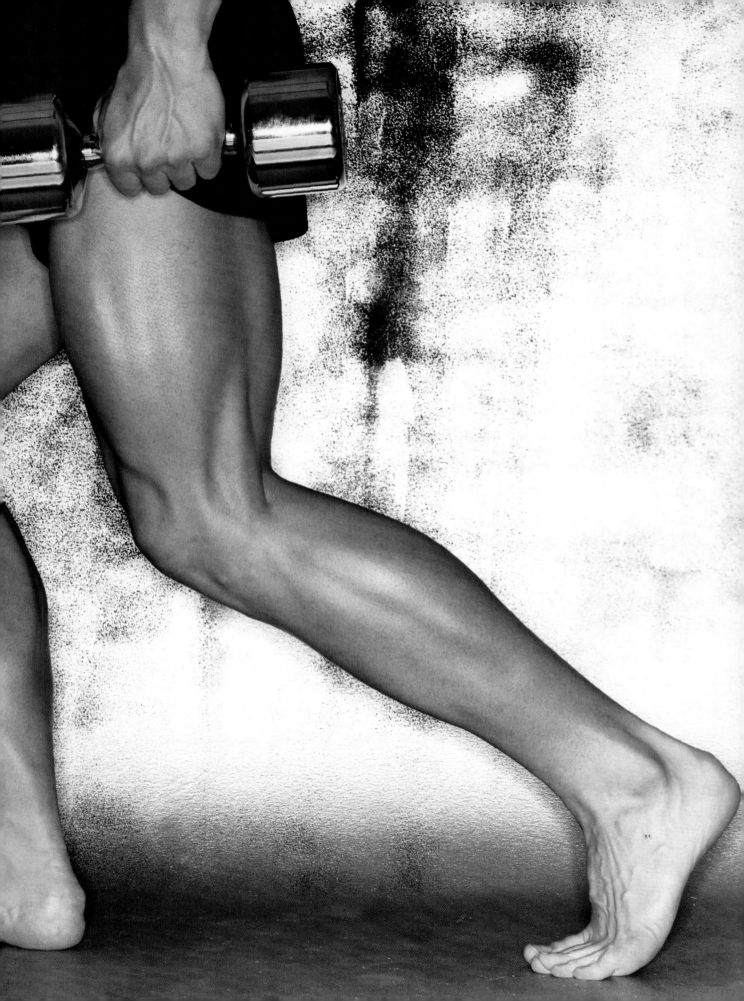

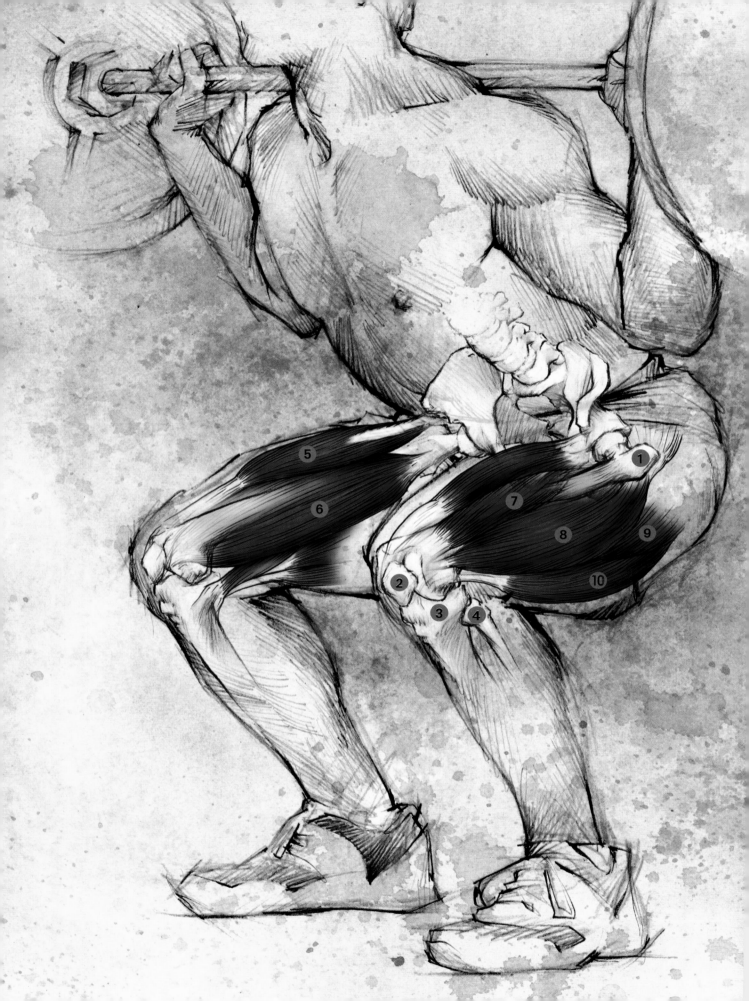

them, as you do in a leg extension, and they show little more growth potential than your abdominals.

We mention this because we never pass up a chance to point out that function rules in the weight room, even though isolation of the targeted muscles seems like a better idea when you first start lifting. Why would all those shiny muscle-isolating machines beckon you if they didn't offer the best path to size and strength?

Machines appear to be more user-friendly than free weights, and they do have their place, especially with beginners (who may lack the coordination and stability to do squats and other heavy-duty lifts) and those recovering from injuries. Once you're past the novice stage, however, it's best to look at the muscles in this chapter in terms of their overall function, rather than what they do in isolation. Of all the muscles on your body, those that act on the knees and ankles may be the ultimate team players.

QUADRICEPS

The four quadriceps muscles are charged with straightening your knee joint once it's bent. That movement is fundamental to running and jumping, which is why this muscle group is capable of both tremendous strength and awe-inspiring endurance. It's just not capable of combining those two qualities in the same person. This is why some marathoners can't jump more than a few inches off the ground and some powerlifters can't run around the block.

Since this book isn't targeting endurance athletes, we'll focus on muscle strength, power, and growth. You'll get all three in spectacular amounts when you put your quadriceps on our programs.

We've already mentioned the **RECTUS FEMORIS**, which is a hip flexor as well as part of the quadriceps group. It's the muscle that splits down the middle of the thigh, originating at the pelvis and ending, along with the other three quad muscles, in the quadriceps tendon, which crosses the kneecap and attaches to the tibia, the larger of your lower-leg bones.

The **VASTUS LATERALIS** is the big boy on the outside front of your thigh. It originates on the outside top of the femur. The **VASTUS MEDIALIS** originates on the inside of the femur, with attachment points running most of the way down the bone. The medialis is very thick near the bottom, forming a teardrop shape just above and to the inside of the knee when it's fully developed. Beneath the rectus femoris and between the lateralis and medialis is the **VASTUS INTERMEDIUS**, with origination points all down the front of the femur.

To develop a particular muscle in the quadriceps group more than the others, you can turn your feet in different directions during leg exercises or emphasize one part of the range of motion over other parts. For instance, the medialis seems to work hardest at the end of the range of motion (near lockout on the squat), so if you want to develop the teardrop shape for aesthetic or functional reasons, you might consider more work in that range of motion. (The medialis has a big role in supporting your kneecap, so exercises that build it selectively are sometimes used to help prevent or rehabilitate knee injuries.) And we've already mentioned that the rectus femoris is a powerful hip flexor, so if you want to preferentially develop that part of your thigh, do ab exercises that involve more hip flexion. Still, it's hard to imagine that those isolation exercises could rival the benefit you'll get from squats.

CALVES

If the quadriceps are simple (although far from easy) to understand and develop, the calf muscles are downright remedial.

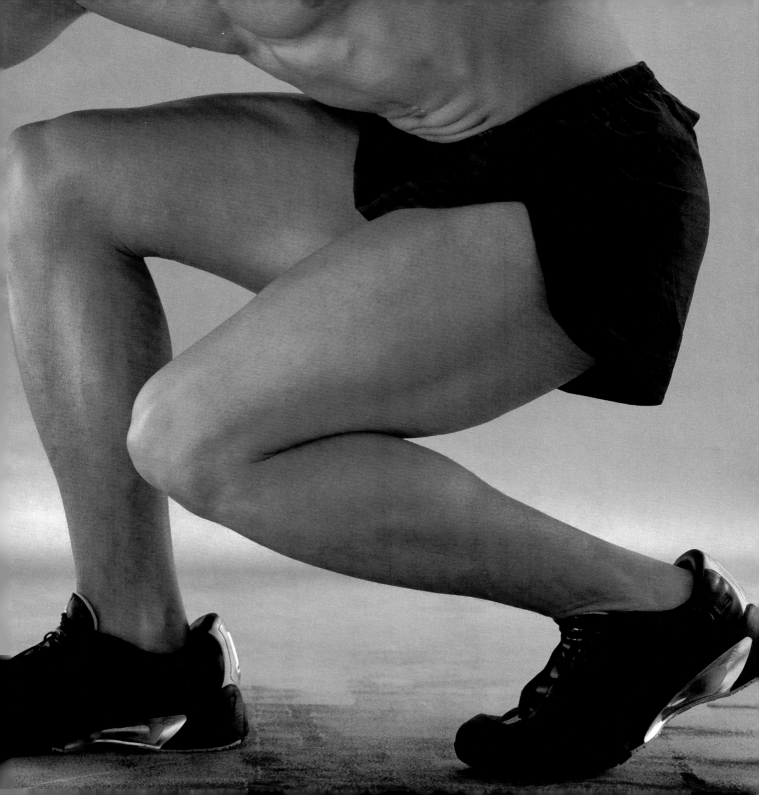

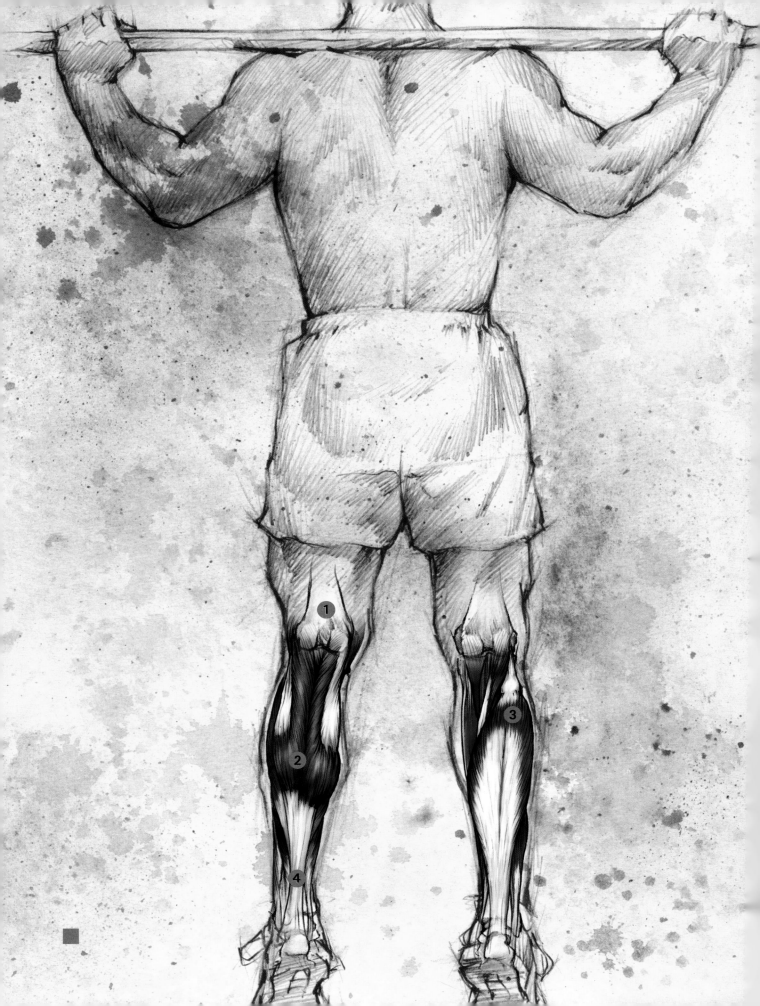

Anyone who's spent a month in a health club knows the two classic calf-developing exercises—standing calf raise and seated calf raise—and can even find the machines without a map.

The biggest and outermost calf muscle is the **GASTROC-NEMIUS**, a two-headed muscle that looks like a split salmon fillet on the back of your leg. The heads originate on the two knobs at the bottom of your femur, which means the gastroc actually crosses your knee joint. So when you do a knee-bending exercise like the leg curl, the gastroc assists the hamstrings.

The **SOLEUS** is a flat sheet of muscle beneath the gastroc. When you watch someone with well-developed calf muscles doing a heel-raise exercise, you can see the soleus from either the side or back. From the side it's one of the thin strips of muscle between the gastroc and the lower-leg bones. (The other strip is the **PER-ONEUS LONGUS**, which has a small role in raising your heels.) From the back, it's the strip of muscle on either side of the Achilles tendon, beneath the gastroc.

The gastroc and soleus combine at the bottom to form the Achilles tendon, which attaches to the heel. This explains why the two muscles generally work together in such exercises as the standing calf raise. When you do a seated calf raise, with your knees bent 90 degrees, you isolate the soleus.

Of course, the calves contain one of those muscle groups that may actually develop better in response to real-life activities than to formal exercise. You can find runners who have better-looking calves than many bodybuilders. And among guys who lift heavy weights, you'll see plenty who have meaty calves even though they don't do any specific calf exercises. That's because all lower-body exercises force the calves to work. One of the authors of this book discovered, upon adding heavy squats to his program for the first time, that his calves grew bigger than they ever had before—

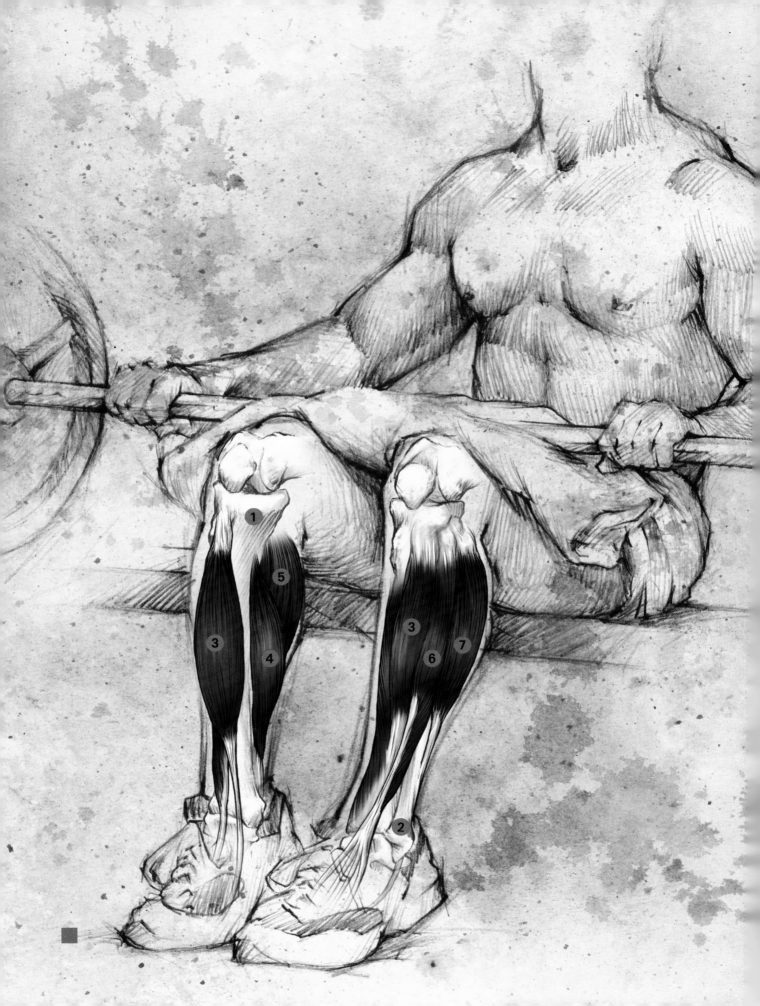

despite the fact that he had stopped doing calf-specific exercises.

This won't happen for everybody, and the calves are such important muscles for sports and aesthetics that it makes sense to do special exercises for them, even if you're a fairly advanced lifter. It's just another example of how exercises that work combinations of large muscle groups can be of greater value than muscle-isolating exercises.

Functionally, the calf muscles are involved in every form of bipedal locomotion, such as walking, running, and jumping. While your big lower-body muscles provide most of the thrusting power for these movements, the calves are the final booster rockets, pushing off from the ankle joints while the quads push off from your knees and your gluteals and hamstrings push from the hip joint.

You have another set of lower-leg muscles, on the front of your shin. While the calves' job is to pull your heel closer to your knee, pushing your toes farther away, the job of the shin muscles is to pull your toes closer to your knee. The largest shin muscle, the **TIBIALIS ANTERIOR**, is still pretty small, or at least thin. It originates on the tibia and attaches to the top of your foot. You can see it by looking at the front of your leg; it's just to the outside of your shinbone. The next muscle to the outside is the **EXTENSOR DIGITORUM LONGUS**, which has a similar role. The next muscles you see, continuing around the outside of the lower leg, are the peroneus longus, soleus, and gastrocnemius, which, of course, are involved in the opposing action.

Few people do specific exercises for the toe-raising muscles, and we don't include any such exercises in our programs. These muscles tend to develop in balance with other lower-leg muscles. During such movements as walking and jogging, they have to raise your toes to keep them from dragging on the ground.

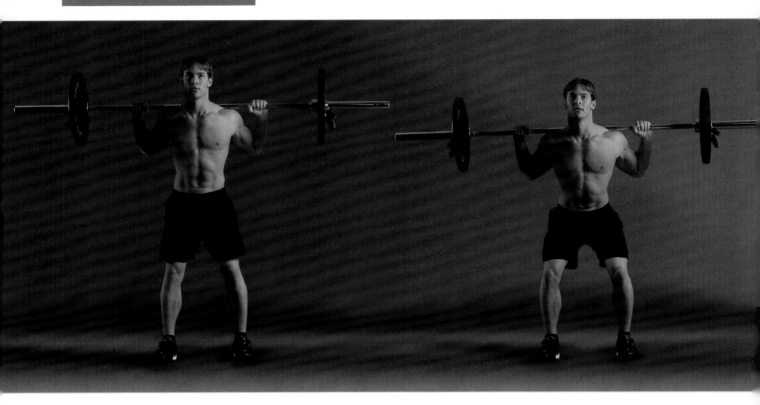

BARBELL SQUAT

Over the past few decades, many have tried to disparage the squat, claiming, among other things, that it destabilizes the knee joint. Such charges never stick. Sure, squats can be tough on the knees, but so are most sports and many other activities. While it's certainly a bad idea to do heavy squats and play full-court basketball on the same day, you can do them safely in the same week, provided you don't have preexisting knee problems.

Some say squats are tough on the lower back, and that rings true for people with preexisting back injuries. These men and women may have abnormal muscle-firing patterns that prevent the back-supporting muscles from working as designed. For lifters with healthy backs and knees, though, the squat is among the best exercises for strength and health. The heavy loads build bone density along with muscle size and strength, and thicker bones will serve you well as you move into your golden years. You probably won't be the guy who breaks his hip and ends up in a nursing home.

Because of the complexity of the squat, we've taken a slightly different approach with its description, as we did with the deadlift in the previous chapter.

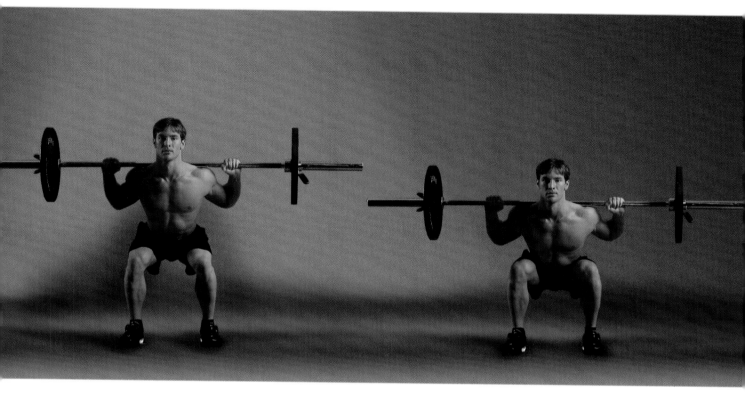

SETUP

■ Set a bar in supports that are just below shoulder height, and load on weight plates.

■ Face the bar and grab it overhand, with your hands just outside your shoulders and your elbows pointing down.

■ Step under the bar and rest it on your back. When you pull your shoulder blades together, your traps will form a nice shelf for the bar to rest upon.

■ Lift the bar off the supports by straightening your body, and step back from the supports (don't step far back, just enough to safely avoid any obstructions).

■ Set your feet shoulder-width apart, bend your knees slightly, pull in your lower abdomen, squeeze your glutes, and set your head in line with your spine—your eyes should be forward or slightly down.

DESCENT

■ Bend your hips and knees simultaneously to lower your body.

■ Keep your belly pulled in to prevent the top of your pelvis from rotating in and forcing your lower back into an exaggerated arch.

■ Squat as deeply as you can without allowing your trunk to move forward more than 45 degrees from a vertical posture.

■ Keep your heels flat on the floor.

PAUSE (if the TEMPO column in your particular workout calls for a pause)

ASCENT

■ Squeeze your glutes together and push them forward to start the ascent.

■ Follow the same path you used on your descent.

■ Keep your knees the same distance apart (your inner-thigh muscles are bigger and stronger than your outer-hip muscles, so the former will try to take over, encouraging your knees to drift inward).

■ Move your hips and shoulders at the same speed—if your hips move faster, you'll increase the trunk angle, risking more strain on your lower back.

■ At the top, keep a slight bend in your knees.

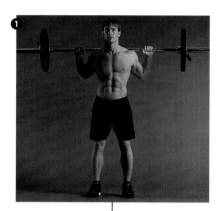

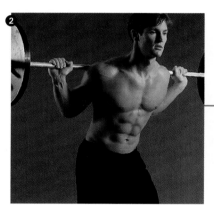

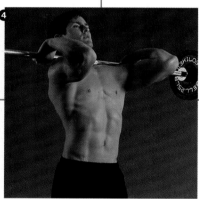

VARIATIONS

① NARROW STANCE: Plant your feet inside shoulder width, putting more emphasis on your outer-hip muscles; they work hard to keep you balanced.

② LOW BAR: In this powerlifting technique, the bar is lower, finding the groove at the base of your rear deltoids. Since the bar is closer to your hips, you can lift more weight. You'll also tend to lean farther forward, creating a flatter surface for the bar. This can be tough on your lower back.

③ HIGH BAR (NOT PICTURED): Rest the bar higher than normal, slightly above your trapezius, on your neck.

④ FRONT: Rest the bar on your front deltoids, holding it with one of two techniques: the Olympic technique, in which you grip the bar with your hands just outside your shoulders (pictured), or the bodybuilding method, in which you cross your arms over the bar and hold it with your hands on opposite shoulders.

With either method, keep your elbows high and your chest up—your upper arms should be parallel to the floor. When using the Olympic technique, avoid wrist strain by opening your hand and allowing the bar to rest on some of your fingers, rather than fully gripping it in your palm. (As long as your elbows are up, the bar will stay in place.)

The front squat emphasizes the same lower-body muscles as the back squat, but the bar position teaches you to use a more upright posture, and some find it easier to get a deeper range of motion with the bar in front.

⑤ BREATHING (NOT PICTURED): This is a 20-rep set meant to fully exhaust your lower-body muscles. For the first 10 reps, pause for 1 second at the top after each rep. For reps 11 through 15, pause for 2 seconds, breathing twice. For reps 16 through 20, pause for 3 seconds, breathing three times. Use a spotter, and at the end of the set, quickly rack the weight and then lean against the bar or squat rack until you're sure you have your equilibrium.

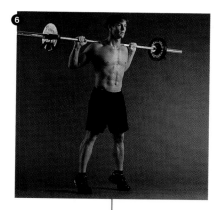

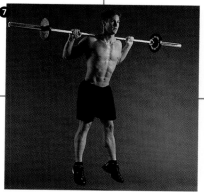

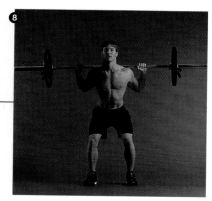

❻ EXPLOSIVE: Use a lighter weight, and on the ascent, come up so hard that you end up on your toes. Don't compromise technique for speed; lower the weight until you're able to come up fast with good form.

❼ JUMP: Use a light weight (or even dumbbells held at arm's length), and do an explosive squat in which you come up so hard and fast that your feet leave the floor. Your goal is to jump as high as you can while holding a weight, not to leave the floor with as much weight as possible. Hold the bar tightly. Land with soft knees and immediately descend for the next rep, staying in control without abruptly stopping—you want a smooth transition from descent to acceleration and from

flight to landing and starting the next descent.

❽ 1/4: Load the bar with 20 to 30 percent more weight than you'd use on full-range squats, and descend one-quarter of your normal range of motion. Be very cautious at first, descending just a few inches, and increase your range of motion slowly until you feel you're close to your "sticking point" (the place where, if you went any farther, you wouldn't come back up).

This variation is designed to get you used to heavier loads, with the idea that you'll someday be able to lift those weights through a full range of motion. So keep your mind on the ultimate goal and tell yourself this is a weight you want

to master. Don't think it will always be more than you can lift.

Because it is more than you can lift right now, you have to play it safe. Use spotters (one at each end of the bar), if you have a couple of willing souls available. Or set up safety bars in a squat rack, positioning them just below the point to which you'll lower the bar. That way, if you can't lift the barbell back up, you can leave it on the safety bars and get out from under it.

KNEE AND ANKLE

QUADRICEPS

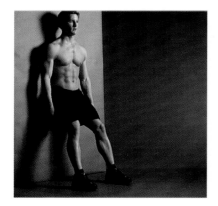

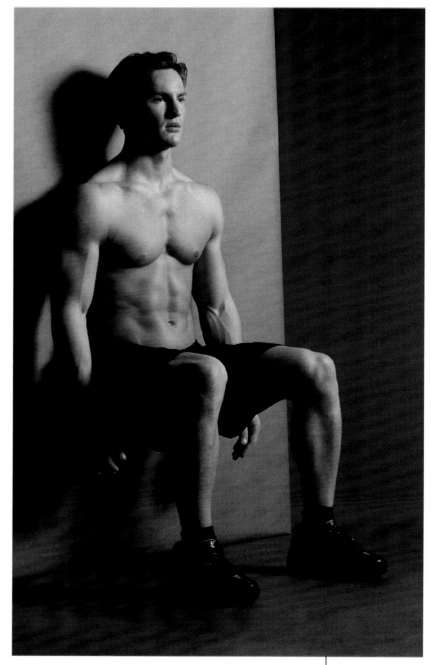

SKI SQUAT

SETUP: Stand with your back against a wall with your feet shoulder-width apart and about 2 feet in front of you.

EXECUTION: Bend your knees to a half-squat position, and hold for the length of time specified in your particular workout. Sink about another 2 inches and hold. Sink yet another 2 inches (the bottoms of your thighs should be about parallel to the floor) and hold. Sink 2 more inches, and hold. Then descend the final 2 inches, at which point your knees should be bent as far as possible. Hold, and stand up—that's your only set.

PROGRESS: You improve by holding each position longer than the one before. Aim to add about 5 seconds per position per workout, so by the third workout you can hold each position 10 seconds longer than you could the first time you tried the exercise.

EXTRA CREDIT: If the exercise is too easy as described, or if you notice that one leg seems to be doing more work than the other, do it on one leg at a time. The challenge here (apart from the obvious issue of having twice as much load on your leg) is keeping your hips parallel to the floor, as they would be in the double-leg version.

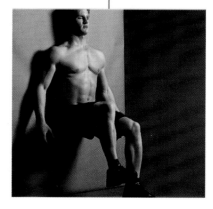

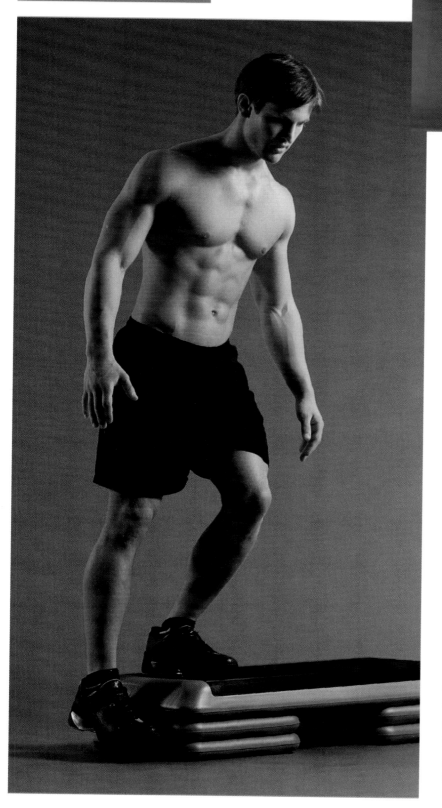

SINGLE-LEG SQUAT, ON LOW BLOCK

SETUP: Find a low block or aerobic step that's 4 to 6 inches high. Stand with one foot on the block, near the edge, and the other off the block entirely. You may want to do this near a wall or column so if you lose your balance, you can catch yourself without falling off the block and terminating the set.

EXECUTION: Bend the knee of your supported leg and slowly lower your body until the other foot brushes—but doesn't rest on—the floor. Pause, then slowly raise yourself to the starting position. Don't pause here; immediately begin the next repetition.

PROGRESS: When you can do 10 smooth repetitions with each leg, use a higher block.

EXTRA CREDIT: If you're astoundingly well-coordinated and endowed with superior muscular endurance in your quadriceps, you may find this exercise too easy. In that case, do as many repetitions as possible with each leg, with this twist: On every 10th rep, pause for 10 seconds in the bottom position.

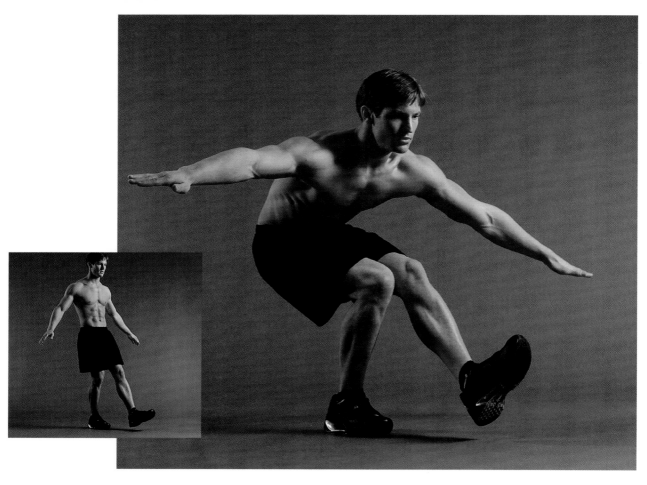

SINGLE-LEG SQUAT, OTHER LEG OUT IN FRONT

SETUP: Find a pole or pillar if you need to hold on to a support for balance. Stand on one leg, with the other leg out in front of your body so its heel is just off the floor at all times. Place one hand (probably the one opposite your working leg) on the supporting structure for balance. (If you can balance without holding on to anything, extend your arms out as stabilizers.)

EXECUTION: Lower yourself as far as you can while keeping your working foot flat on the floor and your nonworking heel hovering just above the floor. Pause, return to the starting position, and finish the set with that leg before repeating with the other.

PROGRESS: Increase your repetitions and range of motion from workout to workout, with range of motion being the most important. When you can do 15 with each leg in a full range of motion (thigh hitting calf), hold a dumbbell in one hand.

IF THE BASIC MOVEMENT IS TOO DIFFICULT: Try the exercise either on a hack squat (using maximum recline) or leaning back against a Swiss ball that's wedged against a wall. The latter variation requires some experimentation so you can find the proper positioning for the ball against your back.

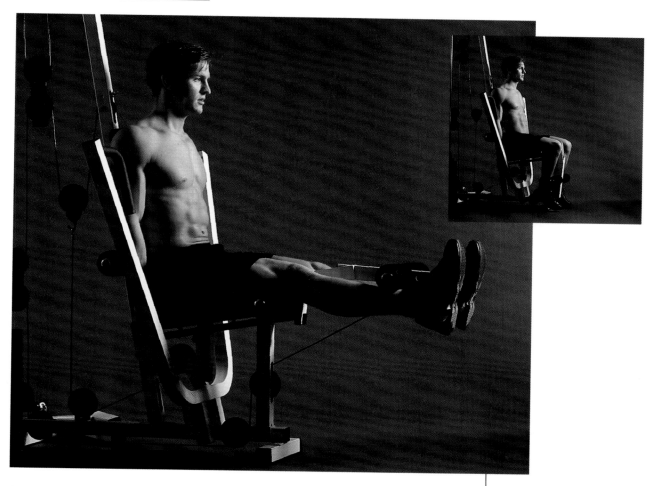

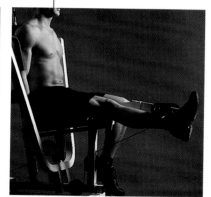

LEG EXTENSION

SETUP: Sit on the leg extension machine with the undersides of your knees firmly braced on the end of the bench. (In other words, don't let your knee joints hang out in space on this exercise.) Place your feet so the machine's pads fit into the curves where the tops of your feet meet your shins.

EXECUTION: Extend your legs at the knees until your legs are straight. Pause, focusing on the contraction of the quadriceps muscle just above and to the inside of the knee joint. You want the "teardrop" part of your quadriceps as tight as possible. Lower the weight with full control, pausing at the bottom without letting the weights in the stack rest together.

VARIATION

SINGLE LEG: Set up the same way, but lift just one leg. This helps resolve strength imbalances from one limb to the other.

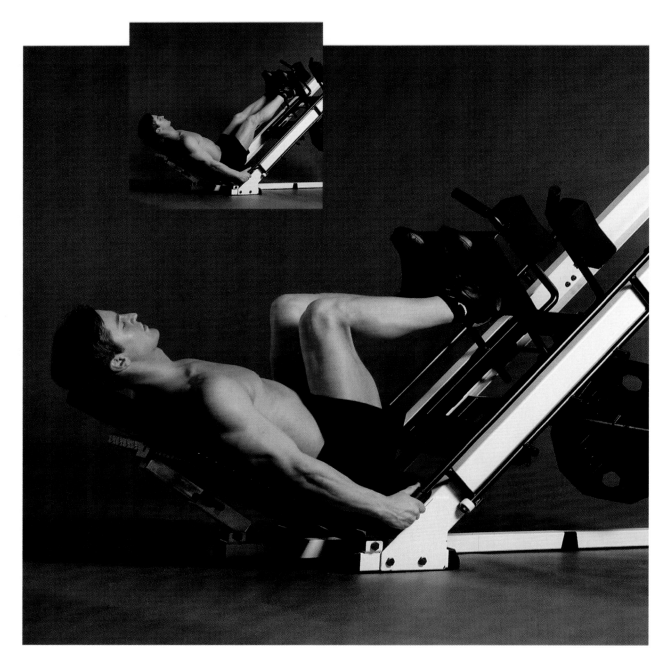

LEG PRESS

SETUP: Sit on the leg press machine with your lower back flat against the back pad, and place your feet about shoulder-width apart on the foot plate. Straighten your legs and release the brakes for the foot plate.

EXECUTION: Lower the foot plate toward you, allowing it to descend as low as is comfortable. Keep your feet flat on the plate and your back flat against the pad. Pause, then push the foot plate back until your knees are nearly straight (but still slightly flexed).

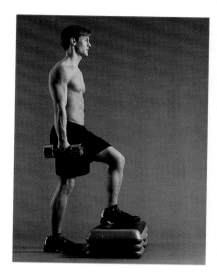

DUMBBELL BLOCK STEP

SETUP: Stand holding a pair of dumbbells and facing a block that's 12 to 18 inches high. Step up onto the bench with one leg.

EXECUTION: Press your heel down against the block to lift your other foot up to the surface of the block. Step down with the second foot, then the first. (This ensures that the first leg does the work going up and coming down.) Repeat with the second leg leading. Repeat until you finish the set.

IF YOU HAVE A STRENGTH IMBALANCE: Do all your reps with your weaker leg first, before working the stronger one.

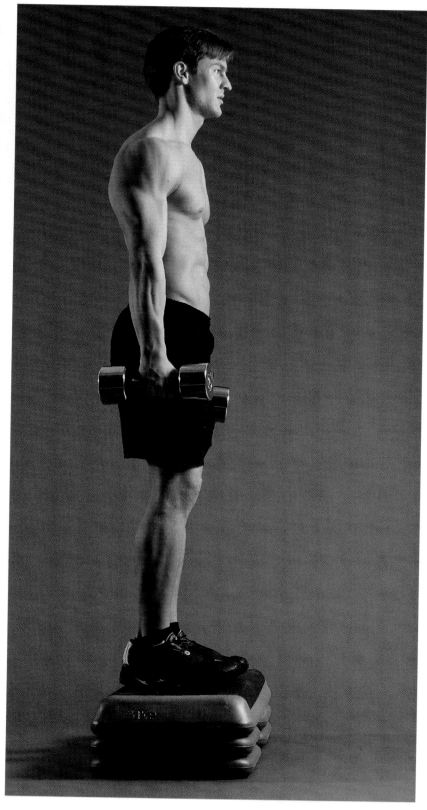

MUSCLES THAT ACT ON THE KNEE AND ANKLE

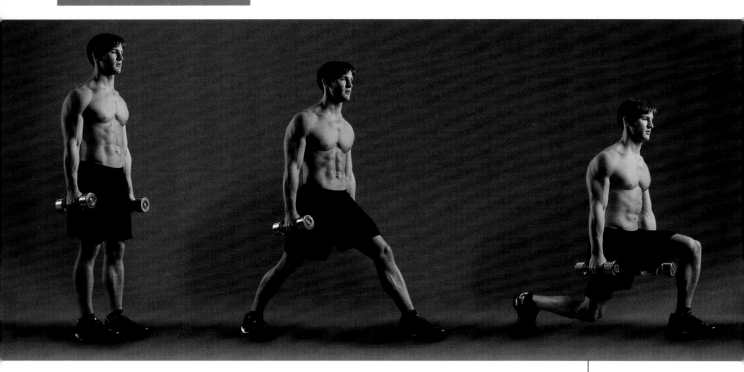

STATIC LUNGE

SETUP: You can do this with a barbell on your back or dumbbells in your hands. Just make sure you do it the same way throughout each particular stage of the workout program. Stand with your feet hip-width apart, then take a long step forward. You want to step far enough so that when you lower your body into the lunge position, the shin of your forward leg is perpendicular to the floor.

EXECUTION: Lower your body until the knee of your rear leg almost touches the floor. Pause, then raise yourself until your front knee is nearly straight. Keep your torso upright throughout the movement. Finish the set, then switch legs and repeat.

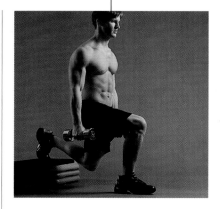

VARIATION
BACK FOOT ON LOW BLOCK: Put your rear foot on a block that's 4 to 6 inches high. Use your body weight only for the warmup set, then hold dumbbells for the work set. The block adds to your range of motion, as you'll feel in the quadriceps of the trailing leg.

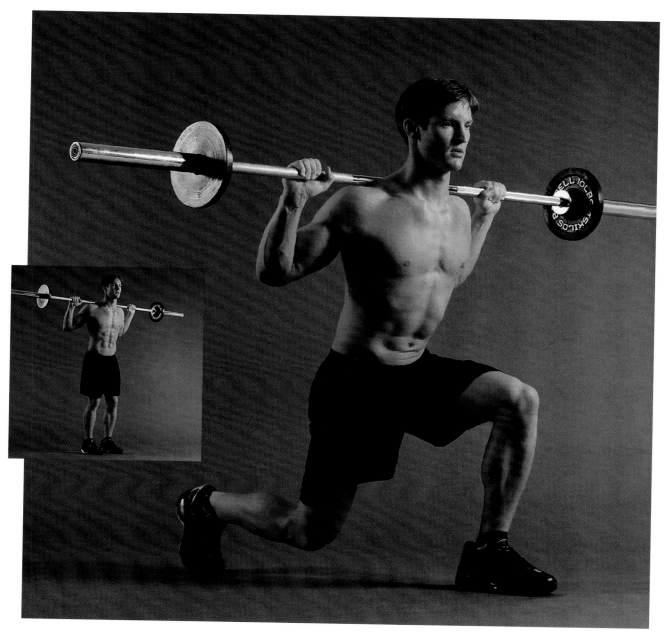

DYNAMIC LUNGE

SETUP: Set a barbell on your shoulders, as you would for a squat, and stand with your feet hip-width apart.

EXECUTION: Step out with one leg, bending both knees until the knee of the back leg is almost on the floor. Without pausing, push back up with the front leg and return to the setup position. Repeat with the other leg. That's 1 repetition.

IF YOU HAVE A STRENGTH IMBALANCE: When one leg is significantly stronger than the other, do 2 consecutive reps on the weak side, then one on the strong side. If the program calls for 10 reps per leg, do 14 on the weak side, 7 on the strong side.

MUSCLES THAT ACT ON THE KNEE AND ANKLE

STANDING CALF RAISE

SETUP: Select a weight, and position yourself in a calf raise machine with your shoulders under the pads, your hands on the supports (wherever they are on the machine you're using), the balls of your feet on the platform, and your heels hanging off.

EXECUTION: Lower your heels as far as you can, then push with the balls of your feet and raise your heels as high as possible.

IF YOU DON'T HAVE A CALF RAISE MACHINE: You can do this with a hack squat and blocks, as pictured. Or you can use a Smith machine (the barbell-on-rails device found in most gyms), with a barbell in a squat rack, or with a heavy dumbbell in one hand while balancing with the other.

VARIATION

EXPLOSIVE (NOT PICTURED): Lift as powerfully and explosively as you can, then lower the weights with control. Keep all other joints, especially the hips and knees, in fixed positions.

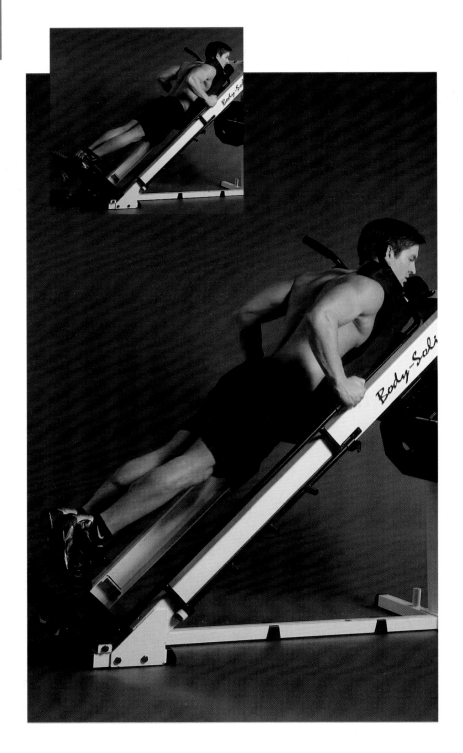

STANDING SINGLE-LEG CALF RAISE

SETUP: Set the ball of one foot on a block or step that puts you at least a few inches off the floor. Let your heel hang off. (You can hold on to a vertical support—a wall, a pillar, a post—for balance, but don't use it to lift yourself up with your arm.)

EXECUTION: Lower your heel until you feel a complete stretch in your calf, then push off the ball of your foot until the calf is fully contracted and the ankle joint is fully extended. Then lower back down to the setup position. Finish the set with that foot, and repeat with the other.

PROGRESS: In most cases, you won't need any load other than your own body weight. However, if it's easy to do all your repetitions with just your body weight, you can perform this movement in a calf raise machine or holding a dumbbell in your nonsupporting hand.

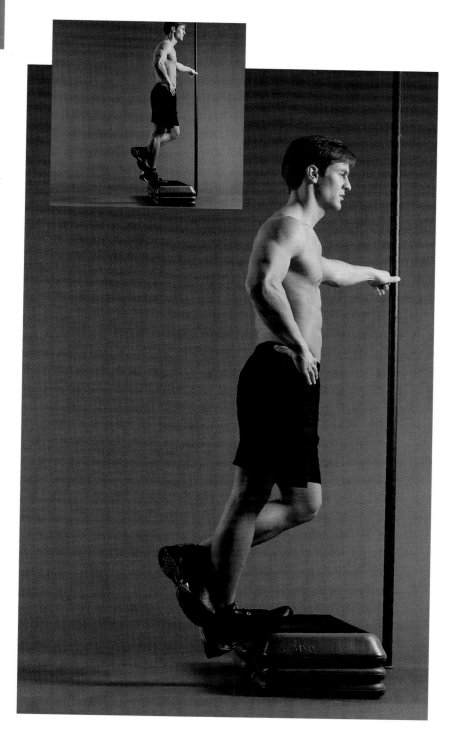

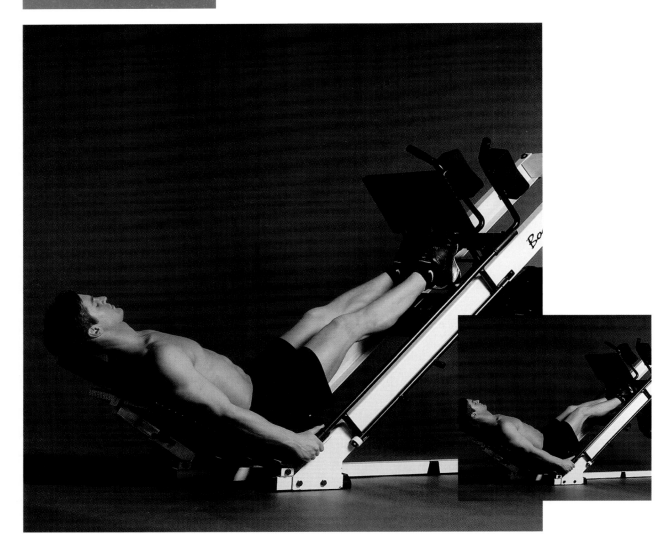

CALF RAISE ON LEG PRESS MACHINE

SETUP: Load the machine and position yourself with the balls of your feet on the platform, about shoulder-width apart. Extend your legs.

EXECUTION: Lower your heels, then raise them.

SAFETY: Don't release the brakes on the leg press machine. Having the brakes engaged won't affect the calf raise, since you don't want to bend your knees and lower the platform. And if you mess up and the weight starts to come down, you won't have to push it back up. (It will probably be more weight than you could use on a leg press.)

VARIATION

SINGLE LEG (NOT PICTURED): Put one foot on the platform and the other on the floor. Always work your weaker leg before your stronger one.

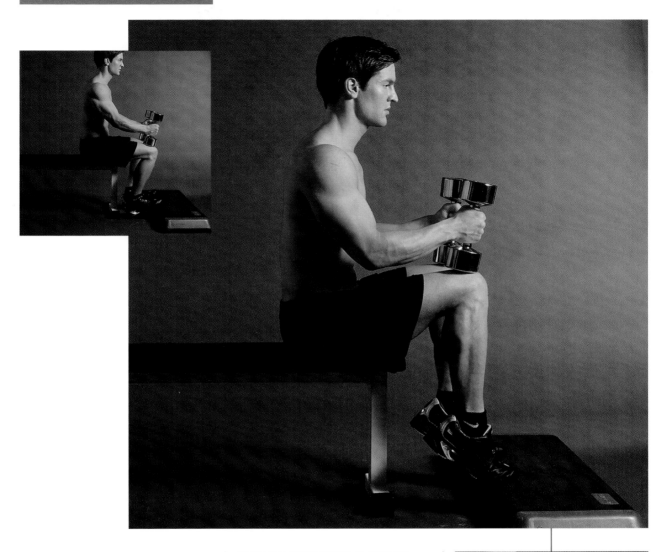

SEATED CALF RAISE

SETUP: Position yourself in the seated calf raise machine (not pictured), with the pad across your knees and the balls of your feet on the platform.

EXECUTION: Lower your heels, then raise them, as described for the calf raise exercises.

IF YOU DON'T HAVE A SEATED CALF RAISE MACHINE: You can use the Smith machine; or place a barbell across your lower thighs, just above your knees (put a towel under the bar to protect your skin); or hold a heavy dumbbell just above each knee (as pictured).

VARIATION
SINGLE LEG: Put one foot on the platform and the other on the floor. Always work your weaker leg before your stronger one.

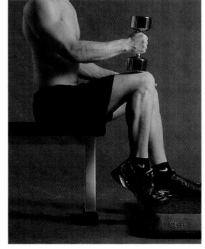

MUSCLES THAT ACT ON THE KNEE AND ANKLE

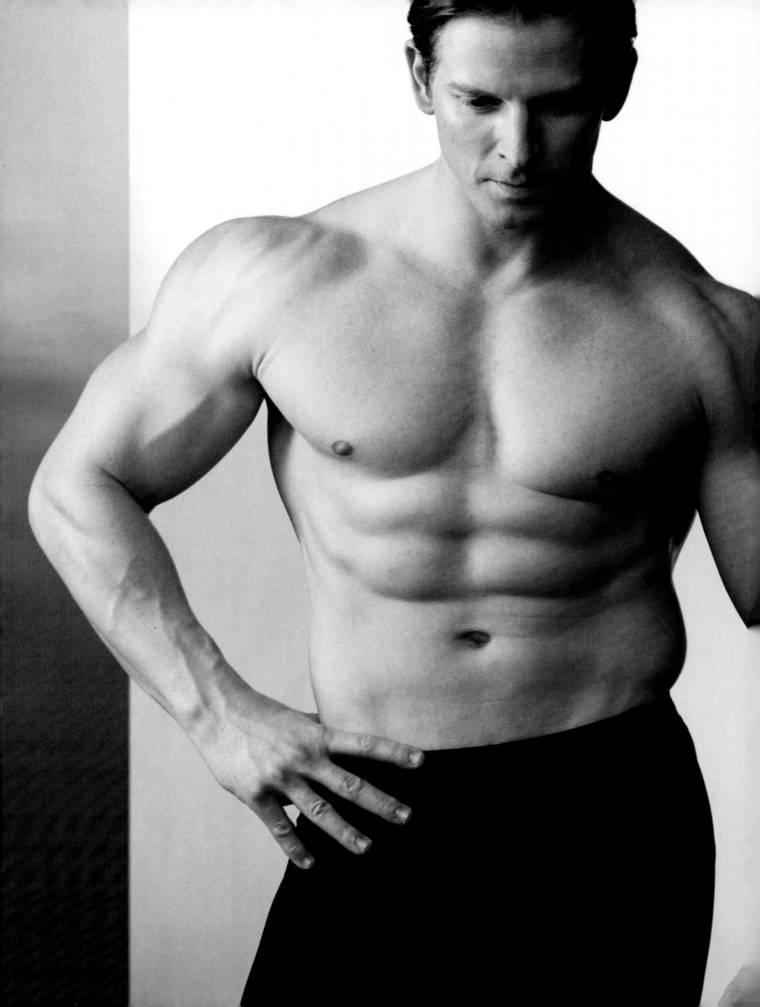

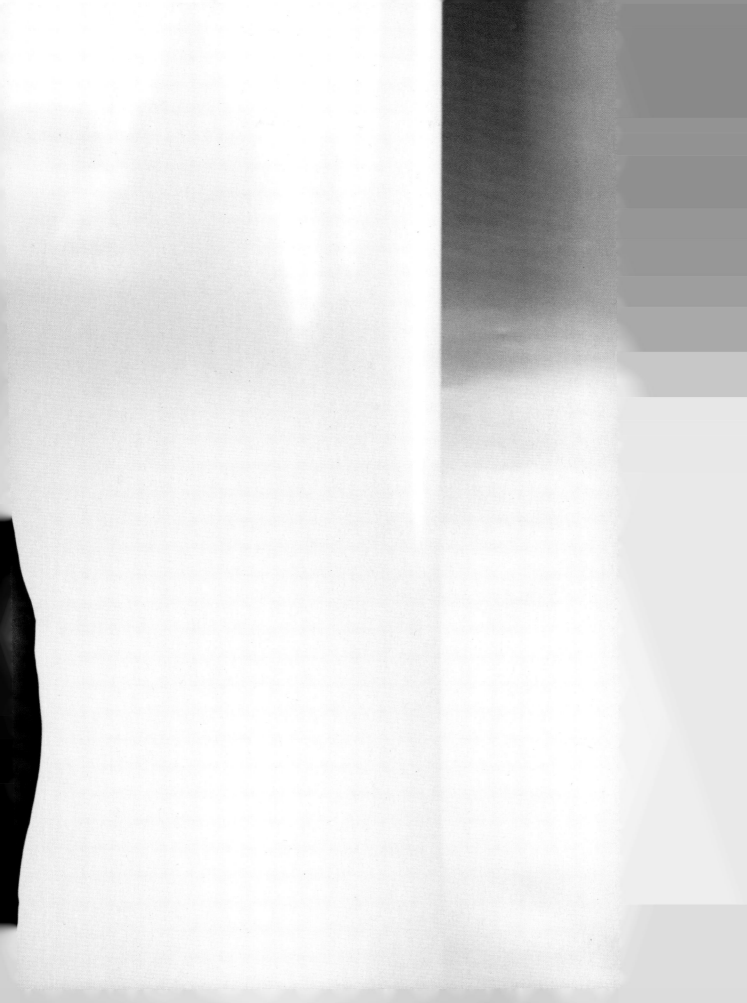

INTRODUCTION TO THE WORKOUTS

THE WORKOUT PROGRAMS IN THIS BOOK are divided into three levels: beginner, intermediate, and advanced. A method that's very effective for a beginner may be of little or no benefit to an intermediate lifter. And a technique that works for an advanced lifter may be dangerous to a beginner or an intermediate whose body hasn't made the adaptations necessary to tolerate the stress of that particular workout system.

So our goal is to give you the safest and most effective workout relative to your training age. *TRAINING AGE* simply refers to the number of years you've been training, and it is one of the most useful ways to determine which program level will work best for you.

It's simple to calculate your training age and thereby determine the skill level you should start with in our workout programs.

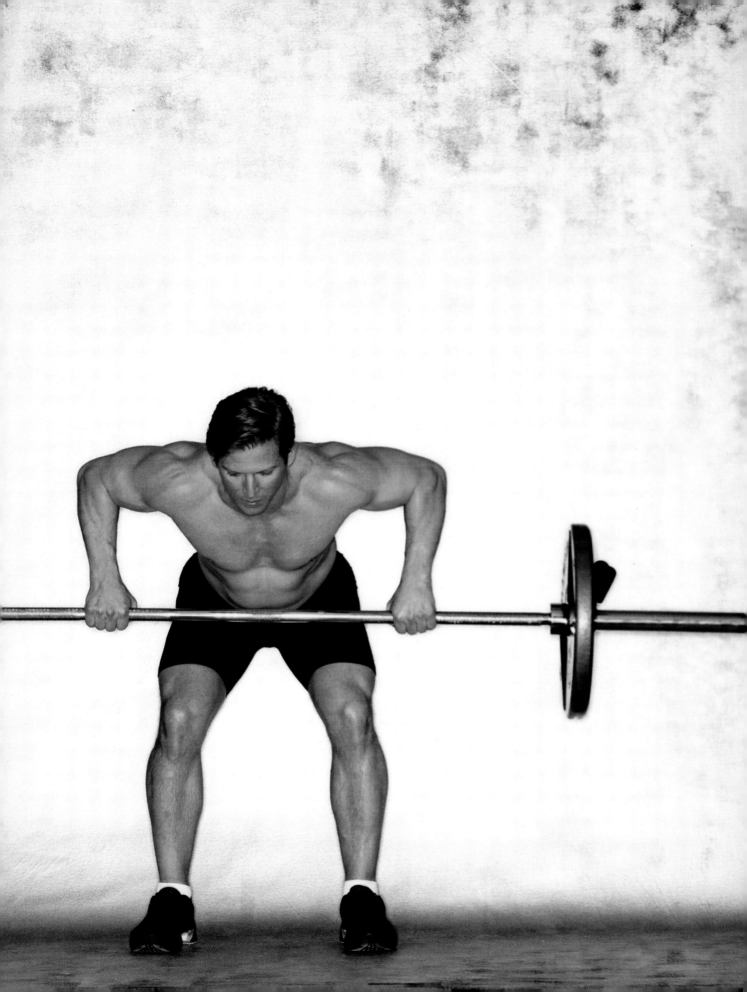

Training age <1 year = Beginner

Training age 1 to 4 years = Intermediate

Training age >4 years = Advanced

Note that your training age refers to your number of *continual* years of training. Once you've laid off the weights for 6 months or more, you should start over at the beginner training level. For instance, if you lifted regularly for 3 years but then quit for 8 months, you should resume with the beginner program.

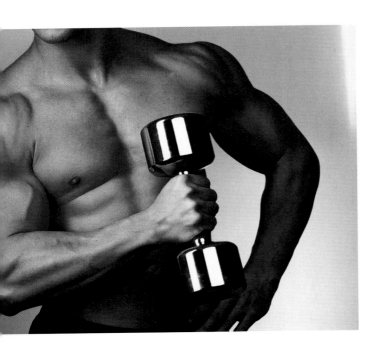

You can do the beginner and intermediate programs back-to-back for a total of about a year's worth of training. You can perform the intermediate and advanced programs consecutively as well. However, we don't expect you to do all three levels back-to-back-to-back. We recommend taking a series of breaks to try out other programs before returning to a third level of our workout system. We hope you keep this book for life and use it as a standard by which to judge the other workout programs you try over the years.

Lifters whose chronological age is under 18 should probably spend extra time at each skill level since their bodies won't make adaptations as quickly. We hope younger readers will also seek advice from coaches and trainers who can assess their progress and help them figure out when they're ready to move up a level.

FROM AGES TO STAGES

Each program level is divided into four stages, with different goals. This style of program design is called **PERIODIZATION**, a polysyllabic way of saying we planned the training progression, rather than letting you figure it out on your own. Here's the sequence.

STAGE	DOMINANT GOAL OR THEME
1	General conditioning and anatomical adaptation; addressing muscle imbalances (when one side of the body is stronger than the other, for example)
2	Hypertrophy (increased muscle size)
3	Strength
4	Maximal strength and power

Each stage is further broken down into two 3-week increments. This is necessary because even though you work toward a single goal in each stage, you won't reach that goal if you do the exact same exercises the exact same way for the full 6-week stage. You need to change things up every 3 weeks to continue making progress.

WORKOUT DURATION

We set up these programs to give you the most training in the least possible time. Your total time for each training session, including flexibility exercise and warmup (both of which we'll tell you more about in the next two chapters), should take no less than 40 minutes and no more than 120. Here's how it breaks down.

WORKOUT COMPONENT	DURATION
Flexibility	10–30 min
Warmup	10–30 min
Workout	20–60 min

We don't expect you to commit to a full 2 hours. Most of the time, you'll spend 40 to 60 minutes exercising, because your stretching and warmup components will generally last just 10 minutes each. You'll make exceptions in deference to injury: If you're recovering from a lower-body injury, for example, you'll devote a full 30 minutes to stretching, and an additional 30 minutes to a general warmup (such as walking on a treadmill or riding an exercise bike at a low intensity). These durations aren't arbitrary—a half-hour is how long it takes to raise your body's core temperature.

The length of your workout—the weight-lifting component—will depend on where you are in each stage of the program. For the beginner program, here's how we see it working out.

WEEK	WORKOUT DURATION
1	20 min
2	20–30 min
3	30–40 min
4	20–30 min
5	30–40 min
6	40–50 min

The intermediate and advanced programs require more time in the early weeks of each stage, but not necessarily in the later weeks. The advanced system, in fact, varies from higher to lower volume throughout the 6-month program. Those of you who try it will probably find that the advanced program is lower in volume than other training systems you've followed. This is one of the most important and appealing ideas behind these workouts: You do the important stuff, and only the important stuff, and then you get on with your life.

Our motto: When in doubt, do less. If you're like most guys, doing more is, at best, a waste of time because you just end up performing repetitive movements. At worst, it's counterproductive because you do so much work that your body can't recover between workouts. Incomplete recovery leads to unsatisfying results.

Make no mistake: These are strenuous programs. You'll push your body in ways it's never been pushed. But you won't push it past its breaking point.

SETS AND REPETITIONS

At each program level, in all stages, we'll tell you how many sets and repetitions of each exercise to perform. We'll do this one of two ways: We'll give you either a fixed number (two sets of 6 repetitions) or a range (one set of 15 to 20).

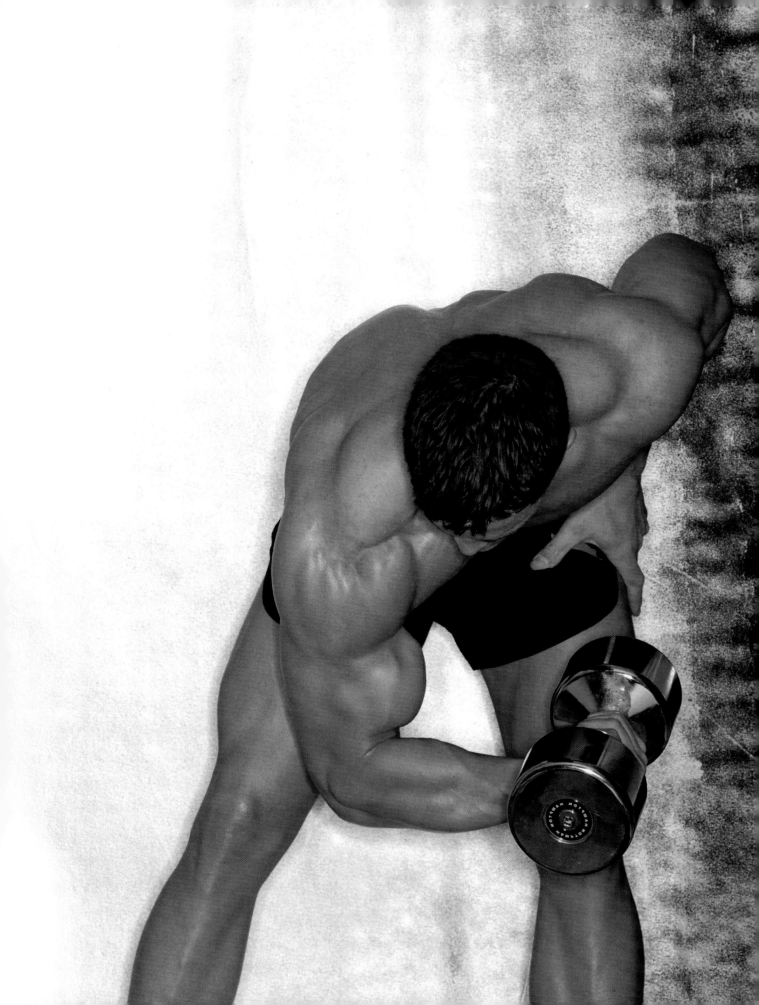

In the case of a fixed number, you should select a weight you're sure you can lift for all the repetitions in a single set (6, in our example). When given a range, pick a weight you're sure you can lift for the lower number of reps (15). Use that same weight from one workout to the next until you're able to complete the higher number of reps (20). Then use a heavier weight in your next workout.

You also have to decide the level of comfort (or discomfort, depending on your viewpoint) you're willing to accept within these parameters. A set of 6 repetitions may be very different for a lifter who wants to push himself on every set than for a lifter who doesn't want to push himself that hard. For the former, a set of 6 may be the most weight he can lift for 6 repetitions, whereas for the other guy, that set of 6 may be performed with a weight he can lift 10 times. Both guys will benefit from the set. The hard pusher will use a heavier weight, relative to his overall strength, than the other guy. The second lifter will use a heavier weight than he would've chosen had we told him to do a set of 10. In that case, he might have selected a weight he could lift 15 times.

In other words, we can tell you which exercise to do and how many times to do it, but we can't pick your level of exertion. (We will say you should never choose a weight that causes you to compromise your lifting form. That's why it's better to err on the side of working with a lower level of intensity, thus assuring that your technique maintains its integrity. Perfect technique is the key to lifting safely and productively over your lifetime.)

TEMPO

If you've lifted before, you've probably just picked up the weights and lifted them at whatever speed felt natural to you. Unfortunately, you've missed out on the benefits of working at different repetition speeds. Deliberately slow lifting speeds help you develop muscular balance and control. Moderately slow speeds allow you to keep your muscles under tension longer, which is thought to help develop muscle mass. Fast speeds help you develop power, which translates to speed and, thus, improved sports performance.

Our workouts include a **TEMPO** designation for each exercise, consisting of three digits: 311, perhaps, or 222.

THE FIRST NUMBER: This is the number of seconds you should take to lower the weight. It comes first because most exercises begin with that part of the movement. Let's say you're doing a bench press: Holding a barbell with straight arms over your chest, you lower it to your chest. Thus, the first number in the tempo column tells you how slowly you should lower the bar. The object is to learn to control the weight without using momentum. You'll lower more slowly early in the programs, and more quickly later, when you're working with heavier weights.

THE SECOND NUMBER: This is the length of the transition between the lowering and lifting parts of the exercise. In other words, it tells you how long to pause. The pause is usually 1 or 2 seconds. When the number is zero, start the lift immediately after lowering the bar, without pausing.

THE THIRD NUMBER: This is the speed of the actual lift. It's usually 1 or 2 seconds. If it's 1, lift as fast as you can while maintaining good form (even though the weight may be so heavy that you won't actually move it fast—the point is to *try* to move it fast). If the third digit is represented by an asterisk (*) instead of a numeral, the exercise is a power movement, so you need to ensure that the weight really does move fast.

For an exercise in which the weight is in the lowered position at the start of the movement—a biceps curl, for example—the tempo numbers will still be listed in the same order. So if the tempo for a biceps curl is 311, start with a 1-second lift (the third number), lower the bar for 3 seconds (the first number), then take a 1-second pause (the second number) before the next 1-second lift.

RECOVERY WEEKS

Our programs are set up with quite a bit of recovery time between workout sessions: You'll always have 48 to 72 hours from one workout to the next since muscles grow bigger and stronger during recovery from lifting, not during the actual process of hoisting and lowering hunks of iron. Still, that isn't always enough rest. So the programs are designed with the idea that you will take regular recovery weeks.

This doesn't necessarily mean you'll take a week off from all exercise or activity. You could play sports, do light lifting (such as calisthenics, or machine work at your gym), hike, or take bike rides with your kids. The point is to give your body a break from formal, serious lifting.

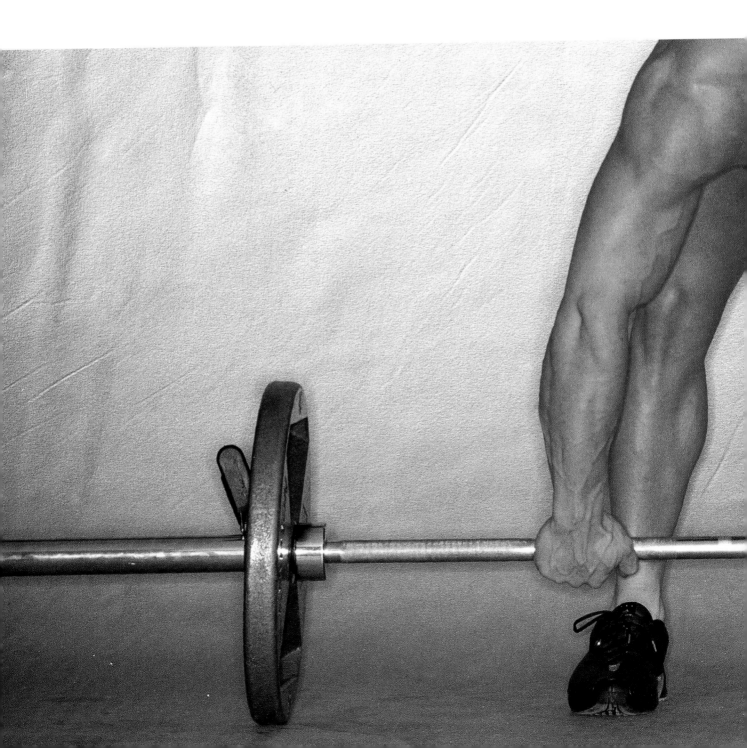

Choose the frequency of your recovery weeks from the following possibilities, all of which are based on the fact that each program level is built in 3-week increments. There are two increments per stage, for a total of eight increments during the four stages.

EVERY 4TH WEEK: You'll train hard for 3 weeks, with the hardest work coming in the 3rd week, then you'll take a week off from heavy lifting. You'll complete each

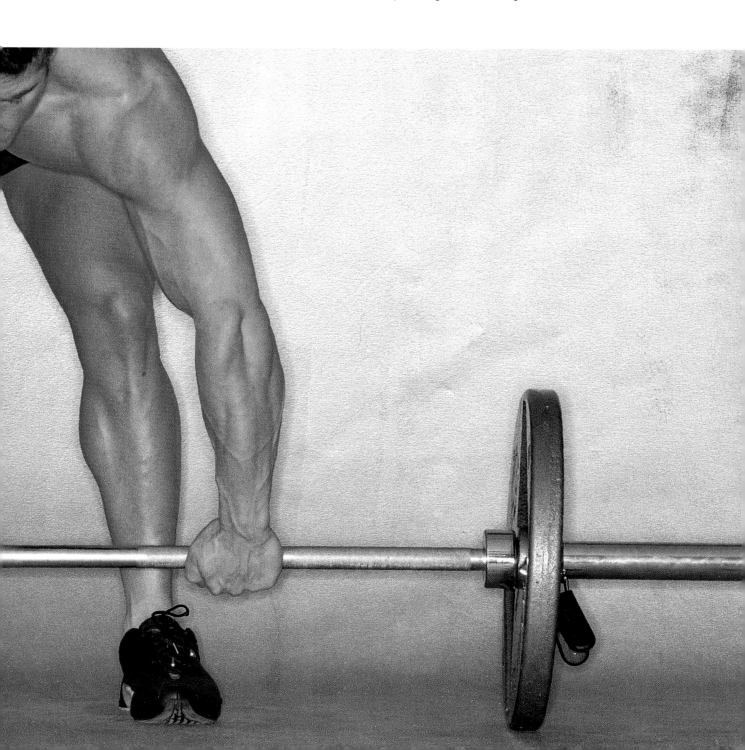

program level in a total of 32 weeks: 24 weeks of lifting and 8 weeks of recovery (including a week of recovery after the entire level is finished, since you'll need it before starting the next level). If you have a demanding job and family life, you may prefer this option.

EVERY 7TH WEEK: You'll do all 6 weeks of a stage, take a week of active recovery, then tackle the next stage. An entire level will take 28 weeks (24 weeks of training, plus 4 weeks of recovery). Most lifters will probably choose this schedule. In fact, the workouts assume you'll go with this option, as you'll see when you jump from a stage designated WEEKS 4–6 to one marked WEEKS 8–10.

EVERY 13TH WEEK: You'll complete two entire stages, take a week off, then tear through the next two stages before taking a final recovery week, completing a level in 26 weeks (24 weeks of lifting, plus 2 weeks of recovery). The youngest and the most experienced lifters will most likely gravitate toward this option.

PROGRESSION

Each workout level is a 6-month program designed so you can make progress every week of training. The two ways in which you can progress are by doing more repetitions with a given weight from one workout to the next, and by using a heavier weight for equal or fewer repetitions.

We want your progression to come in small increments, even when you're sure you could make a big leap from one workout to the next. It's never a mistake to proceed cautiously. Doing so allows your connective tissues more time to adapt to the increasing loads and ensures that your form keeps pace with your strength. So if you have a choice between increasing from 25-pound dumbbells to 30- or 35-pounders the next time you do that workout, choose the 30-pounders, then progress to the 35s the following week.

Sure, there will be times when you'll want to give it everything you have, to absolutely flatten yourself. Just make sure those times come in the final week of a stage, and make sure the following week is a recovery week.

OTHER TYPES OF TRAINING

For physical and mental health, sports may be the best activities you can pursue—particularly start-stop games like basketball, hockey, soccer, and racquet sports. An hour spent playing hoops or soccer is more of a challenge to your muscles and connective tissues than weight lifting or running or just about anything else.

So playing sports while doing our workout programs makes it tough to get all the benefits out of either. The best solution is to play on days when you don't lift and to give yourself an extra day of recovery after playing. We also ask that you give yourself at least 1 full day a week with no exercise at all—no lifting, no sports, no running. (Sex is acceptable, as long as you avoid anything too athletic or vertical.) For example, you could lift on Monday, Wednesday, and Friday, play pickup basketball on Saturday, and take all day Sunday to recover before you lift again on Monday.

If you play sports more often than once a week, you should probably make more radical adjustments. Say you play in a basketball league on Wednesday night and then play a pickup game each Saturday. You could lift weights on Monday and Friday. Your lifting program would be the same; you'd just take a few more weeks to complete it. Let's say you're doing the intermediate program, which has three different workouts: A, B, and C. You need to do each workout three times to finish a 3-week increment of the program. Here's how your training program could work.

	MONDAY	TUESDAY	WEDNESDAY	THURSDAY	FRIDAY	SATURDAY	SUNDAY
Week 1	Workout A	Rest	Basketball	Rest	Workout B	Basketball	Rest
Week 2	Workout C	Rest	Basketball	Rest	Workout A	Basketball	Rest
Week 3	Workout B	Rest	Basketball	Rest	Workout C	Basketball	Rest
Week 4	Workout A	Rest	Basketball	Rest	Workout B	Basketball	Rest
Week 5	Workout C	Rest	Basketball	Rest	Rest	Basketball	Rest

As you see, you'd complete the 3-week increment on Monday of the 5th week. You'd still get all the benefits, assuming you didn't suffer any major injuries from basketball. By the time you'd finish all the stages, your 6-month program would simply become a 9-month program.

A final approach is to play your sport during a specific season—which you may already do anyway, owing to weather or league schedules—and pursue our strength-training programs during the off-season. While playing twice or more a week, you could do lighter, less ambitious, more maintenance-oriented weight workouts.

You might have noted that we've said little about cardiovascular exercise in this book. We assume that a guy who has bought a book with the word *muscle* in the title is primarily interested in building muscle. We don't believe traditional cardiovascular exercise helps you toward that goal. You already know that endurance training doesn't stimulate much muscle growth because it works your smaller, low-growth-potential slow-twitch fibers. (If endurance work did build serious muscle, marathoners would have legs like defensive linemen's, and the streets of Boston and New York City would have to be repaved annually after the cities' signature races.) You may not know that concurrent aerobic and weight exercise produce what's called an *interference effect*. Your body makes all the adaptations you expect in response to the aerobic exercise but only some of the adaptations you expect from strength exercise.

In one study, subjects who did only aerobic exercise saw their type I muscle fibers shrink due to the release of the stress hormone cortisol. Cortisol doesn't want these fibers to get bigger, since such growth would reduce the efficiency of endurance exercise. Study subjects who did only strength training saw growth in both their type I and type II fibers, because strength training reduces resting cortisol levels over time. Though your body still wants cortisol to prevent type I fibers from getting bigger and lowering your aerobic efficiency, in this case might makes right, and lowered resting cortisol levels can't prevent the fibers from growing. But the study subjects who did both aerobic exercise and strength training concurrently experienced only type II growth, without an increase in the size of type I fibers.

That leads to an interesting conclusion: If you want to maximize your muscular growth and fitness, you may want to avoid serious aerobic exercise.

We realize, of course, that you may honestly enjoy running, cycling, rowing or other endurance activities. We would never insist that you give them up. However, we do suggest that you at least reserve them for the days on which you don't lift weights. You don't want any other activity to drain your muscles of the energy they need to perform your weight workouts.

INDIVIDUALIZING THE PROGRAMS

When we design strength-training programs, we know the first question most lifters will have is some variation on "Would it hurt if I changed the exercises around a little bit?" Or, "Is it a problem if I want to do six more sets of bench presses each workout?"

Our answer is: Do whatever you want. It's your life.

These are general programs. They weren't pulled out of thin air—they're the result of decades of experience in training people of all ages, abilities, and goals. That doesn't necessarily make them the perfect programs for you. You may have injuries that dictate modifications of certain exercises. You may be an athlete who has to add sport-specific components to the programs. Or you may just be the kind of guy who likes to get under the hood of a workout, tinkering with sets, repetitions, and exercise selections to eke out better gains—or just amuse yourself.

Assuming none of these descriptions applies to you, we suggest you do the workouts exactly as we present them. You'll almost inevitably get better results by suspending whatever programs you've done in the past and trying it our way, with exercises and techniques you haven't tried before.

RECORDING YOUR RESULTS

Strength training plays tricks on your memory. It causes you to inflate some numbers over time and shrink others. Let's say you were pretty strong in your youth, bench-pressing 315 pounds for one repetition at a body weight of 220 pounds. Now, 10 years later, you distinctly remember benching 335 pounds for two repetitions at a body weight of 180.

This is why recording the results of your workouts is important to you and your descendants. Training logs offer proof of your maximum strength, if you had any. They also provide evidence of your senility to the heirs who wish to gain control of your estate, if you have one.

The more immediate purpose of keeping a training log is even more important. It's difficult—impossible, really—to remember the results of every set of every exercise from one workout to the next. And you can't make steady progress if you're constantly guessing about the point from which you're progressing.

We recommend that you keep a training notebook in your gym bag and make recording your sets, reps, and weight loads as essential as your jockstrap.

CHAPTER

TWELVE

THE TWISTED TRUTH ABOUT FLEXIBILITY

EXERCISE SCIENCE IS PRONE TO THE OCCASIONAL REVERSAL. A belief that's been handed down as absolute truth for years and years can become heresy almost overnight, and heresy can become truth almost as fast. Such is the case with what we like to call the Great Exercise Paradigm Shift, in which the primacy of aerobic exercise was questioned by strength coaches and then renounced by a generation of trainers who learned to do with dumbbells and protein shakes what was once thought possible only with a treadmill.

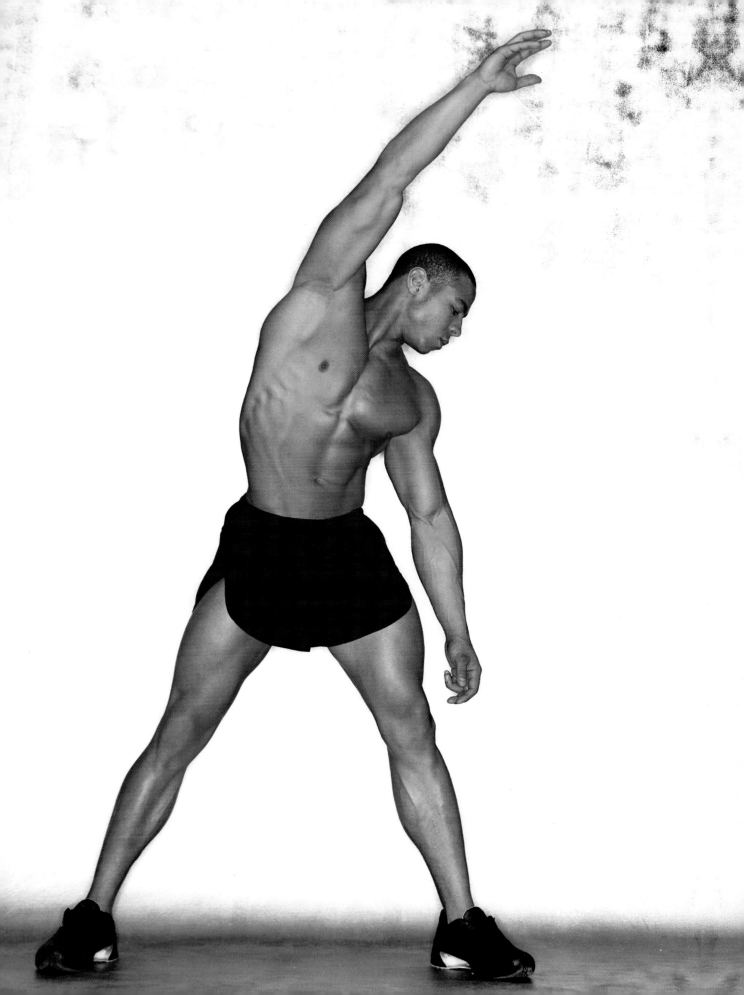

We were all for that reformation. Now comes another shift that we're almost completely against: Emerging research is showing that some of the most fundamental beliefs about flexibility and stretching aren't so fundamental after all.

The scientific research has followed two tracks. First, researchers reviewed studies examining the relationship between pre-exercise stretching and injury rates. Conclusion: Stretching doesn't prevent injuries.

Meanwhile, researchers questioned whether pre-event stretching improves performance. They found that if the event involves a single, all-out burst of power, stretching actually *hinders* performance. One typical study, published in 1998 in *Research Quarterly for Exercise and Sport*, found that 20 minutes of stretching inhibited maximum quadriceps strength by 8.1 percent and maximum hamstring strength by 7.3 percent.

You'd think that in the face of this mounting evidence that stretching is overrated—and perhaps even counterproductive—we'd have lost faith in the practice. We haven't. And we're happy to explain why.

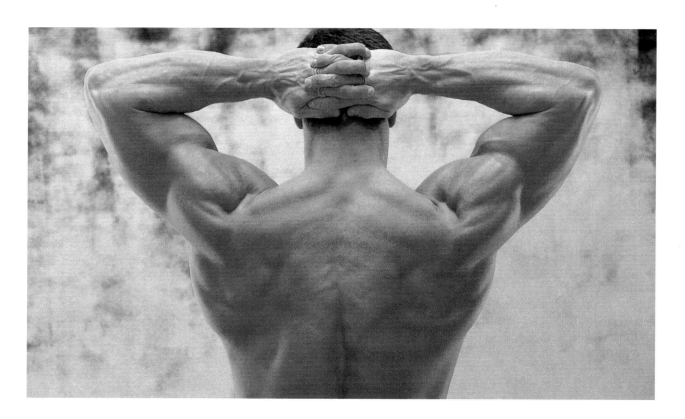

WHY WE STRETCH

When you were a baby, you were capable of feats of flexibility that would put a yogi into traction. Nearly everything that has happened to your body since then has made you less flexible. Your bones have gotten longer and stiffer. Your lowermost vertebrae fused during adolescence, dramatically changing the range of motion in your hips. And any exercise you've performed has most likely shortened and stiffened your muscles and connective tissues.

This last phenomenon may be your body's strategy to provide more thrust: Shorter, stiffer muscles act like tighter springs, creating a better rebound effect. Ironically, this strategy can backfire. The poor flexibility in those short, stiff muscles can prevent you from achieving a full range of motion in your exercises. A compromised range of motion limits the benefits of the exercise. In other words, the price of tight muscles is that you get less muscle growth from the same strength-training effort.

Stretching counteracts tightness, restoring muscles to their proper lengths and tension. So it not only fosters full range of motion during exercise but also helps you recover better and faster after exercise. Quicker recovery means the muscles are ready to repeat a workout sooner.

We base our opinion on pure experience. That experience has shown us that when athletes stretch diligently and rigorously, they train better, perform better, recover faster, and over the long haul, suffer fewer chronic and debilitating injuries.

HOW TO STRETCH

Textbooks will tell you there are three types of stretching exercises:

1. STATIC

2. DYNAMIC

3. PNF (proprioceptive neuromuscular facilitation)

The first is the one that you're most familiar with: You get into a stretched position and hold it. Then you relax into a deeper stretch; or you end the stretch, rest, and then repeat the stretch; or you end the stretch and move on to the next. The bible of this type of flexibility exercise is the book *Stretching*, by Bob Anderson.

Dynamic stretching involves moving your body into stretched positions without holding those postures. An example is a series of martial arts kicks. You may also have heard the term *ballistic stretching*. This refers to dynamic stretching in which you use momentum and muscle power to force your body into a deeper stretch than it might be able to manage without an extra push.

Finally, PNF stretching involves a series of muscle contractions and releases that create a deeper muscle stretch without the dangers of ballistic stretching. You typically hold a PNF stretch for a couple of seconds. The most popular guide to this technique is *The Whartons' Stretch Book*, by Jim and Phil Wharton, who use a PNF variation they call *active-isolated stretching*.

We're going to keep this simple by recommending static stretching. (You'll find upper- and lower-body flexibility routines later in this chapter.) It isn't that the other two approaches don't have their place, particularly for elite athletes. We simply believe, based on our experience, that static stretching is the simplest, easiest, safest, and most universally beneficial type of stretching exercise.

STRETCHING GUIDELINES

WHEN TO STRETCH: We promote a currently unfashionable idea: static stretching before strength training. Ultimately, it probably doesn't matter whether you stretch before training, after training, or only on nontraining days. What counts is that you stretch with some purpose and focus. And you're most likely to have that sort of dedication before a workout, rather than after, when you're tired and hungry.

When you stretch before a weight workout, you must regard it as a separate process from your weight warmup, because stretching actually cools down your muscles. (In the next chapter, we'll discuss the type of warmup that is appropriate before you lift.)

THE TIGHT-SIDE RULE: For strength training, we recommend starting unilateral exercises (in which you work one arm or leg at a time) with your weak-side

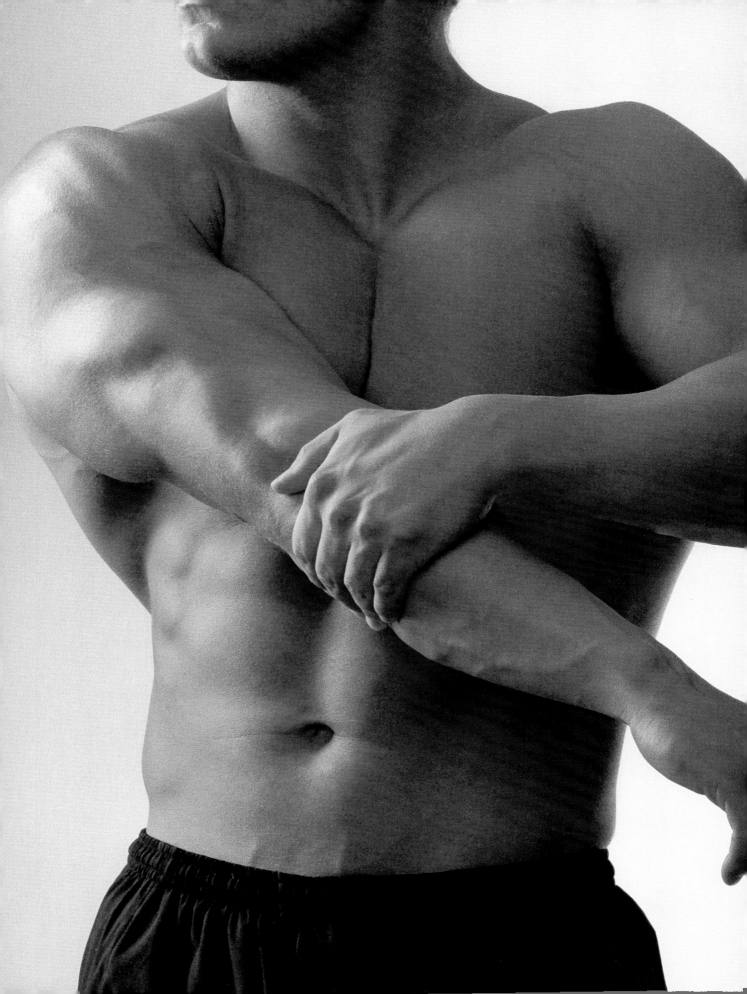

limb before repeating a set with your stronger arm or leg. The same concept applies to stretching, except that it's okay to spend more time and energy stretching your tighter side. (In strength training, you'd almost never consider giving more work to your weaker side, unless you were rehabilitating a serious injury.)

Say one hamstring is tighter than the other. (You don't need any fancy tests to determine this—it will be apparent the first time you do our stretching routine.) Start your routine with the tighter limb. Next, stretch the more flexible side. Then, if you want, return to the tighter one.

You may end up spending more than twice as much time on the tighter side, and that's fine. You could spend the same amount of time on each side; that's fine too. What's absolutely essential is that you start with the tight side. You'll always focus better on the first limb you stretch.

DURATION OF EACH STRETCH: With stretching, more is often better. It's hard to overtrain flexibility. Most likely, at the start of our program you'll hold each stretch for between 10 and 30 seconds, progressing from there. You may hold some stretches for several minutes as you get more comfortable with them.

AVOIDING INAPPROPRIATE PAIN: Toward the end of a good stretch, you'll hit points of mild to moderate discomfort. This is a sign that you're challenging your muscles and connective tissues. You should never feel actual pain when stretching. Pain is a warning that you're on the verge of injury—if you're lucky. If you aren't lucky, pain is a sign that you've already hurt yourself.

So at the beginning of a stretching program, be cautious with discomfort. You can get more aggressive as you figure out your body's limits and learn how to mildly challenge them without pushing past them and injuring your muscles and connective tissues. Remember that if you rush the process and tear something, you'll be worse off than before, because the tear will be repaired with scar tissue that will be even less pliable than the original muscle and collagen.

LENGTH OF STRETCHING WORKOUTS: Start with extremely brief stretching sessions before your regular workouts—5 minutes is plenty for a beginner. From there, progress to perhaps 15 minutes of stretching before upper-body workouts, and as much as 30 minutes before lower-body workouts.

SAFETY: In early 2003, anecdotal reports from doctors and trainers suggested an increase in yoga-related injuries. This sounds like the punch line to a not-even-remotely-funny joke. The fact is any type of exercise can damage muscles and joints if done poorly or overzealously.

Purportedly, the problems with yoga were that classes were too crowded—leaving insufficient room to do all the exercises properly—and instructors were pushing students into more advanced positions before the students were ready for them. So our two safety rules for stretching are pretty basic.

1. Never compromise form, no matter how crowded the gym's stretching area.

2. Progress at your own speed.

Rule number 2 strikes us as less obvious. We'd guess that many a guy will walk into a gym this afternoon, see another fellow reach down with straight legs and put his palms on the floor, and assume he can do that himself. If he can't do it, chances are he'll grab his own ankles and try to pull himself down farther. And he'll become a casualty.

Progress is a process. And there's no guarantee that at the end of that process every guy will be able to put his palms on the floor. Along with exercise and injury history, genetics comes into play. If your father couldn't touch his knees, you may have to concede that you're ahead of the game when you finally reach down and brush your fingers on the floor without straining.

PROGRESSION: Stretching is like any other form of exercise in that most of us hit a "good enough" point. Once you get to that point in your flexibility, we won't judge you. Before you get there, though, you have to make sure you're getting *somewhere*. Our educated guess is that virtually everyone reading this book has less-than-optimal flexibility, including imbalances from one side to the other that could prevent optimal muscle development now or lead to later injuries.

So we think you should track your stretching program the way you track your weight workouts: Time your repetitions of each stretch and your total stretching session. Say you do a hamstring stretch in which you lie on your back with one leg straight up from your hip. Write down the angle of your hip joint—90 degrees, for example (when your hip is perpendicular to your torso and the floor). Over time, try to shorten that angle.

You won't be able to improve flexibility in perpetuity, just as you won't be able to bench-press 1,000 pounds, no matter how hard you try. You don't need to, though. An improvement of just 5 to 10 degrees in your hip flexors can make a huge difference in your squat. You'll be able to go deeper with good form, meaning you'll get more benefit from the exercise.

STRETCHING ROUTINES

The following pages illustrate two sample stretching routines, one for your upper body and another for your lower. Before doing a full-body weight workout, first do both of these routines.

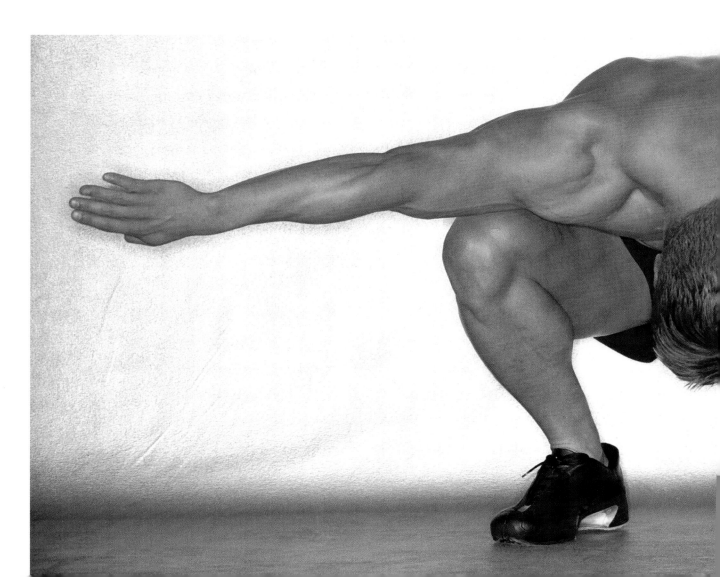

We describe many of the stretches as starting with your right side, with the assumption that you're a right-handed guy whose right side is stronger and tighter than his left. If in fact your left side is tighter, stretch it first.

The bigger the muscle, the longer you should hold a stretch (so the stretches for the largest muscle groups, at the end of each routine, should be held the longest). For all muscle groups, progress from shorter to longer stretches (from 15 to 20 seconds, say) from one workout to the next. Another option is to progress from single to multiple repetitions of stretches: Instead of doing one 15-second stretch for a muscle, do two. Or combine the two strategies by increasing, over the course of several workouts, both the length of each repetition and the number of repetitions for each stretch.

The stretches should flow from one to the next so that each area you loosen makes it easier to stretch the next area targeted.

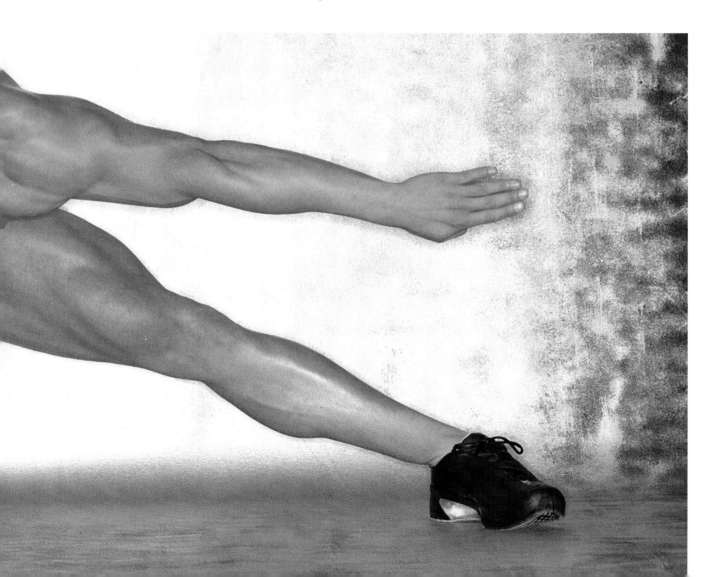

Before an upper-body workout, perform the following routine of six upper-body stretching sequences, holding each stretch for between 5 and 60 seconds.

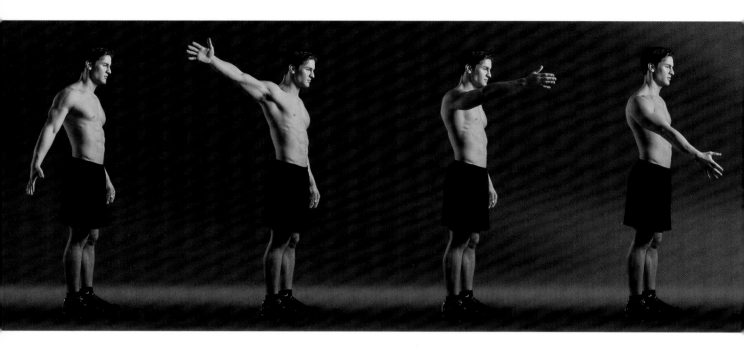

ARM SWING

Swing one arm in circles, from front to back, 10 times. Then swing from back to front 10 times. Repeat with the other arm. If you have arthritic shoulders, start slowly, with small circles, before progressing to a faster movement and bigger circles. Or just swing each arm across the front of your body; this is less stressful on your shoulder joint.

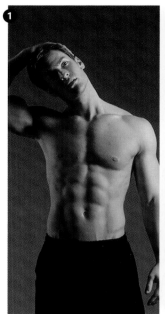
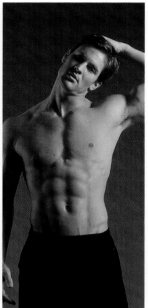
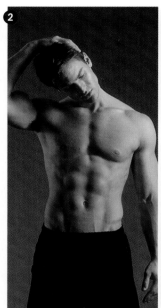
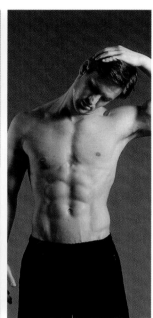

NECK STRETCHES

❶ While standing or kneeling, lower your head to the right, and use your right hand to gently pull your head a little closer toward your right shoulder. Then repeat to your left.

❷ A more aggressive stretch, hitting more of the upper trapezius, is to lower your right ear toward your chest, and then repeat with your left ear.

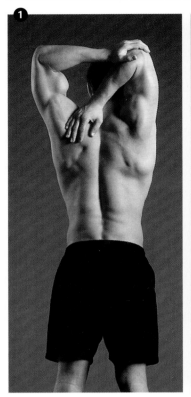
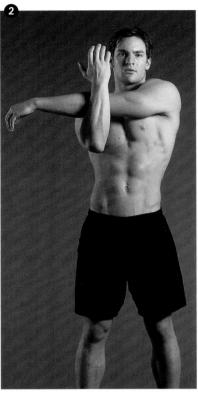

SHOULDER STRETCHES

❶ Lift your right arm up over your head, and with your left hand, gently push back on the right triceps, just above your right elbow. Repeat with your left arm. This stretches the triceps along with the shoulder.

❷ Pull your right arm across your chest, with your left hand pressing against your right triceps, just above your right elbow. Repeat with your left arm. This stretches your rear shoulders.

❸ **NOT PICTURED:** Place your right arm behind your back, your right hand reaching up toward your shoulders. Grab your right wrist with your left hand and gently pull it higher. Repeat with your left arm.

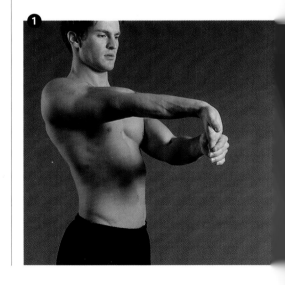

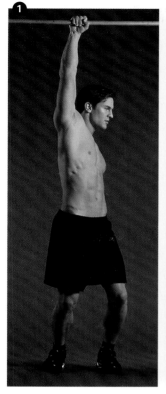

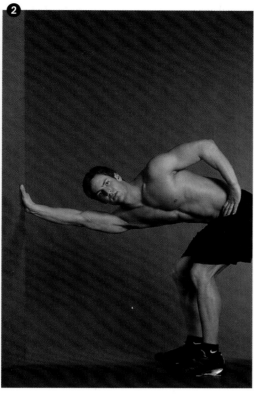

LAT STRETCHES

❶ Stand under a horizontal support such as a chinning bar, and hold it with your right arm (making sure that your feet touch the floor). Lower your body down and push your pelvis to the left to get a good stretch in your lats.

❷ Stand in front of a vertical support, grasp it with your right hand, and lean forward until your upper body is parallel to the floor. Rotate your hips to the left to stretch your lats and upper back.
  Repeat both stretches with your left arm.

FOREARM STRETCHES

Extend your right arm in front of your body, and perform the following three stretches.

❶ With your right palm facing up, use your left hand to pull down on the fingers of your right hand, stretching the forearm flexors.

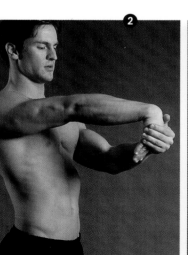

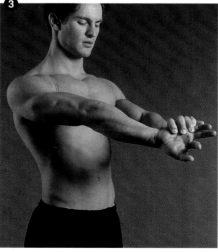

❷ With your right palm facing down, use your left hand to pull down on its fingers, stretching the forearm extensors.

❸ With your right palm facing down, rotate your hand outward, then down. Then use your left hand to push against the back of your right hand. As you push the fingers of your right hand around and up, you stretch your forearm rotators.
  Repeat all three stretches with your left arm.

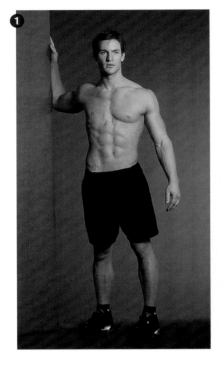

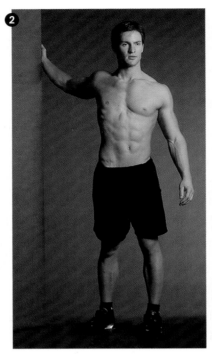

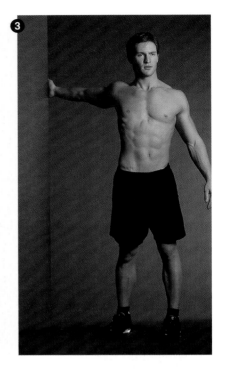

CHEST STRETCHES

Stand close to a wall, door frame, or other vertical support, with your right hand braced against it. Then assume the following four positions.

❶ With your right elbow bent to 90 degrees, your upper arm parallel to the floor, and your forearm in contact with the support, rotate your body to the left, providing a very isolated chest stretch.

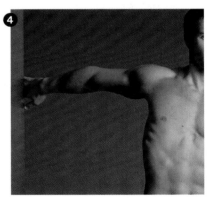

❷ Move a bit farther away from the support, and extend your right arm until the elbow is just bent. Your hand and/or wrist should in contact with the support, with your palm facing forward. Rotate your body to the left. This is a strong chest stretch that you'll also feel in your biceps.

❸ Move a little farther from the support again, and straighten your right arm completely. With your hand/wrist still in contact and your palm facing forward, rotate left. This is an even more intense stretch for your biceps and forearms flexors.

❹ Keeping your right arm straight, rotate your forearm so the back of your hand is against the support. Rotate your body to the left, feeling the stretch in your forearm extensors.

Repeat the four stretches with your left arm.

We recommend doing most of the lower-body stretches on a mat to protect your back and knees. You'll also need a towel, rope, or some other kind of strap for some of the stretches. Hold each stretch for between 15 and 90 seconds.

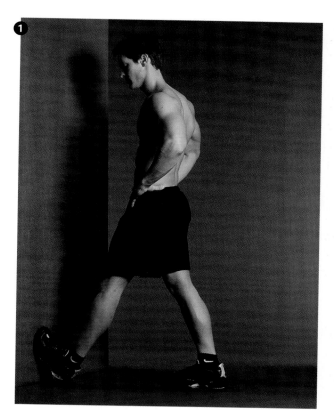 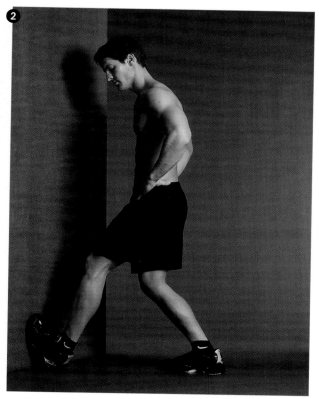

CALF STRETCHES

❶ Stand in front of a wall or another vertical support and place the ball of one foot on the wall keeping that heel in contact with the floor. This forward foot should be at about a 45-degree angle; your rear foot should be flat on the floor. Keeping your forward leg straight, move your hips toward the wall. You should feel this stretch in the middle of your forward calf.

❷ With your forward foot in the same 45-degree angle, bend that knee, lowering your other knee toward the floor if that helps you better feel the stretch. Move your forward knee toward the wall. You should feel this stretch down lower, toward your Achilles tendon and your heel.

Repeat both stretches with your other leg.

THE TWISTED TRUTH ABOUT FLEXIBILITY

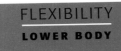
LOWER-BACK STRETCHES

Do all of these stretches while lying faceup on the floor. Do the second and third stretches only if your back is completely healthy and you've had no recent pain or injuries. For all of these positions, come out of the stretch slowly—don't snap back like a rubber band.

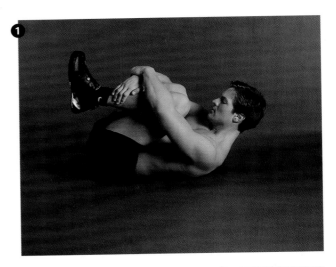

❶ Bring your knees to your chest, wrapping your arms around your lower legs to pull them close. Rock gently.

❷ Extend your legs straight up over your torso, then slowly lower them past your head as far as you can comfortably go. If you feel this more in your upper back or neck, opt for a limited range of motion.

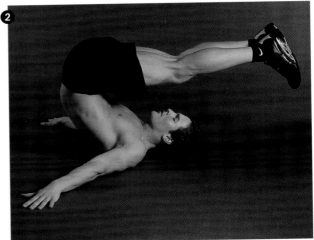

❸ Assuming you haven't experienced any back or neck pain from either of the previous two stretches, bend your knees and lower them toward the floor on either side of your ears. Again, be careful, and cut short the range of motion if you feel pain.

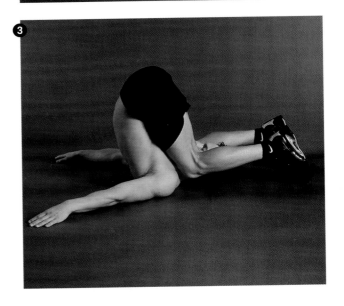

HAMSTRING STRETCHES

❶ Lie faceup on the floor, loop a towel or strap under your right foot like a stirrup, and hold the ends with your hands. Straighten your right leg and raise it as high as you can, gently tugging with the towel toward the end of the stretch to slightly increase the range of motion.

❷ Drop the towel, bend your right knee slightly, grab your ankle with your hands, and pull your right knee as close as you can to your chest.

❸ Wrap your left arm behind your right knee, and grab your right heel with your right hand. Pull your foot as close to your shoulders as you can.

Repeat all three stretches with your left leg.

Remember, these are all hamstring stretches; you shouldn't feel any discomfort at all in your lower back.

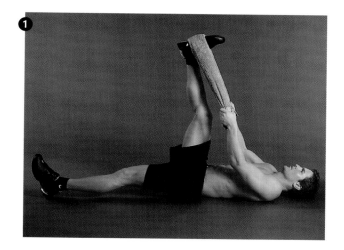

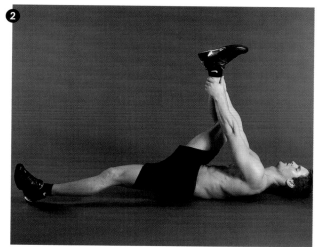

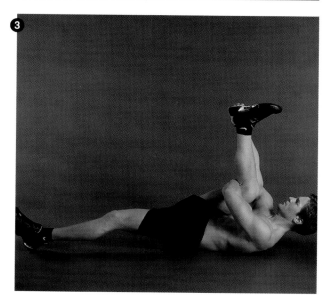

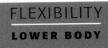

GLUTEAL STRETCHES

❶ Lie faceup on the floor, bend your right knee, and lift your right leg so its calf is across your torso. Push your right knee away with your right hand as you pull your right heel toward your head with your left hand.

❷ Set your right foot on the floor just outside your left hip, holding your right ankle with your left hand. Use your right hand to pull your right knee toward your left shoulder.

❸ Bend your left knee and lift it so your left thigh presses against your right ankle. (If your left leg were straight, your legs would form a backward figure 4.) Reach between your legs with your right hand (yes, we too thought of a bunch of stupid jokes the first time we heard this description) and pull your left lower leg toward your chest to produce the deepest possible stretch in your right glutes. (Your left hand can pull on your right foot.)

Repeat all three stretches with your left leg.

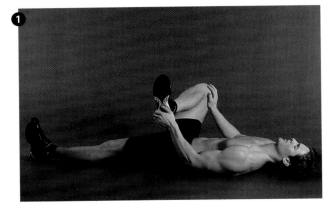

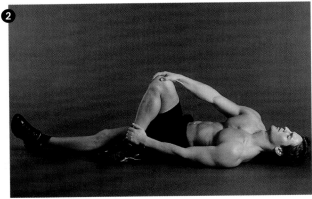

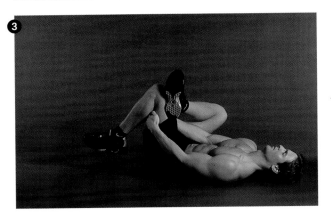

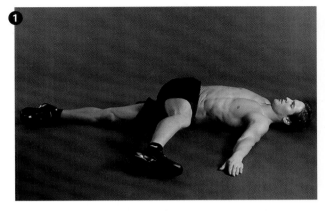

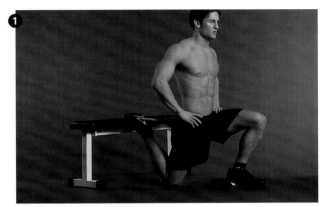

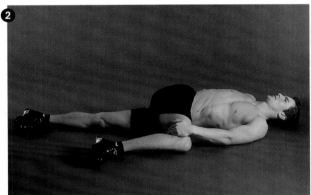

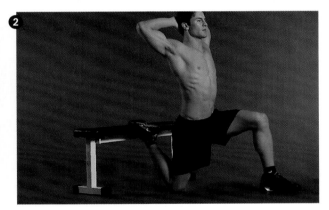

POSTERIOR-CHAIN STRETCHES

Your calves, hamstrings, gluteals, and lower back can work in isolation, but mostly they move as part of a chain. These two moves stretch all of them.

❶ Lie faceup on the floor. Lift your right leg straight up in the air, then lower it down over the left side of your body, keeping the leg straight. Your degree of flexibility will determine where the leg ends up. Over time, you want the leg to get closer to your head.

❷ Bend your right knee, and push it down toward the floor with your left hand.
  Repeat both stretches with your left leg.

HIP FLEXOR/ QUADRICEPS STRETCHES

❶ Kneel on the floor, facing away from a low bench or step, with your right foot on the bench and your left foot flat on the floor in front of you. Your right knee should be on the floor (preferably on a mat or rolled-up towel). Lower your butt toward your right heel. If this is easy, add a pelvic tilt: Pull the top of your pelvis in, or backward, and push the end of your pelvis forward.

❷ Set your left foot farther away from the bench, raise your chest up (try putting your hands on your head), and lower your pelvis down as low as it can go.
  Repeat both stretches with your left foot on the bench.

CHAPTER THIRTEEN

GETTING WARM— AND STAYING WARM

UNLIKE STRETCHING, THE CONCEPT OF WARMING UP is almost entirely without controversy. Just about any expert you talk to is in favor of a warmup of some sort, for both sports and exercise. Most of us instinctively "warm up" before just about anything we do. That's why you see so many guys in the office reading the paper and answering e-mail at 9 A.M., before burying themselves in more challenging tasks by 10 or 11.

Still, a "warmup" means something a little different to almost

grinding-down knee injuries that are common among serious athletes and exercisers.

Before upper-body workouts, we recommend little or no general warmup. Because upper-body muscles are smaller and easily warmed, the specific warmup sets for the individual exercises should suffice.

If you do both upper- and lower-body exercises in the same workout, we suggest a general warmup of at least 10 minutes.

WARMUPS THAT WORK YOU UP, WARMUPS THAT WEAR YOU DOWN

The science behind warmups is still thin, so most of our recommendations are based on experience and common sense. Still, this advice has worked for so many athletes for so long that it's hard to imagine that research could someday invalidate it. Here are the tried-and-true principles upon which we base the specific warmups in our workout programs.

A WARMUP SHOULD INCLUDE A REHEARSAL OF THE ACTUAL EVENT. It's not uncommon for a guy to do a general warmup, then walk right over to the bench-press station or squat rack and load the bar with close to maximal weights. In our view, this is like Barry Bonds's jogging for a quarter-hour before walking up to the plate for an official at-bat. A weight-lifting exercise is an athletic event, and all athletic events require some specific preparation. An athlete will never perform at his peak without first going through the specific motions of his event, whether it's batting, kicking, running, jumping, shooting, or bench-pressing.

THE EVENT SHOULD NOT IMMEDIATELY FOLLOW THE WARMUP. A warmup does deplete some energy from your muscles. For example, it takes your body about 8 minutes to rebuild most of its supply of phosphocreatine—its energy source for very short, near-maximum efforts, including heavy lifts—once that supply has been dented. We don't recommend a full 8-minute lapse between warmup and work sets, but taking it easy for a few minutes between the rehearsal and the event will certainly help.

THE WORKOUT SHOULD DICTATE THE WARMUP. If your workout includes mostly light work sets, you need little or no specific warmups. A light weight won't damage your muscles and joints, and the necessary skill level is low enough that you won't require a rehearsal.

Since the workout charts in part four tell you exactly how many warmup sets to do and how many repetitions to do in those warmup sets, the only question is how much weight to use in your warmup sets. Your warmup-set weight load should be a percentage of the weight you plan to use in your first work set of any given exercise. Here's a quick and easy guide.

# OF WARMUP SETS	% OF WT IN WORK-SET 1
1	60
2	Warmup-Set 1: 40
	Warmup-Set 2: 70
3	Warmup-Set 1: 30
	Warmup-Set 2: 60
	Warmup-Set 3: 80
4	Warmup-Set 1: 20
	Warmup-Set 2: 40
	Warmup-Set 3: 60
	Warmup-Set 4: 80
5	Warmup-Set 1: 10
	Warmup-Set 2: 30
	Warmup-Set 3: 50
	Warmup-Set 4: 70
	Warmup-Set 5: 90

Let's say you're going to do barbell bench presses, and you plan to use 185 pounds in the first work set. If the program calls for doing two warmup sets, you use 40 percent of 185 pounds (75 pounds) in the first one and 70 percent (130 pounds) in the second. Feel free to round up or down to use weights that are easy to combine on the bar. For example, you could go up to 135 pounds for the second warmup set (the bar plus a 45-pound plate on each side), which would be more convenient than stacking up a bunch of smaller plates to total exactly 130.

MODERATE-INTENSITY WARMUPS IMPROVE PERFORMANCE THE MOST. An interesting 1998 study in the *Journal of Orthopaedic Sports and Physical Therapy* (confess: you let your subscription lapse, didn't you?) found that running performance improved most when it was preceded by 15 minutes of jogging at 60 to 70 percent of the subjects' maximal aerobic power (VO_2 max). There was no difference between sprints that

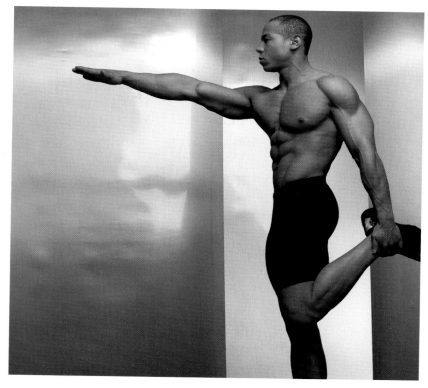

followed 15 minutes of warmup at 80 percent of VO_2 max and those that were done cold, with no warmup at all.

In other words, a warmup that's too intense is a waste of time.

A WARMUP SHOULD NEVER FATIGUE YOUR MUSCLES. This rule has two parts. First, you shouldn't reach muscular fatigue on the actual warmup sets—you should always put away the warmup weights knowing you could've done quite a few more repetitions, had that been your goal. Second (and this follows up on the earlier put-a-little-time-between-warmup-and-event rule), you shouldn't do your work set while still huffing and puffing from your warmups.

WARMUP SETS SHOULD MATCH YOUR GOALS. When you're focused on building muscle size, your workouts will usually have a higher volume of sets and repetitions. In that case, it's okay to do higher-volume warmups—with more repetitions, if not more sets. When you're trying to build pure strength or power, you want to keep everything possible in the tank for the heavy or fast work sets. Your warmups, therefore, will include few repetitions, even though by necessity you'll have to do more sets.

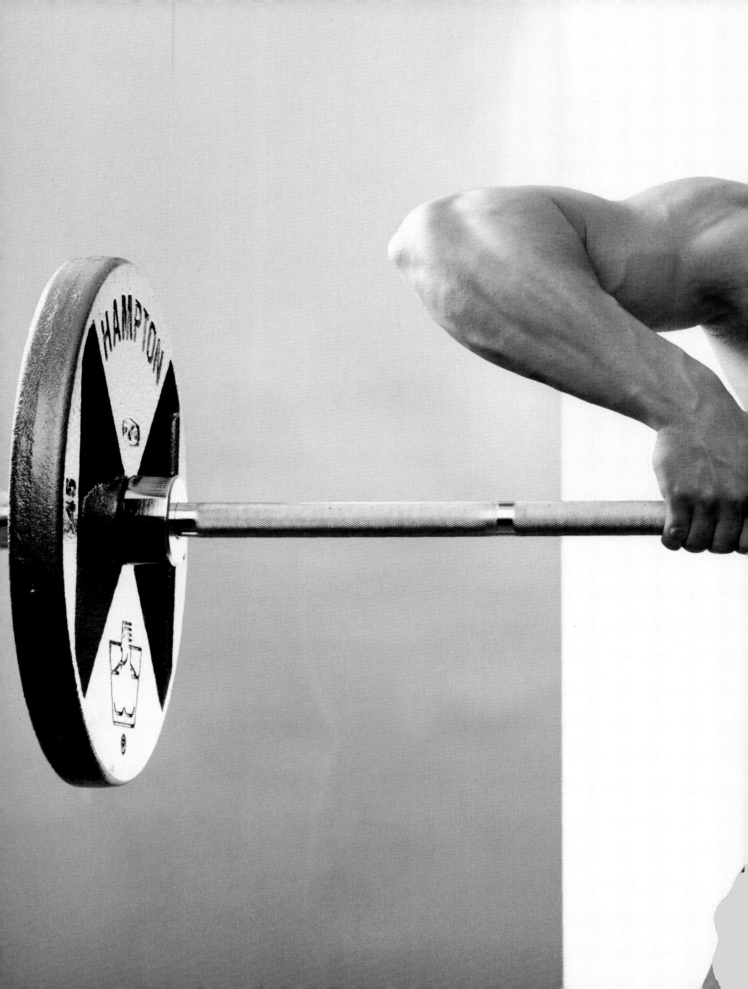

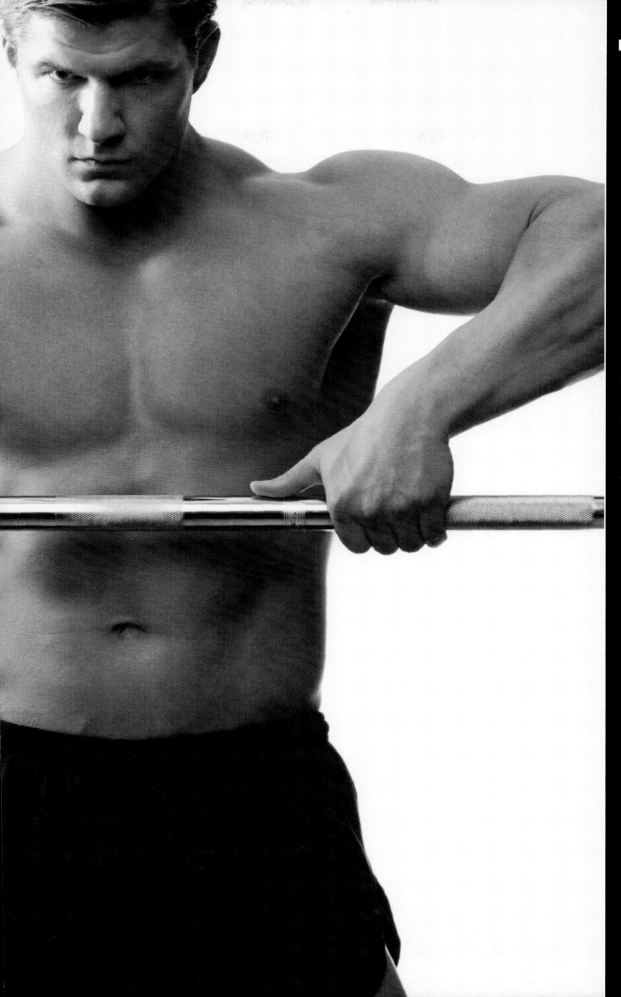

PART 4

THE WORKOUTS

CHAPTER FOURTEEN

THE BEGINNER PROGRAM

THIS 6-MONTH PROGRAM is designed for complete beginners, novices who've been training consistently for less than a year, and more experienced lifters who haven't worked out regularly in recent memory. It is divided into four stages.

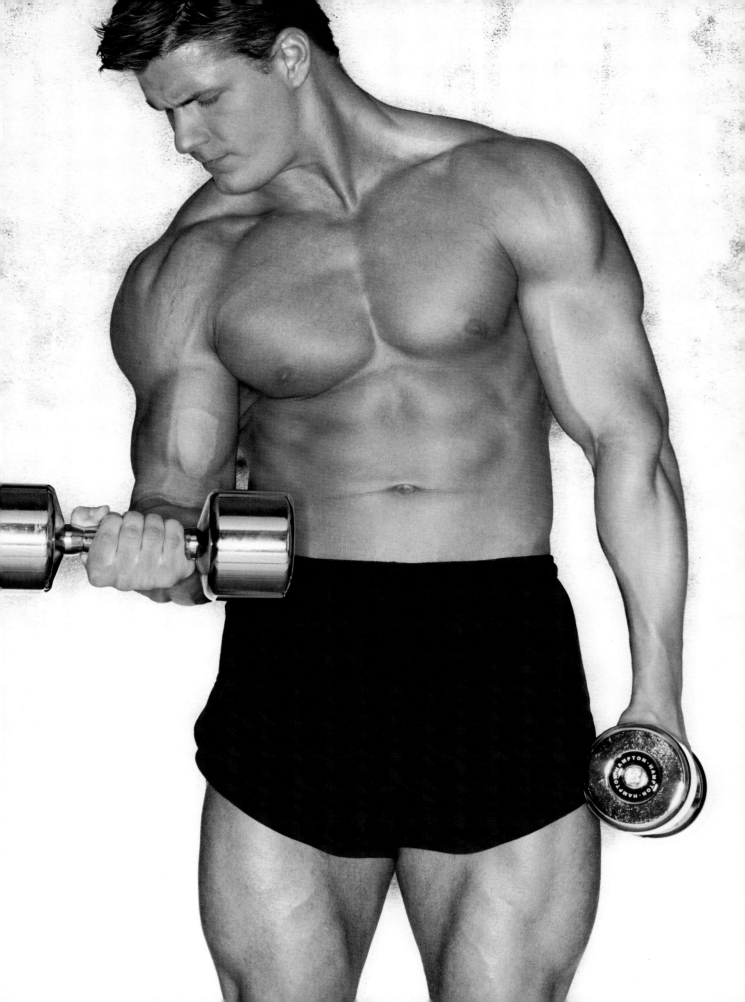

STAGE 1, WEEKS 1 THROUGH 3

This introductory workout is termed a **CIRCUIT ROUTINE** because it calls for you to do a set of each exercise with short rests in between sets. Once you've completed a full circuit of sets, you can either repeat the circuit or end your workout. (Note that the chart below represents a single circuit.)

WEEK 1: Perform one circuit.

WEEK 2: Perform one or two circuits.

WEEK 3: Perform two or three circuits.

When you do multiple circuits, you can rest for 2 to 3 minutes between them.

This is also a **TOTAL-BODY WORKOUT**, meaning it works all the major muscles in your body. Do this workout three times each week.

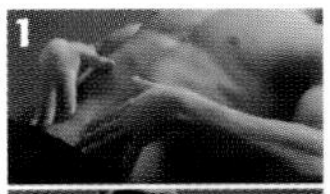

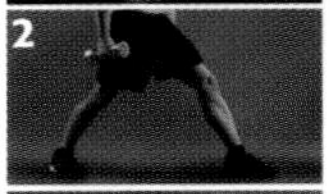

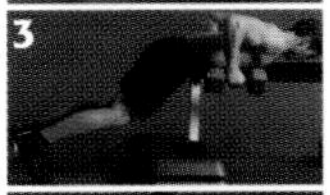

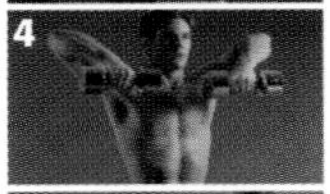

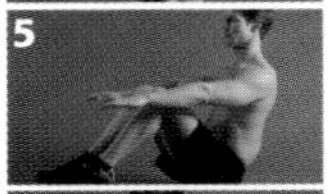

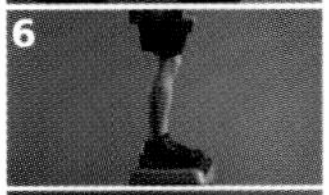

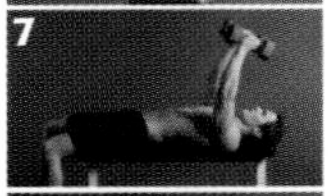

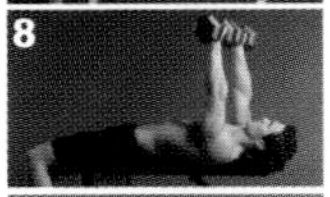

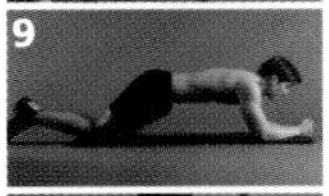

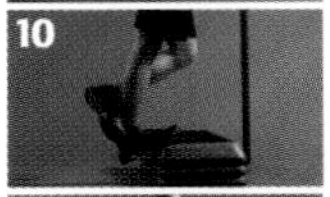

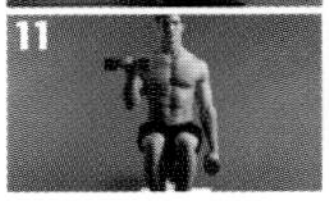

STAGE 1 WEEKS 1–3 EXERCISE	SETS	REPS	TEMPO	REST (SEC)
1 THIN TUMMY	1	15–20	5-sec holds	30
2 STATIC LUNGE	1	15–20	311	30
3 DUMBBELL LYING ROW	1	15–20	311	30
4 DUMBBELL UPRIGHT ROW	1	15–20	311	30
5 CURLUP, CHEAT UP + SLOW LOWER	1	15–20	311	30
6 DUMBBELL BENCH STEP	1	15–20	311	30
7 DUMBBELL LYING PULLOVER	1	15–20	311	30
8 DUMBBELL BENCH PRESS	1	15–20	311	30
9 PUSHUP HOLD	1	15–20	311	30
10 STANDING SINGLE-LEG CALF RAISE	1	15–20	311	30
11 DUMBBELL SEATED HAMMER CURL WITH TWIST, ALTERNATING	1	15–20	311	30
12 DUMBBELL TRICEPS KICKBACK	1	15–20	311	30

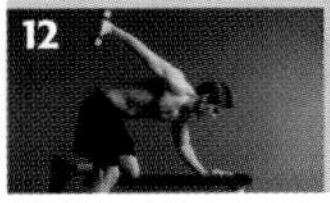

STAGE 1, WEEKS 4 THROUGH 6

This workout uses a variation on the circuit routine. The 12 exercises are divided into three **MINI-CIRCUITS**. Do four of the exercises in a mini-circuit, then either repeat those exercises or move on to the next mini-circuit.

You'll notice some other differences from the previous 3-week workout. Here you work with heavier weights for 10 to 15 repetitions per set, rather than 15 to 20 reps. You rest longer between exercises: 60 seconds instead of 30. And on one exercise—the curlup—you do an exaggeratedly slow movement, taking 5 seconds to raise yourself and another 5 seconds to lower yourself, with a 1-second pause between the two parts of the exercise.

Always rest for 1 to 2 minutes after completing each four-exercise mini-circuit, regardless of whether you repeat that mini-circuit or move on to the next.

In each of the three mini-circuits, the exercises and their respective reps, tempos, and rests remain the same throughout weeks 4, 5, and 6. What changes from week to week is the number of sets per exercise. Here's how many sets you'll do of each exercise.

WEEK 4: Perform one set of each exercise.

WEEK 5: Perform one or two sets of each exercise.

WEEK 6: Perform two or three sets of each exercise.

The number of times you do each mini-circuit also changes from week to week.

WEEK 4: Perform each mini-circuit once.

WEEK 5: Perform each mini-circuit one or two times.

WEEK 6: Perform each mini-circuit two or three times.

Important: When you do a mini-circuit multiple times, repeat each mini-circuit so you finish with it before moving on to the next.

Perform the entire workout three times each week.

We're assuming you'll use our default schedule for recovery weeks and take a week of active rest after each 6-week stage of the program. So after you finish your third workout in week 6, lay off the weights in week 7 before beginning stage 2, week 8.

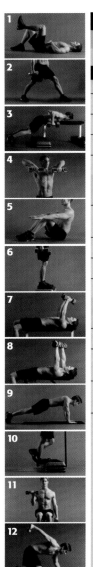

STAGE 1
WEEKS 4–6
MINI-CIRCUIT 1

EXERCISE	SETS			REPS	TEMPO	REST (SEC)
	WEEK 4	WEEK 5	WEEK 6			
1 THIN TUMMY, LIFT ONE LEG	1	1 or 2	2 or 3	10–15	313	60
2 STATIC LUNGE	1	1 or 2	2 or 3	10–15	311	60
3 DUMBBELL LYING ROW	1	1 or 2	2 or 3	10–15	311	60
4 DUMBBELL UPRIGHT ROW	1	1 or 2	2 or 3	10–15	311	60

MINI-CIRCUIT 2

	WEEK 4	WEEK 5	WEEK 6			
5 CURLUP, ARMS STRAIGHT & PARALLEL TO FLOOR	1	1 or 2	2 or 3	10–15	515	60
6 DUMBBELL BENCH STEP	1	1 or 2	2 or 3	10–15	311	60
7 DUMBBELL LYING PULLOVER	1	1 or 2	2 or 3	10–15	311	60
8 DUMBBELL BENCH PRESS	1	1 or 2	2 or 3	10–15	311	60–120

MINI-CIRCUIT 3

	WEEK 4	WEEK 5	WEEK 6			
9 PUSHUP HOLD, HANDS & FEET	1	1 or 2	2 or 3	10–15	311	60
10 STANDING SINGLE-LEG CALF RAISE	1	1 or 2	2 or 3	10–15	311	60
11 DUMBBELL SEATED HAMMER CURL WITH TWIST, ALTERNATING	1	1 or 2	2 or 3	10–15	311	60
12 DUMBBELL TRICEPS KICKBACK	1	1 or 2	2 or 3	10–15	311	60–120

STAGE 2: WEEKS 8 THROUGH 10

At this point, you're past the anatomical-adaptation stage, so here's a more challenging program. The exercises are split into two programs, A and B, that you alternate between.

Workout A contains mostly lower-body exercises, with two exercises for your trapezius at the end. It's no accident that trapezius exercises are included with leg movements. The traps and lower-body muscles work together in hip-dominant movements, such as the deadlift. Since the deadlift is one of the most important exercises for getting bigger and stronger, your mastery of it begins here, with hip-dominant and trap-building exercises combined in the same workout.

Workout B is full of upper-body exercises, including specialized exercises for potential weak links, such as your forearms and rear shoulders.

Abdominal exercises are included in both workouts. Your abdominals will get 20 to 25 percent of your attention in this stage, and you'll work them first in each session.

You can do workout A and workout B four or five times each. It's up to you. If you choose to do each five times, the program will extend into Monday of week 11 of the beginner program; that's when you'll do workout B for the fifth and final time. If you choose to do each four times, you'll finish on Wednesday of week 10. With either option, you can either take the remainder of the final week as a recovery week or go straight into workout A of the program for stage 2's weeks 11 through 13.

Another new feature introduced in this program is that once you get past the abdominal exercises in each workout, you do the exercises as **SUPERSETS**. That means you do pairs of two exercises without resting within each pair. You do rest for 1 to 2 minutes before moving from one superset to another.

These workouts are also arranged as circuits. You progress from one to two to three circuits based on the following parameters.

FIRST TIME YOU DO EACH WORKOUT: Perform one circuit.

SECOND AND THIRD TIMES YOU DO EACH WORKOUT: Perform one or two circuits.

FOURTH AND (OPTIONAL) FIFTH TIMES YOU DO EACH WORKOUT: Perform two or three circuits.

STAGE 2
WEEKS 8–10
WORKOUT A

EXERCISE	SETS	REPS	TEMPO	REST (SEC)
1 THIN TUMMY, LIFT ONE LEG	1	10	313	30
2 CURLUP, ARMS STRAIGHT & PARALLEL TO FLOOR	1	10–20	311	30
3 SIDE RAISE	1	10–15	212	30
4 SEATED THIN TUMMY + CHEEK SQUEEZE	1	10	5-sec holds	60–120
SUPERSET 1				
5 KING DEADLIFT	1	Max	311	0
6 SINGLE-LEG SQUAT, OTHER LEG OUT IN FRONT	1	Max	311	60–120
SUPERSET 2				
7 PRONE HIP-THIGH EXTENSION	1	12–15	311	0
8 STATIC LUNGE, BACK FOOT ON LOW BLOCK	1	12–15	311	60–120
SUPERSET 3				
9 SINGLE-LEG STIFF-LEGGED DEADLIFT	1	Max	311	0
10 SINGLE-LEG SQUAT, ON LOW BLOCK	1	Max	311	60–120
SUPERSET 4				
11 LEG CURL	1	12–15	311	0
12 LEG EXTENSION	1	12–15	311	60–120
SUPERSET 5				
13 SEATED CALF RAISE	1	15–20	311	0
14 STANDING SINGLE-LEG CALF RAISE	1	15–20	311	60–120
SUPERSET 6				
15 DUMBBELL SHRUG, BEHIND BODY	1	12–15	311	0
16 DUMBBELL SHRUG, TO FRONT	1	12–15	311	60–120

STAGE 2
WEEKS 8–10
WORKOUT B

EXERCISE	SETS	REPS	TEMPO	REST (SEC)
1 TOES TO SKY	1	10	313	30
2 CURLUP, LEGS IN AIR, HANDS ON OPPOSITE SHOULDERS, ARMS ACROSS CHEST	1	10–15	311	30
3 LATERAL LEG LOWERING	1	10–15	212	30
4 PUSHUP HOLD, LIFT LEG, THEN ARM	1	10	5-sec holds	60–120
SUPERSET 1				
5 SEATED CABLE ROW	1	12–15	311	0
6 BARBELL BENCH PRESS, FEET ON BENCH	1	12–15	311	60–120
SUPERSET 2				
7 REVERSE DUMBELL FLY	1	12–15	311	0
8 DUMBBELL FLY	1	12–15	311	60–120
SUPERSET 3				
9 LAT PULLDOWN	1	12–15	311	0
10 BARBELL SEATED SHOULDER PRESS, TO FRONT	1	12–15	311	60–120
SUPERSET 4				
11 DUMBBELL LYING PULLOVER, 1 DUMBBELL IN 2 HANDS	1	12–15	311	0
12 DUMBBELL SEATED LATERAL RAISE	1	12–15	311	60–120
SUPERSET 5				
13 DUMBBELL SEATED BICEPS CURL, INCLINE	1	15–20	311	0
14 DUMBBELL SEATED OVERHEAD TRICEPS EXTENSION, 1 DUMBBELL IN 1 HAND	1	15–20	311	60–120
SUPERSET 6				
15 DUMBELL WRIST CURL	1	15–20	311	0
16 DUMBELL WRIST EXTENSION	1	15–20	311	60–120

STAGE 2: WEEKS 11 THROUGH 13

Continue with the A-B-A, B-A-B split routine. Once again, you can decide on your own whether to do each workout four times or five. (Just make sure you do A and B an equal number of times.) Note that the order of exercises has changed, and some of the repetitions are different. This challenges your muscles in new ways and, on the lower-rep sets, allows you to work with heavier weights.

The number of times you perform each circuit remains the same.

FIRST TIME YOU DO EACH WORKOUT: Perform one circuit.

SECOND AND THIRD TIMES YOU DO EACH WORKOUT: Perform one or two circuits.

FOURTH AND (OPTIONAL) FIFTH TIMES YOU DO EACH WORKOUT: Perform two or three circuits.

STAGE 2
WEEKS 11–13
WORKOUT A

EXERCISE	SETS	REPS	TEMPO	REST (SEC)
1 THIN TUMMY, LIFT AND CYCLE OUT ONE LEG	1	10	313	30
2 CURLUP, ARMS STRAIGHT & PARALLEL TO FLOOR	1	10–20	311	30
3 SIDE RAISE, HANDS ON FOREHEAD, ELBOWS IN	1	10–15	212	30
4 SEATED THIN TUMMY + CHEEK SQUEEZE	1	10	5-sec holds	60–120
SUPERSET 1				
5 PRONE HIP-THIGH EXTENSION	1	12–15	311	0
6 KING DEADLIFT	1	Max	311	60–120
SUPERSET 2				
7 STATIC LUNGE, BACK FOOT ON LOW BLOCK	1	12–15	311	0
8 SINGLE-LEG SQUAT, OTHER LEG OUT IN FRONT	1	Max	311	60–120
SUPERSET 3				
9 LEG CURL	1	12–15	311	0
10 SINGLE-LEG STIFF-LEGGED DEADLIFT	1	Max	311	60–120
SUPERSET 4				
11 LEG EXTENSION	1	12–15	311	0
12 SINGLE-LEG SQUAT, ON LOW BLOCK	1	Max	311	60–120
SUPERSET 5				
13 STANDING SINGLE-LEG CALF RAISE	1	15–20	311	0
14 SEATED CALF RAISE	1	15–20	311	60–120
SUPERSET 6				
15 DUMBBELL SHRUG, TO FRONT	1	12–15	311	0
16 DUMBBELL SHRUG, BEHIND BODY	1	12–15	311	60–120

STAGE 2
WEEKS 11–13
WORKOUT B

EXERCISE	SETS	REPS	TEMPO	REST (SEC)
1 TOES TO SKY, ONE KNEE BENT	1	10	313 or 5-sec hold	30
2 CURLUP, LEGS IN AIR, ARMS VERTICAL TOWARD TOES	1	10–15	311	30
3 LATERAL LEG LOWERING	1	10–15	212	30
4 PUSHUP HOLD, LIFT LEG WITH OPPOSITE ARM	1	10	5-sec holds	60–120
SUPERSET 1				
5 REVERSE DUMBELL FLY	1	12–15	311	0
6 SEATED CABLE ROW	1	10–12	311	60–120
SUPERSET 2				
7 DUMBBELL FLY	1	12–15	311	0
8 BARBELL BENCH PRESS, FEET ON BENCH	1	10–12	311	60–120
SUPERSET 3				
9 DUMBBELL LYING PULLOVER, 1 DUMBBELL IN 2 HANDS	1	12–15	311	0
10 LAT PULLDOWN	1	10–12	311	60–120
SUPERSET 4				
11 DUMBBELL SEATED LATERAL RAISE	1	12–15	311	0
12 BARBELL SEATED SHOULDER PRESS, TO FRONT	1	10–12	311	60–120
SUPERSET 5				
13 DUMBBELL WRIST CURL	1	12–15	311	0
14 DUMBBELL SEATED BICEPS CURL, INCLINE	1	10–12	311	60–120
SUPERSET 6				
15 DUMBBELL WRIST EXTENSION	1	12–15	311	0
16 DUMBBELL SEATED OVERHEAD TRICEPS EXTENSION, 1 DUMBBELL IN 1 HAND	1	10–12	311	60–120

STAGE 3, WEEKS 15 THROUGH 17

Now you do fewer exercises—10 instead of 16—with fewer repetitions and heavier weights. Because of those heavier weights—and longer rest periods between sets and exercises—you divide your workout into WARMUP and WORK sets. The nomenclature is easy enough to figure out: A warmup set prepares your muscles and connective tissues for the work sets; the work sets use weights heavy enough to increase your strength and muscle mass. In this part of the program, do a single warmup set of 12 repetitions of each exercise (the ab exercises are excepted), using about 60 percent of the weight you plan to use in your work sets. (Realistically, anything from one-half to two-thirds of your first-set weight will work.) Then rest for 30 to 60 seconds before doing your first (or perhaps only) work set. You decide whether to do one work set per exercise or two. If you're pressed for time or energy on a given day, stick to one. When you feel ready for a more challenging workout, do two sets of each upper- or lower-body exercise.

For the ab exercises in workout A and for all of workout B, do **STRAIGHT SETS**, the system that most of us consider "real" strength training: Do all of your sets of one exercise before you move on to the next exercise.

In workout A, once you finish the ab exercises, you do the upper-body exercises as **ALTERNATED SETS, WITH FULL RECOVERIES BETWEEN SETS**. This means you do them much like supersets in that you do a set of the first exercise followed by a set of the second exercise, alternating between the two until you've completed the prescribed number of sets for both. Unlike in supersets, between sets you should rest for as long as it takes to get your breathing and heart rate back to normal.

In workout B, note the explosive-tempo designation of 10* for the dynamic lunge. This indicates that you should take 1 second to lunge and then, without pausing, push back up as quickly as possible.

Once again, do A-B-A, B-A-B split routines, completing each workout four or five times.

STAGE 3
WEEKS 15–17
WORKOUT A

EXERCISE	WARMUP		WORK		TEMPO	REST (SEC)
	SETS	REPS	SETS	REPS		
STRAIGHT SETS						
1 THIN TUMMY, LIFT AND CYCLE OUT ONE LEG	0	0	1	10	313	30
2 CURLUP, HANDS ON OPPOSITE ELBOWS (NOT PICTURED)	0	0	1	10–15	311	30
3 SIDE RAISE, HANDS ON FOREHEAD, ELBOWS OUT	0	0	1	10–15	212	30
4 SWISS-BALL ALTERNATE-LEG LIFT	0	0	1	10 (each leg)	5-sec holds	60–120
ALTERNATED, WITH FULL RECOVERIES BETWEEN SETS						
5 SEATED CABLE ROW	1	12	1 or 2	10–12	321	Full recovery
6 BARBELL BENCH PRESS, FEET ON BENCH	1	12	1 or 2	10–12	321	Full recovery
ALTERNATED, WITH FULL RECOVERIES BETWEEN SETS						
7 LAT PULLDOWN, BEHIND NECK	1	12	1 or 2	10–12	321	Full recovery
8 BARBELL SEATED SHOULDER PRESS	1	12	1 or 2	10–12	321	Full recovery
ALTERNATED, WITH FULL RECOVERIES BETWEEN SETS						
9 EZ-BAR BICEPS CURL, REVERSE GRIP	1	12	1 or 2	10–12	321	Full recovery
10 EZ-BAR LYING TRICEPS EXTENSION	1	12	1 or 2	10–12	321	Full recovery

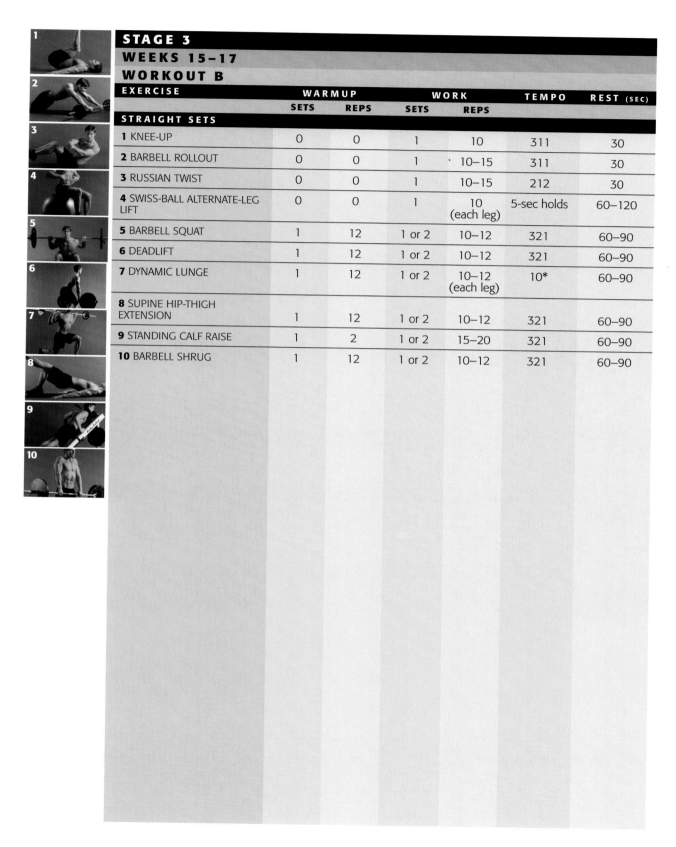

STAGE 3
WEEKS 15–17
WORKOUT B

EXERCISE	WARMUP		WORK		TEMPO	REST (SEC)
	SETS	REPS	SETS	REPS		
STRAIGHT SETS						
1 KNEE-UP	0	0	1	10	311	30
2 BARBELL ROLLOUT	0	0	1	10–15	311	30
3 RUSSIAN TWIST	0	0	1	10–15	212	30
4 SWISS-BALL ALTERNATE-LEG LIFT	0	0	1	10 (each leg)	5-sec holds	60–120
5 BARBELL SQUAT	1	12	1 or 2	10–12	321	60–90
6 DEADLIFT	1	12	1 or 2	10–12	321	60–90
7 DYNAMIC LUNGE	1	12	1 or 2	10–12 (each leg)	10*	60–90
8 SUPINE HIP-THIGH EXTENSION	1	12	1 or 2	10–12	321	60–90
9 STANDING CALF RAISE	1	2	1 or 2	15–20	321	60–90
10 BARBELL SHRUG	1	12	1 or 2	10–12	321	60–90

STAGE 3, WEEKS 18 THROUGH 20

The changes here are subtle: some new, more-challenging variations on the abdominal exercises; fewer repetitions on the lifts, which means lifting heavier weights; and a slightly faster tempo (311, instead of 321) on most exercises.

STAGE 3 WEEKS 18–20 WORKOUT A						
EXERCISE	WARMUP		WORK		TEMPO	REST (SEC)
	SETS	REPS	SETS	REPS		
STRAIGHT SETS						
1 THIN TUMMY, BOTH LEGS UP, CYCLE OUT ONE LEG	0	0	1	10	313	30
2 CURLUP, HANDS ON OPPOSITE ELBOWS + TWIST (NOT PICTURED)	0	0	1	10–15	311	30
3 SIDE RAISE, ON ROMAN CHAIR	0	0	1	10–15	212	30
4 SWISS BALL ALTERNATE LEG LIFT, LYING	0	0	1	10 (each leg)	5-sec holds	30
ALTERNATED, WITH FULL RECOVERIES BETWEEN SETS						
5 SEATED CABLE ROW	1	10	1 or 2	8–10	311	Full recovery
6 BARBELL BENCH PRESS	1	10	1 or 2	8–10	311	Full recovery
ALTERNATED, WITH FULL RECOVERIES BETWEEN SETS						
7 LAT PULLDOWN, BEHIND NECK	1	10	1 or 2	8–10	311	Full recovery
8 BARBELL SEATED SHOULDER PRESS	1	10	1 or 2	8–10	311	Full recovery
ALTERNATED, WITH FULL RECOVERIES BETWEEN SETS						
9 EZ-BAR BICEPS CURL, REVERSE GRIP	1	10	1 or 2	8–10	311	Full recovery
10 EZ-BAR LYING TRICEPS EXTENSION	1	10	1 or 2	8–10	311	Full recovery

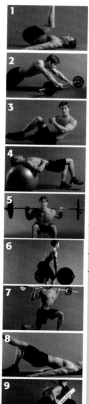

STAGE 3
WEEKS 18–20
WORKOUT B

EXERCISE	WARMUP		WORK		TEMPO	REST (SEC)
	SETS	REPS	SETS	REPS		
1 KNEE-UP	0	0	1	10	311	30
2 BARBELL ROLLOUT	0	0	1	10–15	311	30
3 RUSSIAN TWIST, LEG CYCLE	0	0	1	10–15	212	30
4 SWISS-BALL ALTERNATE-LEG LIFT, LYING	0	0	1	10 (each leg)	5-sec holds	60–120
5 BARBELL SQUAT	1	10	1 or 2	8–10	311	90–120
6 DEADLIFT	1	10	1 or 2	8–10	311	90–120
7 DYNAMIC LUNGE	1	10	1 or 2	8–10	311	90–120
8 SUPINE HIP-THIGH EXTENSION	1	10	1 or 2	8–10	311	90–120
9 STANDING CALF RAISE	1	10	1 or 2	12–15	321	60–90
10 BARBELL SHRUG	1	10	1 or 2	8–10	321	60–90

STAGE 4, WEEKS 22 THROUGH 24

If the straight sets in stage 3 could be called "real" weight lifting, stage 4 is *really* real weight lifting. It features not only heavy weights but also three distinct workouts (designated A, B, and C) a week, rather than the A-B-A, B-A-B split routine.

In workout A, you do what many gym rats consider their favorite exercises: the barbell bench press (horizontal push) and seated cable row (horizontal pull). Workout B is your lower-body routine, with squats and deadlifts. Workout C is your vanity program, hitting your lats (vertical pull), delts (vertical push), and arms.

You start right off by performing three work sets of each of the first two exercises, with heavier weights and fewer repetitions. Take, for instance, the barbell bench press. Your warmup might be 10 repetitions with the 45-pound Olympic barbell. Then your three work sets might be 75 pounds for 10 reps, 85 for 8, and 95 for 6. You say you're stronger than that? Okay, you might warm up with 85 pounds for 10, then work with 135 for 10 reps, 155 for 8, and 175 for 6.

As for the subsequent exercises in each workout, you do just one work set for each nonabdominal move. This remains fixed throughout weeks 22 through 24.

So the overall volume of each workout is low. You do just 10 work sets (and 6 warmup sets) of the six nonabdominal exercises.

The abdominal exercises are also a little different this time around. You still work your abs with four exercises each workout, but this time the ab moves come at the end of the workouts. And you do them as a circuit, with no rest between exercises. You have the option of doing the circuit twice. If you choose to do a second circuit, rest for 60 to 120 seconds before starting it.

Because the aim of this stage is to help you develop maximum power and strength, you perform explosive exercises. Workout B features explosive calf raises and shrugs. Note the tempo designation for each: 10* for the calf raises and 20* for the shrugs. Those tempos mean that you should take 1 or 2 seconds to lower the weight, don't pause, and then lift as quickly and explosively as possible. This isn't a call to get sloppy and sling weights around. Your form still has to be perfect. Just be perfect and fast.

There's no ambiguity about how many times to do each workout: In 3 weeks, perform workouts A, B, and C three times each.

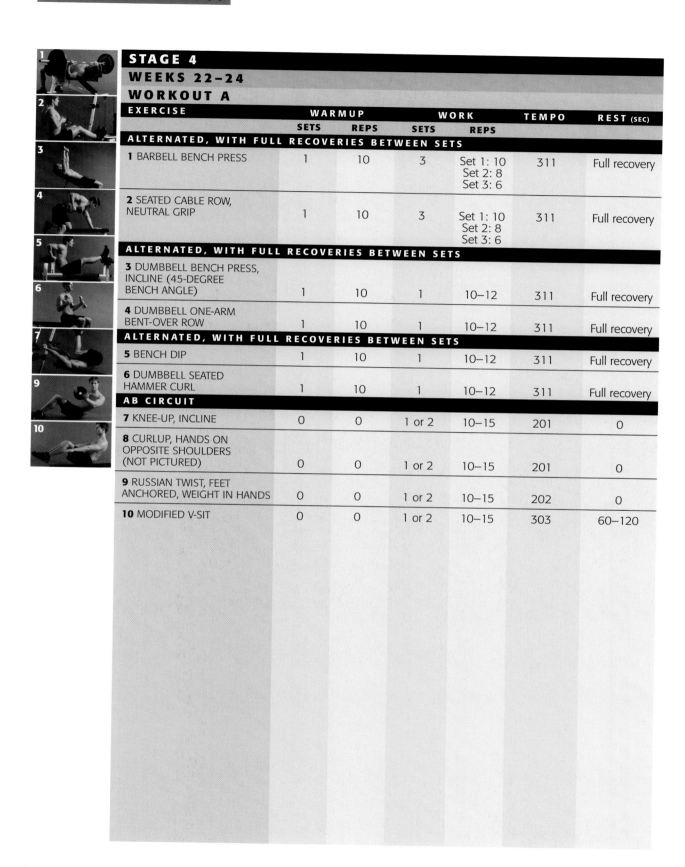

STAGE 4
WEEKS 22–24
WORKOUT A

EXERCISE	WARMUP		WORK		TEMPO	REST (SEC)
	SETS	REPS	SETS	REPS		
ALTERNATED, WITH FULL RECOVERIES BETWEEN SETS						
1 BARBELL BENCH PRESS	1	10	3	Set 1: 10 Set 2: 8 Set 3: 6	311	Full recovery
2 SEATED CABLE ROW, NEUTRAL GRIP	1	10	3	Set 1: 10 Set 2: 8 Set 3: 6	311	Full recovery
ALTERNATED, WITH FULL RECOVERIES BETWEEN SETS						
3 DUMBBELL BENCH PRESS, INCLINE (45-DEGREE BENCH ANGLE)	1	10	1	10–12	311	Full recovery
4 DUMBBELL ONE-ARM BENT-OVER ROW	1	10	1	10–12	311	Full recovery
ALTERNATED, WITH FULL RECOVERIES BETWEEN SETS						
5 BENCH DIP	1	10	1	10–12	311	Full recovery
6 DUMBBELL SEATED HAMMER CURL	1	10	1	10–12	311	Full recovery
AB CIRCUIT						
7 KNEE-UP, INCLINE	0	0	1 or 2	10–15	201	0
8 CURLUP, HANDS ON OPPOSITE SHOULDERS (NOT PICTURED)	0	0	1 or 2	10–15	201	0
9 RUSSIAN TWIST, FEET ANCHORED, WEIGHT IN HANDS	0	0	1 or 2	10–15	202	0
10 MODIFIED V-SIT	0	0	1 or 2	10–15	303	60–120

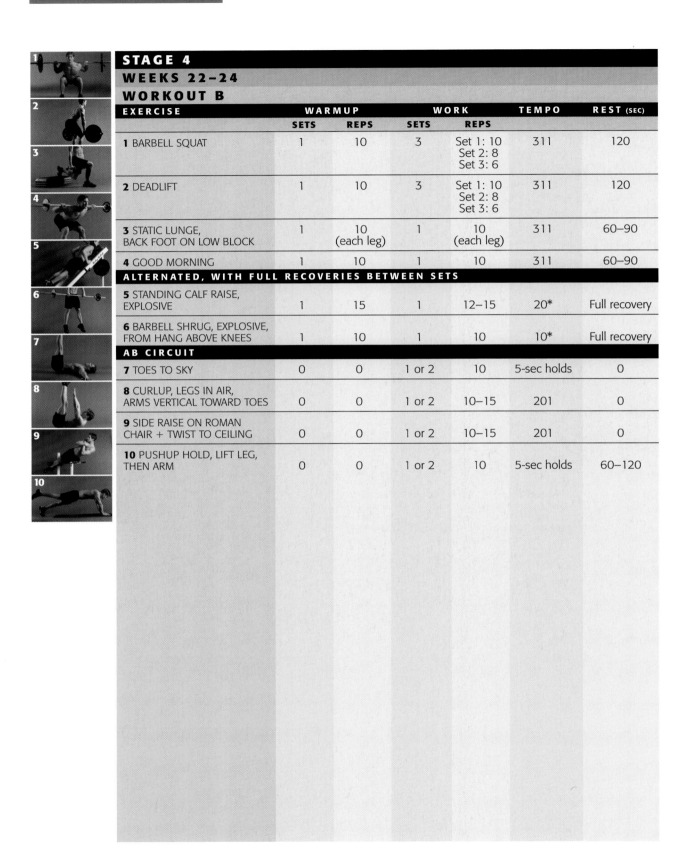

STAGE 4
WEEKS 22–24
WORKOUT B

EXERCISE	WARMUP		WORK		TEMPO	REST (SEC)
	SETS	REPS	SETS	REPS		
1 BARBELL SQUAT	1	10	3	Set 1: 10 Set 2: 8 Set 3: 6	311	120
2 DEADLIFT	1	10	3	Set 1: 10 Set 2: 8 Set 3: 6	311	120
3 STATIC LUNGE, BACK FOOT ON LOW BLOCK	1	10 (each leg)	1	10 (each leg)	311	60–90
4 GOOD MORNING	1	10	1	10	311	60–90
ALTERNATED, WITH FULL RECOVERIES BETWEEN SETS						
5 STANDING CALF RAISE, EXPLOSIVE	1	15	1	12–15	20*	Full recovery
6 BARBELL SHRUG, EXPLOSIVE, FROM HANG ABOVE KNEES	1	10	1	10	10*	Full recovery
AB CIRCUIT						
7 TOES TO SKY	0	0	1 or 2	10	5-sec holds	0
8 CURLUP, LEGS IN AIR, ARMS VERTICAL TOWARD TOES	0	0	1 or 2	10–15	201	0
9 SIDE RAISE ON ROMAN CHAIR + TWIST TO CEILING	0	0	1 or 2	10–15	201	0
10 PUSHUP HOLD, LIFT LEG, THEN ARM	0	0	1 or 2	10	5-sec holds	60–120

STAGE 4
WEEKS 22–24
WORKOUT C

EXERCISE	WARMUP		WORK		TEMPO	REST (SEC)
	SETS	REPS	SETS	REPS		
ALTERNATED, WITH FULL RECOVERIES BETWEEN SETS						
1 LAT PULLDOWN, REVERSE GRIP	1	10	3	Set 1: 10 Set 2: 8 Set 3: 6	311	Full recovery
2 BARBELL SEATED SHOULDER PRESS	1	10	3	Set 1: 10 Set 2: 8 Set 3: 6	311	Full recovery
ALTERNATED, WITH FULL RECOVERIES BETWEEN SETS						
3 DUMBBELL LYING PULLOVER, 1 DUMBBELL IN 2 HANDS	1	10	1	10–12	311	Full recovery
4 DUMBBELL SEATED LATERAL RAISE	1	10	1	10–12	311	Full recovery
ALTERNATED, WITH FULL RECOVERIES BETWEEN SETS						
5 EZ-BAR BICEPS CURL	1	12	1	10–12	311	Full recovery
6 TRICEPS PUSHDOWN	1	10	1	10–12	311	Full recovery
AB CIRCUIT						
7 KNEE-UP, INCLINE	0	0	1 or 2	10–15	201	0
8 CURLUP, ARMS STRAIGHT & PARALLEL TO FLOOR + TWIST (NOT PICTURED)	0	0	1 or 2	10–15	201	0
9 RUSSIAN TWIST, FEET ANCHORED, WEIGHT IN HANDS	0	0	1 or 2	10–15	202	0
10 MODIFIED V-SIT	0	0	1 or 2	10–15	303	60–120

STAGE 4, WEEKS 25 THROUGH 27

The big switch here is that you do another new, even more challenging muscle-building technique. For the first two exercises in each workout, instead of progressing from moderate weights and moderate reps to heavy weights and low reps, do the opposite: Start with two warmup sets, then work with your heaviest weight in the first work set. In subsequent work sets, use progressively lighter weights and higher reps.

Even before you begin, give yourself a pat on the back. You're technically still a beginner, but the heavy-to-light system is a pretty damned advanced workout configuration. All your energy, muscular and emotional, must be focused on that first work set, in which you work with the most weight you've ever used in this program—and probably in your life.

Also, note that the tempos for the big-muscle exercises are quicker in this program. On most exercises, you do 211 tempos, meaning that you take just 2 seconds to lower the weight. (On squats and deadlifts, the tempo is 201, so you do not pause between lowering and raising the weight.)

Finally, do fewer repetitions of the "assistance" exercises following the big boys. Keep doing one work set of each move, but work with heavier weights, fewer reps, and slightly faster tempos.

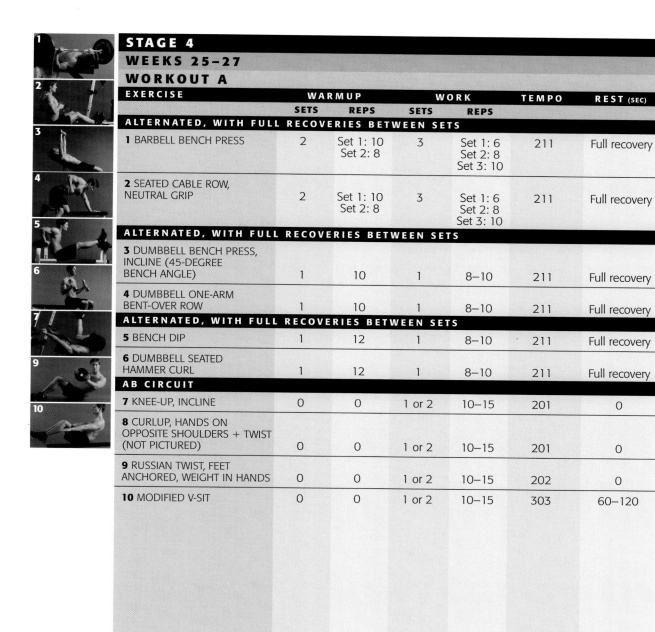

STAGE 4
WEEKS 25–27
WORKOUT A

EXERCISE	WARMUP		WORK		TEMPO	REST (sec)
	SETS	REPS	SETS	REPS		
ALTERNATED, WITH FULL RECOVERIES BETWEEN SETS						
1 BARBELL BENCH PRESS	2	Set 1: 10 Set 2: 8	3	Set 1: 6 Set 2: 8 Set 3: 10	211	Full recovery
2 SEATED CABLE ROW, NEUTRAL GRIP	2	Set 1: 10 Set 2: 8	3	Set 1: 6 Set 2: 8 Set 3: 10	211	Full recovery
ALTERNATED, WITH FULL RECOVERIES BETWEEN SETS						
3 DUMBBELL BENCH PRESS, INCLINE (45-DEGREE BENCH ANGLE)	1	10	1	8–10	211	Full recovery
4 DUMBBELL ONE-ARM BENT-OVER ROW	1	10	1	8–10	211	Full recovery
ALTERNATED, WITH FULL RECOVERIES BETWEEN SETS						
5 BENCH DIP	1	12	1	8–10	211	Full recovery
6 DUMBBELL SEATED HAMMER CURL	1	12	1	8–10	211	Full recovery
AB CIRCUIT						
7 KNEE-UP, INCLINE	0	0	1 or 2	10–15	201	0
8 CURLUP, HANDS ON OPPOSITE SHOULDERS + TWIST (NOT PICTURED)	0	0	1 or 2	10–15	201	0
9 RUSSIAN TWIST, FEET ANCHORED, WEIGHT IN HANDS	0	0	1 or 2	10–15	202	0
10 MODIFIED V-SIT	0	0	1 or 2	10–15	303	60–120

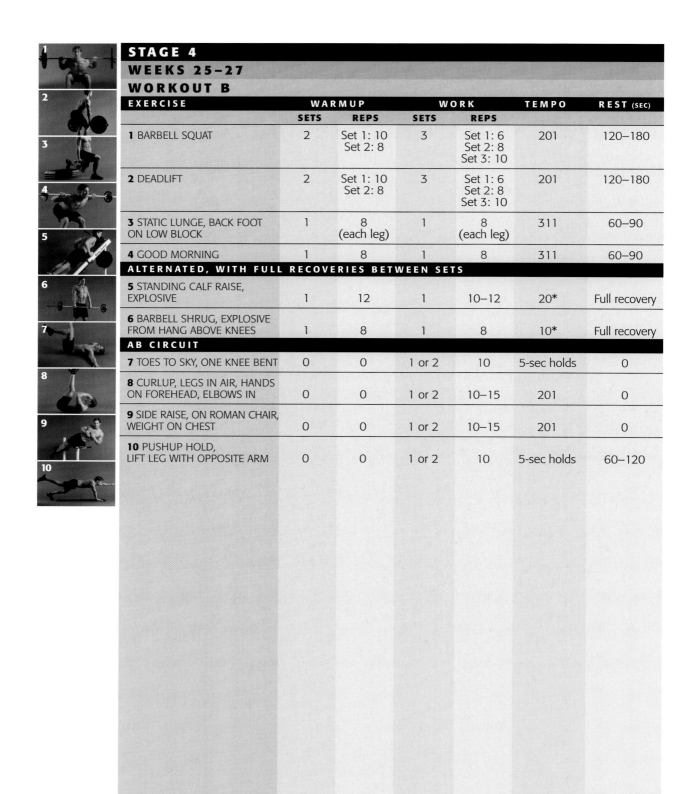

STAGE 4
WEEKS 25–27
WORKOUT B

EXERCISE	WARMUP		WORK		TEMPO	REST (SEC)
	SETS	REPS	SETS	REPS		
1 BARBELL SQUAT	2	Set 1: 10 Set 2: 8	3	Set 1: 6 Set 2: 8 Set 3: 10	201	120–180
2 DEADLIFT	2	Set 1: 10 Set 2: 8	3	Set 1: 6 Set 2: 8 Set 3: 10	201	120–180
3 STATIC LUNGE, BACK FOOT ON LOW BLOCK	1	8 (each leg)	1	8 (each leg)	311	60–90
4 GOOD MORNING	1	8	1	8	311	60–90
ALTERNATED, WITH FULL RECOVERIES BETWEEN SETS						
5 STANDING CALF RAISE, EXPLOSIVE	1	12	1	10–12	20*	Full recovery
6 BARBELL SHRUG, EXPLOSIVE FROM HANG ABOVE KNEES	1	8	1	8	10*	Full recovery
AB CIRCUIT						
7 TOES TO SKY, ONE KNEE BENT	0	0	1 or 2	10	5-sec holds	0
8 CURLUP, LEGS IN AIR, HANDS ON FOREHEAD, ELBOWS IN	0	0	1 or 2	10–15	201	0
9 SIDE RAISE, ON ROMAN CHAIR, WEIGHT ON CHEST	0	0	1 or 2	10–15	201	0
10 PUSHUP HOLD, LIFT LEG WITH OPPOSITE ARM	0	0	1 or 2	10	5-sec holds	60–120

STAGE 4
WEEKS 25–27
WORKOUT C

EXERCISE	WARMUP		WORK		TEMPO	REST (SEC)
	SETS	REPS	SETS	REPS		
ALTERNATED, WITH FULL RECOVERIES BETWEEN SETS						
1 LAT PULLDOWN, REVERSE GRIP	2	Set 1: 10 Set 2: 8	3	Set 1: 6 Set 2: 8 Set 3: 10	211	Full recovery
2 BARBELL SEATED SHOULDER PRESS	2	Set 1: 10 Set 2: 8	3	Set 1: 6 Set 2: 8 Set 3: 10	211	Full recovery
ALTERNATED, WITH FULL RECOVERIES BETWEEN SETS						
3 DUMBBELL LYING PULLOVER, 1 DUMBBELL IN 2 HANDS	1	10	1	8–10	211	Full recovery
4 DUMBBELL SEATED LATERAL RAISE	1	10	1	8–10	211	Full recovery
ALTERNATED, WITH FULL RECOVERIES BETWEEN SETS						
5 EZ-BAR BICEPS CURL	1	12	1	8–10	211	Full recovery
6 TRICEPS PUSHDOWN	1	12	1	8–10	211	Full recovery
AB CIRCUIT						
7 KNEE-UP, INCLINE	0	0	1 or 2	10–15	201	0
8 CURLUP, HANDS ON OPPOSITE SHOULDERS (NOT PICTURED)	0	0	1 or 2	10–15	201	0
9 RUSSIAN TWIST, FEET ANCHORED, WEIGHT IN HANDS	0	0	1 or 2	10–15	202	0
10 MODIFIED V-SIT	0	0	1 or 2	10–15	303	60–120

CHAPTER FIFTEEN

THE INTERMEDIATE PROGRAM

THIS 6-MONTH PROGRAM is for lifters who have been training continuously for a year or more or who have just completed the beginner program in the previous chapter. Advanced lifters who have never done an Ian King–designed program may also want to start here before moving up to the advanced workout. Like the beginner program, this one is divided into four stages.

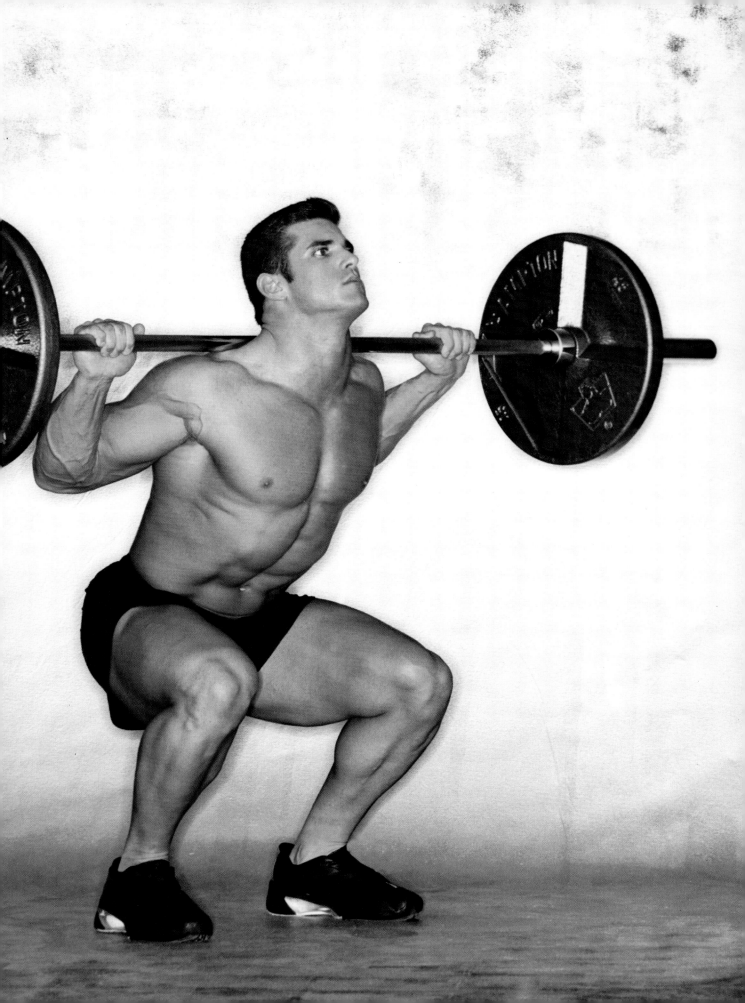

STAGE 1, WEEKS 1 THROUGH 3

You could call this initial segment a bottom-up proposition. Its purpose is to shore up your weakest links, so the best place to start is your feet and hands—or at least your calves and forearms. It's divided up into three workouts, A, B, and C, each of which you do once a week.

The exercises within each workout are grouped as **CIRCUITS**, **SUPERSETS**, or **TRISETS**. In the circuits, there's no designated rest period between the exercises because the time it takes to set up for each exercise is plenty of recovery time. A superset means you do pairs of two exercises without rest within each pair. Rest for 1 to 2 minutes before moving from one pair to another. A triset is three consecutive exercises without rest. A warmup for a superset or triset should itself be done in the same form—that is, do a warmup set of the first exercise immediately followed by a warmup set of the subsequent exercise(s).

Workouts A, B, and C end with the lat pulldown, barbell squat, and barbell bench press, respectively. Do each of these exercises with an exaggeratedly slow tempo, working with much less weight than you're used to. If you have hidden weaknesses in these lifts, they won't stay hidden for long. As you gradually work your way up to faster tempos and place more emphasis on these big-muscle movements, you'll build strength faster because you'll have exposed and corrected your weaknesses.

STAGE 1
WEEKS 1–3
WORKOUT A

EXERCISE	REPS		TEMPO	REST (SEC)
	WARMUP	WORK		
CONTROLLED AB CIRCUIT				
1 THIN TUMMY	0	10	5-sec holds	0
2 CURLUP, CHEAT UP + SLOW LOWER, *OR* CURLUP, ARMS STRAIGHT & PARALLEL TO FLOOR	0	10	5–15-sec lowering or 515	0
3 RUSSIAN TWIST	0	15–30	303	0
4 PUSHUP HOLD, HANDS & FEET	0	10	5-sec holds	60–120
CALF TRISET				
5 STANDING SINGLE-LEG CALF RAISE	Optional 10–15	15–20	321	0
6 CALF RAISE ON LEG PRESS MACHINE, SINGLE LEG	Optional 10–15	15–20	321	0
7 SEATED CALF RAISE, SINGLE LEG	Optional 10–15	15–20	321	60–120
SUPERSET 1				
8 DUMBBELL WRIST CURL	Optional 10–15	15–20	321	0
9 DUMBBELL WRIST EXTENSION	Optional 10–15	15–20	321	60–120
SUPERSET 2				
10 DUMBBELL LYING PULLOVER	12	12–15	321	0
11 DUMBBELL SEATED LATERAL RAISE	12	12–15	321	60–120
SUPERSET 3				
12 DUMBBELL SEATED SHOULDER PRESS, PALMS IN	10	10–12	321	0
13 LAT PULLDOWN, BEHIND NECK	10	10–12	321	60–120
SUPERSET 4				
14 BARBELL SEATED SHOULDER PRESS	8	8	613	0
15 LAT PULLDOWN	8	8	613	60–120

STAGE 1
WEEKS 1–3
WORKOUT B

EXERCISE	REPS		TEMPO	REST (SEC)
	WARMUP	WORK		
CONTROLLED AB STRAIGHT SETS				
1 TOES TO SKY	0	10	5-sec holds	30
2 CURLUP, LEGS IN AIR, HANDS ON OPPOSITE SHOULDERS, ARMS ACROSS CHEST	0	10–15	313	30
3 SIDE RAISE	0	10–15	313	30
4 SEATED THIN TUMMY + CHEEK SQUEEZE	0	10	5-sec holds	30
BICEPS TRISET				
5 EZ-BAR BICEPS CURL, WIDE GRIP	10	10	321	0
6 EZ-BAR BICEPS CURL, REVERSE GRIP	10	10	321	0
7 EZ-BAR BICEPS CURL, CLOSE GRIP	10	10	321	60–120
TRICEPS TRISET				
8 TRICEPS PUSHDOWN, REVERSE GRIP	10	10	321	0
9 TRICEPS PUSHDOWN, WIDE GRIP	10	10	321	0
10 TRICEPS PUSHDOWN, NEUTRAL GRIP	10	10	321	60–120
LOWER-BODY SUPERSET 1				
11 LEG CURL, SINGLE LEG	15	12–15	321	0
12 LEG EXTENSION, SINGLE LEG	15	12–15	321	60–120
LOWER-BODY SUPERSET 2				
13 SINGLE-LEG STIFF-LEGGED DEADLIFT	0	5–20	321	0
14 SINGLE-LEG SQUAT, ON LOW BLOCK	0	10–20	321	60–120
LOWER-BODY SUPERSET 3				
15 KING DEADLIFT	8	5–20	311	0
16 SINGLE-LEG SQUAT, OTHER LEG OUT IN FRONT	8	5–20	311	60–120
LOWER-BODY SUPERSET 4				
17 DEADLIFT	Optional 10–15	8	316	0
18 BARBELL SQUAT	Optional 10–15	8	613	60–120

STAGE 1
WEEKS 1–3
WORKOUT C

EXERCISE	REPS		TEMPO	REST (SEC)
	WARMUP	WORK		
CONTROLLED AB CIRCUIT				
1 THIN TUMMY	0	10	313 or 5-sec holds	0
2 CURLUP, CHEAT UP + SLOW LOWER, *OR* CURLUP, ARMS STRAIGHT & PARALLEL TO FLOOR	0	10	5–15-sec lowering or 515	0
3 RUSSIAN TWIST	0	15–30	303	0
4 PUSHUP HOLD, HANDS & FEET	0	10	5-sec holds	60–120
DUMBBELL SHRUG TRISET				
5 DUMBBELL SHRUG, BEHIND BODY	10	10	321	0
6 DUMBBELL SHRUG	10	10	321	0
7 DUMBBELL SHRUG, TO FRONT	10	10	321	60–120
SUPERSET 1				
8 BARBELL WRIST EXTENSION	Optional 10–15	15–20	321	0
9 BARBELL WRIST CURL	Optional 10–15	15–20	321	60–120
SUPERSET 2				
10 REVERSE DUMBBELL FLY	12	12–15	321	0
11 DUMBBELL FLY	12	12–15	321	60–120
SUPERSET 3				
12 DUMBBELL ONE-ARM BENT-OVER ROW	10	10–12	321	0
13 DUMBBELL BENCH PRESS, INCLINE, NEUTRAL GRIP	10	10–12	321	60–120
SUPERSET 4				
14 SEATED CABLE ROW	8	8	613	0
15 BARBELL BENCH PRESS, FEET ON BENCH	8	8	613	60–120

STAGE 1, WEEKS 4 THROUGH 6

Once again, you do three workouts—A, B, and C—weekly. You continue working on weak links—you just concentrate on links that are a little higher on the chain. You do intensely exhausting work on many muscle groups, from large (quadriceps, hamstrings, and lats) to small (biceps, triceps, and rear delts). You also do abdominal exercises, with a repetition range of 10 to 30 and tempo ranges that feel pretty natural for those exercises. The idea is to establish a rhythmic tempo and just knock out the reps with good form and no rest between exercises.

Speaking of rest: There isn't any between most of the exercises. Go from one exercise to the next, taking no more time than you need to set up. For several exercises, you perform two sets of 10 reps—in those cases, rest for 2 minutes between those two sets, and use the same weight or a slightly heavier weight in the second set.

Finally, learn the following new techniques.

STRIP SETS: These are designated as 10+10+10. Lift as much weight as you can for 10 repetitions. Decrease the weight and do 10 more reps. Then decrease the weight one more time and do 10 more. Don't worry about choosing the right amounts of weight the first time—chances are you won't get them perfect until the third time through each workout. Our advice: Start with less weight than you think you can handle. That way, you can improve a bit each workout.

1.5 REPS: Some of the more conventional big-muscle exercises feature the designation 1.5 in the TEMPO column. This means "one and a half" reps. Say you do an upright row with a barbell. You pull the bar up to the top position, in which your shoulder muscles are fully contracted. Then you lower it halfway, pause, and lift it back to the top. Then lower it all the way to the starting position so that your arms are completely straight. This doubles the work you do in the toughest part of the exercise. In a set of 10, you do 10 full reps and 10 half reps.

BREATHING SQUAT: As noted in chapter nine, choose a weight you think you can lift 12 times with good form. Do 10 reps the way you normally would, taking one breath per repetition. On the next 5 reps, take two breaths per rep. (That is, at the end of a rep, exhale, inhale, exhale, then inhale and do your next rep.) For the final 5 reps of the 20-rep set, breathe three times.

STAGE 1
WEEKS 4–6
WORKOUT A

EXERCISE	WARMUP		WORK		TEMPO	REST (SEC)
	SETS	REPS	SETS	REPS		
ENDURANCE AB CIRCUIT						
1 THIN TUMMY, LIFT ONE LEG	0	0	1	10–30	313	0
2 CURLUP, ARMS STRAIGHT & PARALLEL TO FLOOR	0	0	1	10–30	311	0
3 RUSSIAN TWIST	0	0	1	10–30	202	0
4 MODIFIED V-SIT	0	0	1	10–30	301	60–120
SUPERSET						
5 DUMBBELL SEATED BICEPS CURL WITH TWIST	1	10	Strip	10+10+10	311	0
6 EZ-BAR BICEPS CURL, REVERSE GRIP	1	10	1	10	311	60–120
SUPERSET						
7 REVERSE DUMBBELL FLY	1	10	Strip	10+10+10	311	0
8 SEATED CABLE ROW, REVERSE GRIP	1	10	1	10	1.5	60–120
STRAIGHT SETS						
9 SEATED CABLE ROW	1	10	2	10	311	120
SUPERSET						
10 DUMBBELL LYING PULLOVER, 1 DUMBBELL IN 2 HANDS, ACROSS BENCH	1	10	Strip	10+10+10	311	0
11 LAT PULLDOWN, WIDE GRIP	1	10	1	10	1.5	60–120
STRAIGHT SETS						
12 LAT PULLDOWN, NEUTRAL GRIP	1	10	2	10	311	120

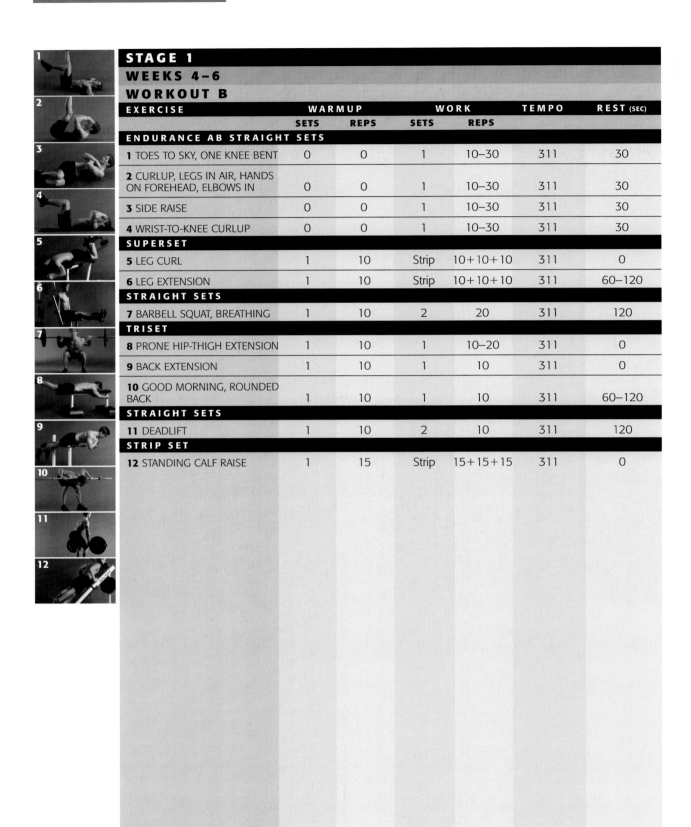

STAGE 1
WEEKS 4–6
WORKOUT B

EXERCISE	WARMUP		WORK		TEMPO	REST (SEC)
	SETS	REPS	SETS	REPS		
ENDURANCE AB STRAIGHT SETS						
1 TOES TO SKY, ONE KNEE BENT	0	0	1	10–30	311	30
2 CURLUP, LEGS IN AIR, HANDS ON FOREHEAD, ELBOWS IN	0	0	1	10–30	311	30
3 SIDE RAISE	0	0	1	10–30	311	30
4 WRIST-TO-KNEE CURLUP	0	0	1	10–30	311	30
SUPERSET						
5 LEG CURL	1	10	Strip	10+10+10	311	0
6 LEG EXTENSION	1	10	Strip	10+10+10	311	60–120
STRAIGHT SETS						
7 BARBELL SQUAT, BREATHING	1	10	2	20	311	120
TRISET						
8 PRONE HIP-THIGH EXTENSION	1	10	1	10–20	311	0
9 BACK EXTENSION	1	10	1	10	311	0
10 GOOD MORNING, ROUNDED BACK	1	10	1	10	311	60–120
STRAIGHT SETS						
11 DEADLIFT	1	10	2	10	311	120
STRIP SET						
12 STANDING CALF RAISE	1	15	Strip	15+15+15	311	0

STAGE 1
WEEKS 4–6
WORKOUT C

EXERCISE	WARMUP		WORK		TEMPO	REST (SEC)
	SETS	REPS	SETS	REPS		
ENDURANCE AB CIRCUIT						
1 THIN TUMMY, LIFT ONE LEG	0	0	1	10–30	313	0
2 CURLUP, HANDS ON OPPOSITE ELBOWS (NOT PICTURED)	0	0	1	10–30	311	0
3 RUSSIAN TWIST	0	0	1	10–30	202	0
4 MODIFIED V-SIT	0	0	1	10–30	301	60–120
SUPERSET						
5 DUMBBELL SEATED OVERHEAD TRICEPS EXTENSION, 1 DUMBBELL IN 2 HANDS	1	10	Strip	10+10+10	311	0
6 BARBELL BENCH PRESS, VERY CLOSE GRIP	1	10	1	10	311	60–120
SUPERSET						
7 DUMBBELL SEATED LATERAL RAISE	1	10	Strip	10+10+10	311	0
8 BARBELL UPRIGHT ROW	1	10	1	10	1.5	60–120
STRAIGHT SETS						
9 BARBELL SEATED SHOULDER PRESS	1	10	2	10	311	120
SUPERSET						
10 DUMBBELL FLY, THUMBS IN	1	10	Strip	10+10+10	311	0
11 BARBELL BENCH PRESS, INCLINE, WIDE GRIP	1	10	1	10	1.5	60–120
STRAIGHT SETS						
12 BARBELL BENCH PRESS	1	10	2	10	311	120

STAGE 2, WEEKS 8 THROUGH 10

By this point, your arms, deltoids, and calves have toughened up. That extra endurance comes into play now, as you start emphasizing compound, multi-joint exercises.

This phase also introduces a technique called *21*. Start with seven repetitions in the most difficult part of the range of the motion—for example, in the case of lateral raises do seven reps in the top half of the movement. Then do seven reps through the full range of motion, and finish with seven in the bottom half of the range. When warming up for 21, do each warmup rep through a full range of motion.

In workout B, you do some of your biceps and triceps exercises as *ALTERNATED SETS, WITH FULL RECOVERIES BETWEEN SETS*. This means you do them much like supersets in that you do a set of the first exercise followed by a set of the second exercise, alternating between the two until you've completed the prescribed number of sets for both. Unlike in supersets, between sets you should rest for as long as it takes to get your breathing and heart rate back to normal.

The goal of your ab exercises is strength. You do more challenging exercises, faster and for fewer repetitions. In workout B, you do a modified V-sit with an explosive tempo (10*): Lower for 1 second, forgo a pause, and then raise as fast as possible.

STAGE 2
WEEKS 8–10
WORKOUT A

EXERCISE	WARMUP		WORK		TEMPO	REST (SEC)
	SETS	REPS	SETS	REPS		
STRENGTH AB STRAIGHT SETS						
1 KNEE-UP, INCLINE	0	0	1	10–15	201	60
2 CURLUP, WEIGHTED (NOT PICTURED)	0	0	1	10–15	201	60
3 SIDE RAISE, HANDS ON FOREHEAD, ELBOWS OUT	0	0	1	10–15	201	60
4 SWISS-BALL ALTERNATE-LEG LIFT	0	0	1	10 (each leg)	5-sec holds	60
STRAIGHT SETS						
5 BARBELL SEATED SHOULDER PRESS, WIDE GRIP	1	10	2	10	321	120
6 DUMBBELL SEATED SHOULDER PRESS	1	10	1	10	1.5	60–120
7 DUMBBELL SEATED LATERAL RAISE	1	10 (full range of motion)	1	21	311	60
8 DEADLIFT, WIDE GRIP	1	10	2	10	311	120
9 STIFF-LEGGED DEADLIFT, CHEST UP, WIDE GRIP	1	10	1	10	1.5	60–120
10 GOOD MORNING, ROUNDED BACK	1	10 (full range of motion)	1	21	311	60
11 SEATED CALF RAISE	1	10	1	12–15	311	60
12 STANDING CALF RAISE	0	0	1	15–20	311	60
13 STANDING SINGLE-LEG CALF RAISE	0	0	1	20+ (each leg)	311	60

STAGE 2
WEEKS 8–10
WORKOUT B

EXERCISE	WARMUP		WORK		TEMPO	REST (SEC)
	SETS	REPS	SETS	REPS		
STRENGTH AB STRAIGHT SETS						
1 TOES TO SKY, KNEES TO SKY	0	0	1	10	5-sec holds	60
2 BARBELL ROLLOUT	0	0	1	10–15	201	60
3 RUSSIAN TWIST, FEET ANCHORED, WEIGHT IN HANDS	0	0	1	10–15	202	60
4 MODIFIED V-SIT	0	0	1	10–15	10*	60
STRAIGHT SETS						
5 BARBELL BENT-OVER ROW, WIDE GRIP	1	10	2	10	321	120
6 SEATED CABLE ROW, REVERSE GRIP	1	10	1	10	1.5	60–120
7 DUMBBELL ONE-ARM BENT-OVER ROW	1	10 (full range of motion)	1	21	311	60
8 BARBELL BENCH PRESS, INCLINE, WIDE GRIP	1	10	2	10	321	120
9 BARBELL BENCH PRESS, WIDE GRIP, TO NECK, FEET ON BENCH (NOT PICTURED)	1	10	1	10	1.5	60–120
10 DUMBBELL BENCH PRESS, DECLINE	1	10 (full range of motion)	1	21	311	60
ALTERNATED, WITH FULL RECOVERIES BETWEEN SETS						
11 DUMBBELL SEATED HAMMER CURL, INCLINE	1	10	1 or 2	Set1: 10 Optional set 2:15	311	Full recovery
12 DIP/BENCH DIP	1	10 (bench dip)	1or 2	Set 1: 10 Optional set 2: 15	311	Full recovery

STAGE 2
WEEKS 8–10
WORKOUT C

EXERCISE	WARMUP		WORK		TEMPO	REST (SEC)
	SETS	REPS	SETS	REPS		
STRENGTH AB STRAIGHT SETS						
1 KNEE-UP, INCLINE	0	0	1	10	201	60
2 CURLUP, LEGS IN AIR, WEIGHT ON CHEST	0	0	1	10–15	201	60
3 RUSSIAN TWIST, LEG CYCLE	0	0	1	15–30	212	60
4 SWISS-BALL ALTERNATE-LEG LIFT	0	0	1	10 (each leg)	5-sec holds	60
STRAIGHT SETS						
5 CHINUP	1	10 (on lat-pulldown machine)	2	10	321	120
6 LAT PULLDOWN	1	10	1	10	1.5	60–120
7 DUMBBELL LYING PULLOVER, 1 DUMBBELL IN 2 HANDS, ACROSS BENCH	1	10 (full range of motion)	1	21	311	60
8 BARBELL SQUAT, HIGH BAR, NARROW STANCE	1	10	2	10	311	120
9 STATIC LUNGE, BACK FOOT ON LOW BLOCK	1	10	1	10	1.5	60–120
10 LEG PRESS, SINGLE LEG	1	10 (full range of motion)	1	21	311	60
11 BARBELL SHRUG, REVERSE GRIP	1	10	1	10	311	60
12 BARBELL SHRUG	0	0	1	10	311	60
13 BARBELL SHRUG, WIDE GRIP	0	0	1	10	311	60

STAGE 2, WEEKS 11 THROUGH 13

Up to now, you've prepared your body for heavy lifting by shoring up weak areas, building muscular endurance, and generally gearing up for hard work. It's finally time to do some of that heavy lifting. This is a dramatic shift that's been a long time coming—you've done 9 full weeks of preparation. Once you start and see how much strength you gain and how fast you gain it, you'll be glad you did all that prep work.

Focus on two major strength exercises per workout—with three weekly workouts, that's six heavy exercises in all. For each, do two warmup sets, three work sets, and one **BACK-OFF SET**. The back-off set is a decades-old concept that has aged gracefully. Back in the day, old-timers did low-rep sets followed by high-rep sets under the assumption that this would flush the muscles with blood and drive out lactic acid. They believed that this would prevent soreness (it won't) and jump-start the recovery process (another myth—more work causes muscles to recover more slowly). Today, we do low reps followed by high reps for a completely different reason: neural disinhibition. That's a lot of syllables (seven—count 'em) that simply mean you can use heavier weights for a high-rep set when it follows several low-rep sets.

The benefit of lifting heavier weights should be obvious by now. You develop more muscle than you would with lighter weights for the same number of reps, and you induce a deeper level of fatigue in your muscles. Yes, fatigue is something you have to use judiciously when training—too little and you get disappointing results; too much and you overtrain and get injured or see diminishing returns. But when you use it wisely—as you will in this stage of the program—the deeper fatigue leads to better muscle development. The idea is that you take muscles that have been pushed to the max by heavy-weight, low-rep sets, then flush them with blood with a low-weight, high-rep set. (Make sure you have some protein before your workout, if you want to get the best results from this technique. The blood will bring nutrients with it, and jump-start the recovery process.)

At the end of each workout, do one **ASSISTANCE EXERCISE**, a move that will help get your body ready for the next stage, with even more emphasis on strength and power.

The chinups in workout C may be a bit confusing. The warmups, as noted, should be done on the lat-pulldown machine, using the same underhand grip you'll use on chinups. The three work sets are weighted—that is, you use some kind of load in addition to your body weight. (If you can't chin your body weight for more than eight reps—the number in the first work set—you needn't use extra weight for that set.) You can use a weight belt designed for chinups, with a chain in front to hold dumbbells or weight plates. Or you can use a weighted vest, if you have one, or a backpack with weights in it. For the back-off set, go back to the lat-pulldown machine, unless you're one of those super-athletes who can knock off 12 to 15 chinups with your arms and back almost completely fried. (If you are that strong, you probably should be doing the advanced program.)

The ab routines in this segment are also different. Workouts A, B, and C each has a different goal. Workout A aims for speed and power (fast movements, including some with explosive tempos indicated by 10* or 20*). Workout B is all about control (slow movements, with some holds). And Workout C builds strength (loaded movements). Each workout also includes five ab exercises, instead of four. In workouts A and B, you have the option of doing a second set of each exercise. (If you opt for a second set, do the exercises circuit-style, completing sets of all five, with no rest in between, before doing the second circuit. You can rest for a minute or two between circuits.) In workout C, in which you use weights for the ab exercises, do a warmup circuit followed by a work circuit.

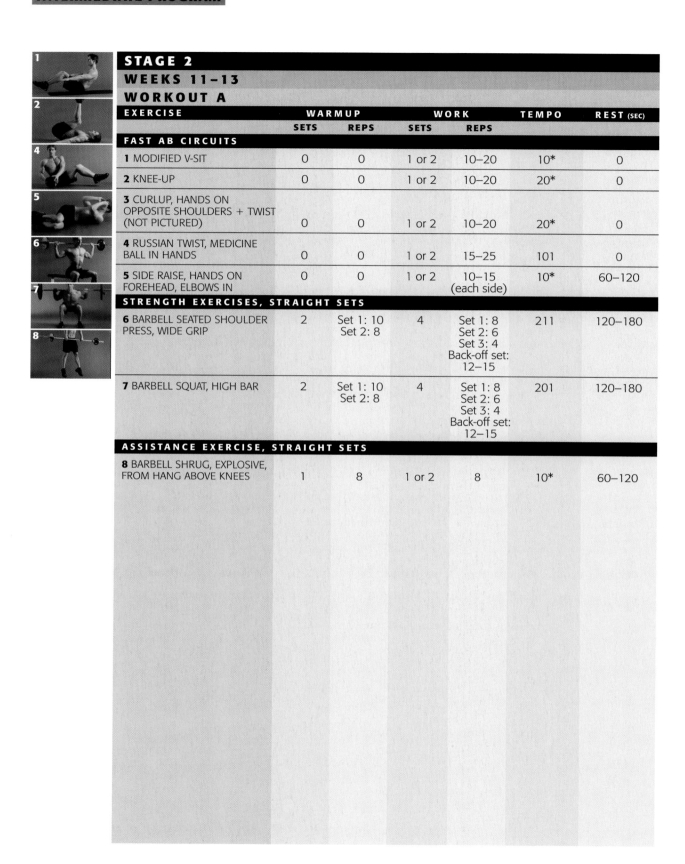

STAGE 2
WEEKS 11–13
WORKOUT A

EXERCISE	WARMUP		WORK		TEMPO	REST (SEC)
	SETS	REPS	SETS	REPS		
FAST AB CIRCUITS						
1 MODIFIED V-SIT	0	0	1 or 2	10–20	10*	0
2 KNEE-UP	0	0	1 or 2	10–20	20*	0
3 CURLUP, HANDS ON OPPOSITE SHOULDERS + TWIST (NOT PICTURED)	0	0	1 or 2	10–20	20*	0
4 RUSSIAN TWIST, MEDICINE BALL IN HANDS	0	0	1 or 2	15–25	101	0
5 SIDE RAISE, HANDS ON FOREHEAD, ELBOWS IN	0	0	1 or 2	10–15 (each side)	10*	60–120
STRENGTH EXERCISES, STRAIGHT SETS						
6 BARBELL SEATED SHOULDER PRESS, WIDE GRIP	2	Set 1: 10 Set 2: 8	4	Set 1: 8 Set 2: 6 Set 3: 4 Back-off set: 12–15	211	120–180
7 BARBELL SQUAT, HIGH BAR	2	Set 1: 10 Set 2: 8	4	Set 1: 8 Set 2: 6 Set 3: 4 Back-off set: 12–15	201	120–180
ASSISTANCE EXERCISE, STRAIGHT SETS						
8 BARBELL SHRUG, EXPLOSIVE, FROM HANG ABOVE KNEES	1	8	1 or 2	8	10*	60–120

STAGE 2
WEEKS 11–13
WORKOUT B

EXERCISE	WARMUP		WORK		TEMPO	REST (SEC)
	SETS	REPS	SETS	REPS		
CONTROLLED AB CIRCUITS						
1 KNEE-UP	0	0	1 or 2	10	303	0
2 CURLUP, ARMS STRAIGHT & PARALLEL TO FLOOR	0	0	1 or 2	10	303	0
3 LATERAL LEG LOWERING	0	0	1 or 2	10 (each side)	303	0
4 SIDE RAISE	0	0	1 or 2	10	303	0
5 PUSHUP HOLD, LIFT LEG, THEN ARM	0	0	1 or 2	10	5-sec holds	60–120
ALTERNATED, WITH FULL RECOVERIES BETWEEN SETS						
6 BARBELL BENT-OVER ROW, WIDE GRIP	2	Set 1: 10 Set 2: 8	4	Set 1: 8 Set 2: 6 Set 3: 4 Back-off set: 12–15	211	Full recovery
7 BARBELL BENCH PRESS, INCLINE	2	Set 1: 10 Set 2: 8	4	Set 1: 8 Set 2: 6 Set 3: 4 Back-off set: 12–15	211	Full recovery
ASSISTANCE EXERCISE, STRAIGHT SETS						
8 DUMBBELL SEATED HAMMER CURL	1	10	1 or 2	8	211	60–120

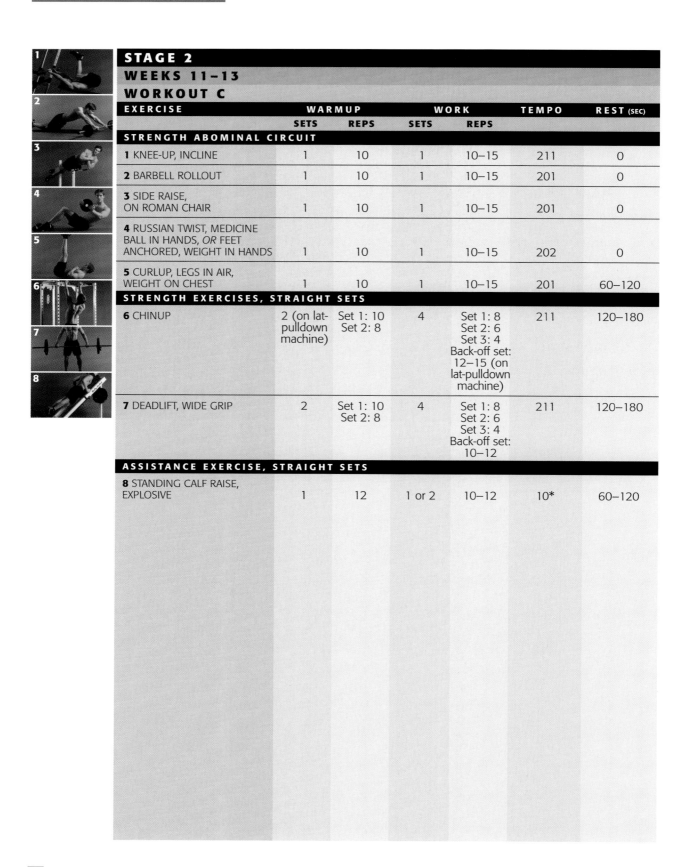

STAGE 2
WEEKS 11–13
WORKOUT C

EXERCISE	WARMUP		WORK		TEMPO	REST (SEC)
	SETS	REPS	SETS	REPS		
STRENGTH ABOMINAL CIRCUIT						
1 KNEE-UP, INCLINE	1	10	1	10–15	211	0
2 BARBELL ROLLOUT	1	10	1	10–15	201	0
3 SIDE RAISE, ON ROMAN CHAIR	1	10	1	10–15	201	0
4 RUSSIAN TWIST, MEDICINE BALL IN HANDS, *OR* FEET ANCHORED, WEIGHT IN HANDS	1	10	1	10–15	202	0
5 CURLUP, LEGS IN AIR, WEIGHT ON CHEST	1	10	1	10–15	201	60–120
STRENGTH EXERCISES, STRAIGHT SETS						
6 CHINUP	2 (on lat-pulldown machine)	Set 1: 10 Set 2: 8	4	Set 1: 8 Set 2: 6 Set 3: 4 Back-off set: 12–15 (on lat-pulldown machine)	211	120–180
7 DEADLIFT, WIDE GRIP	2	Set 1: 10 Set 2: 8	4	Set 1: 8 Set 2: 6 Set 3: 4 Back-off set: 10–12	211	120–180
ASSISTANCE EXERCISE, STRAIGHT SETS						
8 STANDING CALF RAISE, EXPLOSIVE	1	12	1 or 2	10–12	10*	60–120

STAGE 3, WEEKS 15 THROUGH 17

This stage offers yet another shock to your body. It shifts to a different system, in which you tackle the six strength exercises you did in weeks 11 through 13 from some different directions. You do the exercises in different sequences, with various grips and loads. The two exercises focusing on your back muscles—chinups and rows—are paired in the same workout, as are the deadlift and squat, and the bench press and shoulder press. This is a very serious challenge to the endurance of your weak-link muscles—arms, deltoids, lower back, calves. Remember all those strip sets and 21s you did for these muscles? Here's the payoff.

The ab exercises are now at the end of each workout, instead of the beginning. You're back to single sets, rather than multiple sets with a warmup; and you focus on one goal—control—instead of the three goals you worked toward in the previous 3 weeks.

STAGE 3
WEEKS 15–17
WORKOUT A

EXERCISE	WARMUP		WORK		TEMPO	REST (SEC)
	SETS	REPS	SETS	REPS		
STRAIGHT SETS						
1 WIDE-GRIP PULLUP	2 (use lat-pulldown machine, if needed)	Set 1: 10 Set 2: 8	2	6	311	180
2 CHINUP *OR* LAT PULLDOWN, REVERSE GRIP	0	0	1	12	311	120
3 NEUTRAL-GRIP PULLUP *OR* LAT PULLDOWN, NEUTRAL GRIP	0	0	1	15–20	311	60
4 BARBELL BENT-OVER ROW	2	Set 1: 8 Set 2: 6	2	6	311	180
5 BARBELL BENT-OVER ROW, REVERSE GRIP	0	0	1	12	311	120
6 BARBELL BENT-OVER ROW, WIDE GRIP	0	0	1	15–20	311	60
7 EZ-BAR PREACHER CURL	1	8	2	Set 1: 6–8 Set 2: 10–12	311	60–120
CONTROLLED AB CIRCUIT						
8 THIN TUMMY, LIFT & CYCLE OUT 1 LEG	0	0	1	10	313	0
9 CURLUP, ARMS STRAIGHT & PARALLEL TO FLOOR	0	0	1	10	515	0
10 RUSSIAN TWIST, LEG CYCLE	0	0	1	15–30	303	0
11 PUSHUP HOLD, LIFT LEG WITH OPPOSITE ARM	0	0	1	10	5-sec holds	0

STAGE 3
WEEKS 15–17
WORKOUT B

EXERCISE	WARMUP		WORK		TEMPO	REST (SEC)
	SETS	REPS	SETS	REPS		
STRAIGHT SETS						
1 DEADLIFT	2	Set 1: 10 Set 2: 8	2	6	311	180
2 DEADLIFT, WIDE GRIP	0	0	1	10	10*	120
3 DEADLIFT, WIDE GRIP, STANDING ON BLOCKS	0	0	1	15	10*	60
4 BARBELL SQUAT, FRONT	2	Set 1: 8 Set 2: 6	2	6	301	180
5 BARBELL SQUAT, HIGH BAR (NOT PICTURED)	0	0	1	10	301	120
6 BARBELL SQUAT, HIGH BAR, NARROW STANCE	0	0	1	15	301	60
7 BARBELL SHRUG, JUMP, FROM HANG ABOVE KNEES	1	8	1 or 2	8	10*	60
CONTROLLED AB STRAIGHT SETS						
8 TOES TO SKY, ONE KNEE BENT	0	0	1	10	5-sec holds	30
9 CURLUP, LEGS IN AIR, HANDS ON FOREHEAD, ELBOWS IN	0	0	1	10–15	313	30
10 SIDE RAISE, HANDS ON FOREHEAD, ELBOWS IN	0	0	1	10–15	313	30
11 SEATED THIN TUMMY + CHEEK SQUEEZE	0	0	1	10	5-sec holds	30

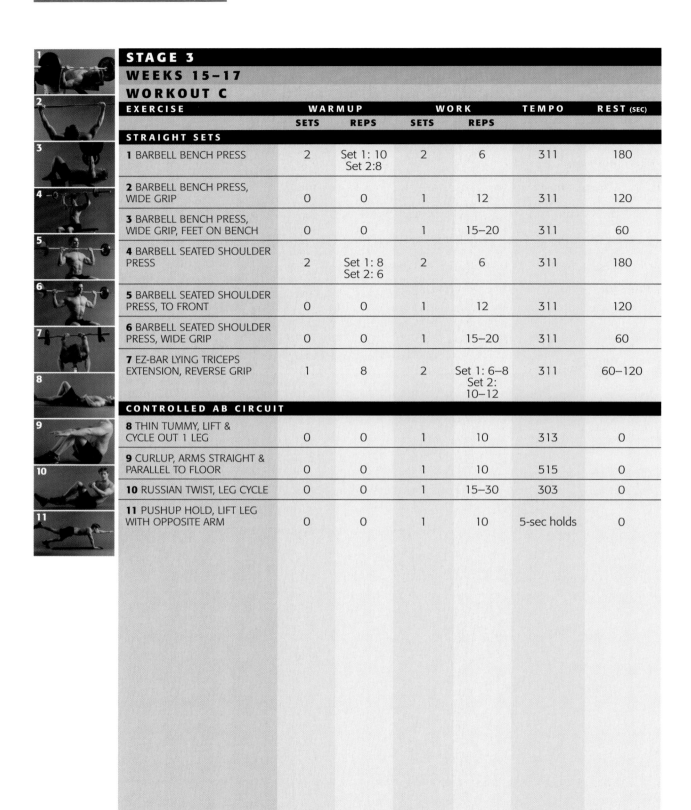

STAGE 3
WEEKS 15–17
WORKOUT C

EXERCISE	WARMUP		WORK		TEMPO	REST (SEC)
	SETS	REPS	SETS	REPS		
STRAIGHT SETS						
1 BARBELL BENCH PRESS	2	Set 1: 10 Set 2:8	2	6	311	180
2 BARBELL BENCH PRESS, WIDE GRIP	0	0	1	12	311	120
3 BARBELL BENCH PRESS, WIDE GRIP, FEET ON BENCH	0	0	1	15–20	311	60
4 BARBELL SEATED SHOULDER PRESS	2	Set 1: 8 Set 2: 6	2	6	311	180
5 BARBELL SEATED SHOULDER PRESS, TO FRONT	0	0	1	12	311	120
6 BARBELL SEATED SHOULDER PRESS, WIDE GRIP	0	0	1	15–20	311	60
7 EZ-BAR LYING TRICEPS EXTENSION, REVERSE GRIP	1	8	2	Set 1: 6–8 Set 2: 10–12	311	60–120
CONTROLLED AB CIRCUIT						
8 THIN TUMMY, LIFT & CYCLE OUT 1 LEG	0	0	1	10	313	0
9 CURLUP, ARMS STRAIGHT & PARALLEL TO FLOOR	0	0	1	10	515	0
10 RUSSIAN TWIST, LEG CYCLE	0	0	1	15–30	303	0
11 PUSHUP HOLD, LIFT LEG WITH OPPOSITE ARM	0	0	1	10	5-sec holds	0

STAGE 3, WEEKS 18 THROUGH 20

Here's where it gets heavy—really heavy. You do just two strength exercises per workout, using a technique called **WAVE LOADING**. The concept is more complex, physiologically, than the others you've been exposed to so far. Here's how it works: After a thorough warmup (three sets with increasingly heavy weights), do a set of six repetitions, followed by a set of one rep with a weight that's much heavier—but not so heavy that you won't be able to increase it in the next two sets. Next, do another set of six with a heavier weight than you used the first time. Follow that with another set of one, with a weight that is much heavier than you used in the first set of one but that is less than your one-rep max. (Ideally, use a weight that you could lift once or even twice more.) Finish with a back-off set.

End each workout with a circuit of four ab exercises focusing on endurance, using a rhythmic tempo.

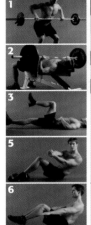

STAGE 3
WEEKS 18–20
WORKOUT A

EXERCISE	WARMUP		WORK		TEMPO	REST (SEC)
	SETS	REPS	SETS	REPS		
ALTERNATED, WITH FULL RECOVERIES BETWEEN SETS						
1 BARBELL BENT-OVER ROW	3	Set 1: 10 Set 2: 8 Set 3: 6	5	Wave set 1: 6 Wave set 2: 1[†] Wave set 3: 6[‡] Wave set 4: 1[§] Back-off set: 10–15	211	Full recovery
2 BARBELL BENCH PRESS	3	Set 1: 10 Set 2: 8 Set 3: 6	5	Wave set 1: 6 Wave set 2: 1[†] Wave set 3: 6[‡] Wave set 4: 1[§] Back-off set: 10–15	211	Full recovery
ENDURANCE AB CIRCUIT						
3 THIN TUMMY, BOTH LEGS UP, CYCLE OUT ONE LEG	0	0	1	10–30	313	0
4 CURLUP, HANDS ON OPPOSITE ELBOWS (NOT PICTURED)	0	0	1	10–30	311	0
5 RUSSIAN TWIST, FEET ANCHORED	0	0	1	10–30	202	0
6 MODIFIED V-SIT	0	0	1	10–30	301	0

† Much heavier
‡ Heavier than wave set 1
§ Heavier than wave set 2

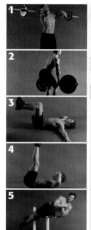

STAGE 3
WEEKS 18–20
WORKOUT B

EXERCISE	WARMUP		WORK		TEMPO	REST (SEC)
	SETS	REPS	SETS	REPS		
WAVE SETS						
1 BARBELL SQUAT, FRONT	3	Set 1: 10 Set 2: 8 Set 3: 6	5	Wave set 1: 6 Wave set 2: 1† Wave set 3: 6‡ Wave set 4: 1§ Back-off set: 10–15	201	180–240
2 DEADLIFT	2	Set 1: 8 Set 2: 6	5	Wave set 1: 6 Wave set 2: 1† Wave set 3: 6‡ Wave set 4: 1§ Back-off set: 10–15	211	180–240
ENDURANCE AB STRAIGHT SETS						
3 TOES TO SKY, KNEES TO SKY	0	0	1	10–30	311	30
4 CURLUP, LEGS IN AIR, HANDS ON FOREHEAD, ELBOWS OUT	0	0	1	10–30	311	30
5 SIDE RAISE, ON ROMAN CHAIR	0	0	1	10–30	311	30
6 WRIST-TO-KNEE CURLUP, FULL LYING POSITION (NOT PICTURED)	0	0	1	10–30	311	30

† Much heavier
‡ Heavier than wave set 1
§ Heavier than wave set 2

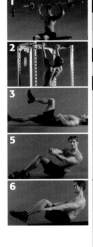

STAGE 3
WEEKS 18–20
WORKOUT C

EXERCISE	WARMUP		WORK		TEMPO	REST (SEC)
	SETS	REPS	SETS	REPS		
WAVE SETS, ALTERNATED, WITH FULL RECOVERIES BETWEEN SETS						
1 BARBELL SEATED SHOULDER PRESS	3	Set 1: 10 Set 2: 8 Set 3: 6	5	Wave set 1: 6 Wave set 2: 1† Wave set 3: 6‡ Wave set 4: 1§ Back-off set: 10–15	211	Full recovery
2 CHINUP	3 (use lat-pulldown machine)	Set 1: 10 Set 2: 8 Set 3: 6	5	Wave set 1: 6 Wave set 2: 1† Wave set 3: 6‡ Wave set 4: 1§ Back-off set: 10–15 (use lat-pulldown machine)	211	Full recovery
ENDURANCE AB CIRCUIT						
3 THIN TUMMY, BOTH LEGS UP, CYCLE OUT ONE LEG	0	0	1	10–30	313	0
4 CURLUP, HANDS ON OPPOSITE ELBOWS (NOT PICTURED)	0	0	1	10–30	311	0
5 RUSSIAN TWIST, FEET ANCHORED	0	0	1	10–30	202	0
6 MODIFIED V-SIT	0	0	1	10–30	301	0

† Much heavier
‡ Heavier than wave set 1
§ Heavier than wave set 2

STAGE 4, WEEKS 22 THROUGH 24

Now you do wave loading with a more straightforward progression, using slightly heavier weights in each of the three work sets of each strength exercise. Another interesting switch is that in the barbell bench press in workout A you bring the bar down to a lower-than-normal point on your chest. This is a powerlifting technique that helps greater utilize your triceps and lats in the lift and also shortens the distance the bar has to travel. It'll take you a workout or two to get used to it, but you should notice a quick strength increase after that.

In workout B, you do some support work for your biceps and triceps using heavy weights and performing alternated sets with full recoveries. (If, by some wild chance, you're concerned about the size and appearance of your arms, you'll really like what these exercises do for you.)

You've already done ab exercises for stability and control and for rhythm and endurance. This time, you use weights, to develop strength.

STAGE 4 — WEEKS 22–24 — WORKOUT A

EXERCISE	WARMUP		WORK		TEMPO	REST (SEC)
	SETS	REPS	SETS	REPS		
WAVE SETS						
1 BARBELL BENCH PRESS, TO LOWER CHEST	3	Set 1: 10 Set 2: 8 Set 3: 6	4	Wave set 1: 6 Wave set 2: 5† Wave set 3: 4‡ Back-off set: 10–15	211 211 211 211	Up to 240
2 DEADLIFT	3	Set 1: 8 Set 2: 6 Set 3: 4	4	Wave set 1: 6 Wave set 2: 5† Wave set 3: 4‡ Back-off set: 10–15	211 211 211 211	Up to 240
STRENGTH AB STRAIGHT SETS						
3 KNEE-UP, VERTICAL	0	0	1	10–15	201	60
4 CURLUP, WEIGHTED (NOT PICTURED)	0	0	1	10–15	201	60
5 SIDE RAISE, ON ROMAN CHAIR, WEIGHT ON CHEST	0	0	1	10–15	201	60
6 SWISS-BALL ALTERNATE LEG LIFT, LYING	0	0	1	10 (each leg)	5-sec holds	60

† Use slightly more weight than in wave set 1
‡ Use slightly more weight than in wave set 2

STAGE 4
WEEKS 22–24
WORKOUT B

EXERCISE	WARMUP		WORK		TEMPO	REST (SEC)
	SETS	REPS	SETS	REPS		
ALTERNATED, WITH FULL RECOVERIES BETWEEN SETS						
1 PULLUP	3 (on lat-pulldown machine)	Set 1: 10 Set 2: 8 Set 3: 6	3	Set 1: 6 Set 2: 5 Set 3: 4	211	Full recovery
2 BARBELL SEATED SHOULDER PRESS, TO FRONT	3	Set 1: 10 Set 2: 8 Set 3: 6	3	Set 1: 6 Set 2: 5 Set 3: 4	211	Full recovery
ALTERNATED, WITH FULL RECOVERIES BETWEEN SETS						
3 EZ-BAR BICEPS CURL	1	8	2 or 3	Set 1: 6 Set 2: 6 Optional back-off set: 10	211	Full recovery
4 BARBELL BENCH PRESS, CLOSE GRIP	1	8	2 or 3	Set 1: 6 Set 2: 6 Optional back-off set: 10	211	Full recovery
STRENGTH AB STRAIGHT SETS						
5 KNEE-UP, VERTICAL	0	0	1	10–15	201	60
6 BARBELL ROLLOUT	0	0	1	10–15	201	60
7 RUSSIAN TWIST, FEET ANCHORED, WEIGHT IN HANDS	0	0	1	10–15	202	60
8 FULL V-SIT	0	0	1	10–15	10*	60

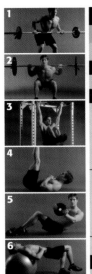

STAGE 4
WEEKS 22–24
WORKOUT C

EXERCISE	WARMUP		WORK		TEMPO	REST (SEC)
	SETS	REPS	SETS	REPS		
STRAIGHT SETS						
1 BARBELL BENT-OVER ROW, REVERSE GRIP	3	Set 1: 10 Set 2: 8 Set 3: 6	4	Set 1: 6 Set 2: 5 Set 3: 4 Back-off set: 10–15	211	Up to 240
2 BARBELL SQUAT	3	Set 1: 8 Set 2: 6 Set 3: 4	4	Set 1: 6 Set 2: 5 Set 3: 4 Back-off set: 10–15	201	Up to 240
3 KNEE-UP, VERTICAL	0	0	1	10	201	60
STRENGTH AB STRAIGHT SETS						
4 CURLUP, LEGS IN AIR, WEIGHT ON CHEST	0	0	1	10–15	311	60
5 RUSSIAN TWIST, FEET ANCHORED, WEIGHT IN HANDS	0	0	1	10–15	212	60
6 SWISS-BALL ALTERNATE LEG LIFT, LYING	0	0	1	10 (each leg)	5-sec holds	60

STAGE 4, WEEKS 25 THROUGH 27

Given the range of techniques you've used and the amount of weight you've lifted, you're probably wondering how we're going to send you off. With a bang, that's how. It's time to lift the heaviest damn weights you've ever lifted for four reps; perform three new power exercises (jump squat, clean pull, and high pull) in workout B; and do circuits of five ab exercises each workout, with different goals each time: speed, strength, and control.

Also, add a new element to your bench press: an arched back. We don't mean lift your butt off the bench—in a powerlifting meet, doing that would disqualify you. We mean arch between your butt and shoulders to raise your torso higher off the bench. The bar then has even less distance to travel. Use this technique cautiously; if you have a history of back problems, it's probably not a good idea. (Then again, if you have a history of back problems, you probably haven't gotten this far in the program, given the emphasis on bent-over rows, squats, and deadlifts, all of which would probably be more than a compromised lower back could handle.)

On the squat, hold the bar lower on your back (as per the "low bar" designation). Powerlifters do this to lower their centers of gravity. You also have the option of using a weight belt during your squats and deadlifts. Though you don't have to use one, you'll probably find that a belt helps your confidence when you use maximum weights on these lifts. The back support probably adds to the lifts themselves. (Belts are legal in powerlifting competition, so using one isn't cheating.)

On your major lifts, do two sets of four reps. For the second set, use heavier weight than for the first. The longer rest periods between these sets—up to 5 minutes—make this possible. Resting that long takes some getting used to. Old-time powerlifters used to sit down and read the newspaper between sets. While that's a bit excessive, we do suggest you recover fully between these max-weight sets. These should be the heaviest weights you've ever lifted, and you don't want to blow your chance to set new personal bests. You've waited almost 6 months to get to this point—don't jeopardize it just so you can get to the shower a couple of minutes earlier. After the two max-weight sets, do one or two back-off sets.

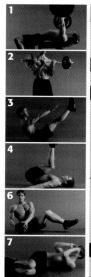

STAGE 4
WEEKS 25–27
WORKOUT A

EXERCISE	WARMUP		WORK		TEMPO	REST (SEC)
	SETS	REPS	SETS	REPS		
ALTERNATED, WITH FULL RECOVERIES BETWEEN SETS						
1 BARBELL BENCH PRESS, TO LOWER CHEST, ARCHED BACK	3	Set 1: 10 Set 2: 8 Set 3: 6	4	Set 1: 4 Set 2: 4 Back-off set 1: 8–10 Back-off set 2: 12–15	211	Full recovery
2 EZ-BAR BICEPS CURL, CLOSE GRIP	3	Set 1: 10 Set 2: 8 Set 3: 6	4	Set 1: 4 Set 2: 4 Set 3: 8–10 Back-off set: 12–15	211	Full recovery
FAST AB CIRCUIT						
3 FULL V-SIT	0	0	1 or 2	10–20	10*	0
4 KNEE-UP	0	0	1 or 2	10–20	20*	0
5 CURLUP, HANDS ON FOREHEAD, ELBOWS OUT + TWIST (NOT PICTURED)	0	0	1 or 2	10–20	20*	0
6 RUSSIAN TWIST, MEDICINE BALL IN HANDS	0	0	1 or 2	15–25	101	0
7 SIDE RAISE, HANDS ON FOREHEAD, ELBOWS IN	0	0	1 or 2	10–15 (each side)	10*	0

STAGE 4
WEEKS 25–27
WORKOUT B

EXERCISE	WARMUP		WORK		TEMPO	REST (SEC)
	SETS	REPS	SETS	REPS		
STRAIGHT SETS						
1 BARBELL SQUAT, LOW BAR	3	Set 1: 8 Set 2: 6 Set 3: 4	2	4	211	Up to 300
2 BARBELL SQUAT, EXPLOSIVE	0	0	1 or 2	6–8	20*	180–240
3 BARBELL SQUAT, JUMP	1	6	1	8–10	10*	120–180
4 DEADLIFT	2	Set 1: 6 Set 2: 4	2	4	211	Up to 300
5 CLEAN PULL	1	6	1 or 2	6	10*	180–240
6 HIGH PULL	1	8	1	8	10*	120–180
CONTROLLED AB CIRCUIT						
7 KNEE-UP	0	0	1 or 2	10	303	0
8 CURLUP, HANDS ON OPPOSITE ELBOWS (NOT PICTURED)	0	0	1 or 2	10	303	0
9 LATERAL LEG LOWERING	0	0	1 or 2	10 (each side)	303	0
10 SIDE RAISE, ON ROMAN CHAIR, HANDS ON FOREHEAD	0	0	1 or 2	10	303	0
11 PUSHUP HOLD, LIFT LEG WITH OPPOSITE ARM	0	0	1 or 2	10	5-sec holds	0

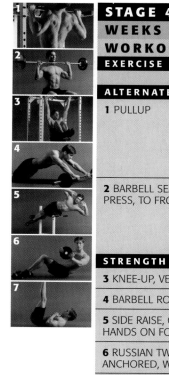

STAGE 4
WEEKS 25–27
WORKOUT C

EXERCISE	WARMUP		WORK		TEMPO	REST (SEC)
	SETS	REPS	SETS	REPS		
ALTERNATED, WITH FULL RECOVERIES BETWEEN SETS						
1 PULLUP	3 (on lat-pulldown machine)	Set 1: 10 Set 2: 8 Set 3: 6	4	Set 1: 4 Set 2: 4† Back-off set 1: 8–10 Back-off set 2: 12–15	211	Full recovery
2 BARBELL SEATED SHOULDER PRESS, TO FRONT	3	Set 1: 10 Set 2: 8 Set 3: 6	4	Set 1: 4 Set 2: 4† Back-off set 1: 8–10 Back-off set 2: 12–15	211	Full recovery
STRENGTH AB CIRCUIT						
3 KNEE-UP, VERTICAL	1	10	1	10–15	211	0
4 BARBELL ROLLOUT	1	10	1	10–15	201	0
5 SIDE RAISE, ON ROMAN CHAIR, HANDS ON FOREHEAD	1	10	1	10–15	201	0
6 RUSSIAN TWIST, FEET ANCHORED, WEIGHT IN HANDS	1	10	1	10–15	202	0
7 CURLUP, LEGS IN AIR, WEIGHT ON CHEST	1	10	1	10–15	201	0

† Use more weight

CHAPTER SIXTEEN

THE ADVANCED PROGRAM

THIS IS A 6-MONTH PROGRAM for lifters who have been training continuously for at least 4 years and who have completed the intermediate program in the previous chapter. Less experienced lifters may also attempt it if they've just finished the intermediate program. This program is divided into four stages, and each stage is further segmented into two 3-week increments. Finally, each 3-week segment offers three workouts—A, B, and C. Do each workout once a week for the duration of the 3 weeks.

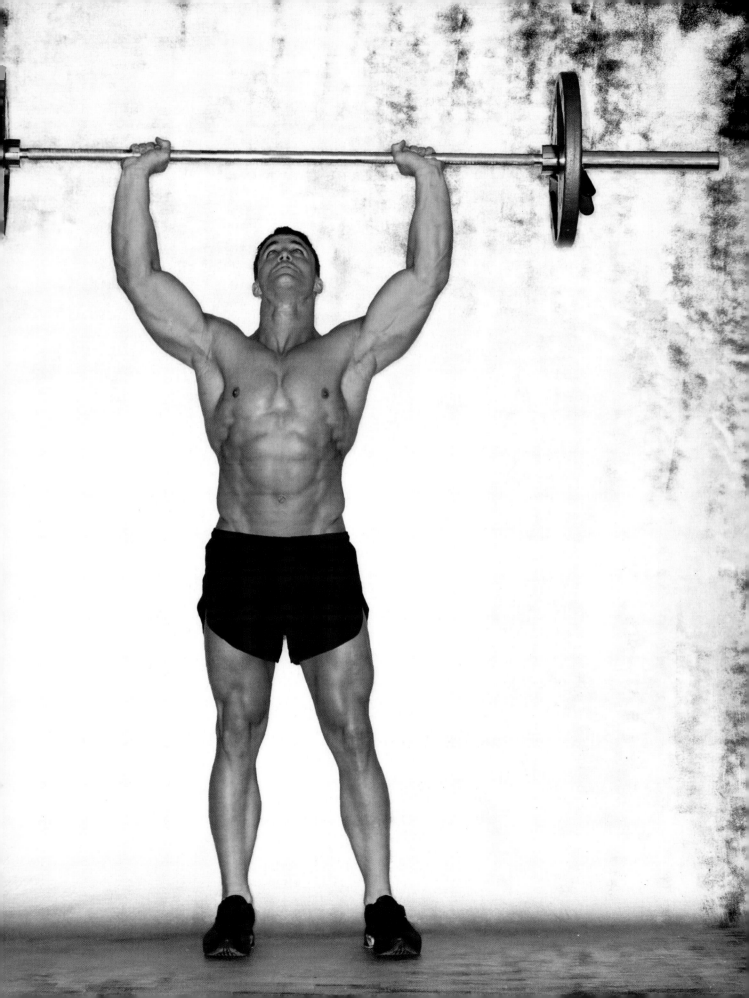

STAGE 1, WEEKS 1 THROUGH 3

Prepare to leave your ego in your locker with your deodorant and jock-itch powder. These first 3 weeks, you develop muscular control and shore up weak links. You also address potential muscle and strength imbalances.

Here are a few definitions and reminders.

10+10 or 10+10+10: This notation indicates a strip set. Start with an appropriate weight for a 10-rep set, do the reps, quickly strip enough weight off the bar to do another 10 reps, and then repeat one more time (if indicated).

SUPERSET: This is two consecutive exercises without rest. A warmup for a superset should itself be done in superset form.

TRISET: This is three consecutive exercises without rest. A warmup for a triset should itself be done in triset form.

1.5 REPS: If you see this in the TEMPO column, do a rep, pause, go halfway back to the starting position, pause, go back to the finishing position, and pause again before going all the way back to the starting position. Twelve 1.5 reps actually include 24 reps in the toughest part of the motion. Load the barbell appropriately.

804 OR 408 TEMPO: You know that the first number in the TEMPO column represents the speed of the lowering phase, the middle number is the length of the pause, and the third number is the duration of the actual lifting of the weight. For a deadlift, use a 408 tempo, taking 4 seconds to lower the weight and immediately, without pausing, taking 8 seconds to lift it. Most other big-muscle exercises in this workout should be done at a tempo of 804: 8 seconds of lowering the weight and 4 seconds of lifting it, again with no pause in between.

5 STOPS: This is the tempo for ski squats in workout B. Stop five times on the way down, and hold each position for 10 to 40 seconds per stop.

SUPERSET STRIP SET: Do a set of one exercise followed by a set of a second exercise, followed by a two-set strip set of the first exercise, followed by a two-set strip set of the second exercise.

21: Do seven reps in the toughest half of the range of motion, followed by seven full-range reps, followed by seven in the easiest half of the range.

STAGE 1
WEEKS 1–3
WORKOUT A

EXERCISE	WARMUP		WORK		TEMPO	REST (SEC)
	SETS	REPS	SETS	REPS		
CONTROLLED AB CIRCUIT						
1 THIN TUMMY	0	0	1	10	5-sec holds	0
2 CURLUP, CHEAT UP & SLOW LOWER, *OR* CURLUP, ARMS STRAIGHT & PARALLEL TO FLOOR	0	0	1	10	5–15-sec lowering or 515	0
3 RUSSIAN TWIST	0	0	1	15–30	303	0
4 PUSHUP HOLD, HANDS & FEET	0	0	1	10	5-sec holds	0
STRIP SET						
5 BARBELL WRIST EXTENSION	1	10	1	10+10+10	311	0
BICEPS TRISET						
6 DUMBBELL SEATED BICEPS CURL, INCLINE	1	10	1	10	422	0
7 EZ-BAR PREACHER CURL, REVERSE GRIP	1	10	1	10	422	0
8 DUMBBELL SEATED HAMMER CURL + TWIST	1	10	1	10	422	60–120
SUPERSET						
9 DUMBBELL LYING PULLOVER	1	12	1	12	1.5s	0
10 DUMBBELL SEATED LATERAL RAISE	1	12	1	12	1.5s	60–120
SUPERSET						
11 LAT PULLDOWN, NEUTRAL GRIP	1	10	1	21	311	0
12 DUMBBELL SEATED SHOULDER PRESS, ARNOLD PRESS	1	10	1	21	311	60–120
SUPERSET						
13 WIDE-GRIP PULLUP	1	6 (on lat-pulldown machine at 311 tempo)	1	4–6	804	0
14 BARBELL SEATED SHOULDER PRESS, WIDE GRIP	1	6 (at 311 tempo)	1	4–6	804	60–120

STAGE 1
WEEKS 1–3
WORKOUT B

EXERCISE	WARMUP		WORK		TEMPO	REST (SEC)
	SETS	REPS	SETS	REPS		
CONTROLLED AB CIRCUIT						
1 TOES TO SKY	0	0	1	10	5-sec holds	30
2 CURLUP, LEGS IN AIR, HANDS ON OPPOSITE SHOULDERS, ARMS ACROSS CHEST	0	0	1	10–15	313	30
3 SIDE RAISE	0	0	1	10–15	313	30
4 SEATED THIN TUMMY + CHEEK SQUEEZE	0	0	1	10	5-sec holds	30
CALF SUPERSET STRIP SET						
5 SEATED CALF RAISE, SINGLE LEG	1	10	1	10	311	0
6 STANDING SINGLE-LEG CALF RAISE	1	10	1	10	311	0
7 SEATED CALF RAISE, SINGLE LEG	1	10	1	10+10	311	0
8 STANDING SINGLE LEG CALF RAISE	1	10	1	10+10	311	60–120
SUPERSET						
9 LEG CURL, SINGLE LEG	0	0	1	15–20	1.5s	0
10 LEG EXTENSION, SINGLE LEG	0	0	1	15–20	1.5s	60–120
SUPERSET						
11 SUPINE HIP-THIGH EXTENSION	0	0	1	10–20	311	0
12 SKI SQUAT	0	0	1	5 stops	10–40 sec per stop	60–120
SUPERSET						
13 SINGLE-LEG STIFF-LEGGED DEADLIFT	0	0	1	5–10	422	0
14 STATIC LUNGE, BACK FOOT ON LOW BLOCK	0	0	1	8–10	422	60–120
SUPERSET						
15 DEADLIFT	1	6 at 311 tempo (optional)	1	6	408	0
16 BARBELL SQUAT	1	6 at 311 tempo (optional)	1	6	804	60–120
SHRUG TRISET						
17 BARBELL SHRUG, WIDE GRIP	1	10	1	10	311	0
18 BARBELL SHRUG	1	10	1	10	311	0
19 BARBELL SHRUG, REVERSE GRIP	1	10	1	10	311	60–120

STAGE 1
WEEKS 1–3
WORKOUT C

EXERCISE	WARMUP		WORK		TEMPO	REST (SEC)
	SETS	REPS	SETS	REPS		
CONTROLLED AB CIRCUIT						
1 THIN TUMMY	0	0	1	10	313 or 5-sec holds	0
2 CURLUP, CHEAT UP & SLOW LOWER, *OR* ARMS STRAIGHT & PARALLEL TO FLOOR	0	0	1	10	5–15-sec lowering or 515	0
3 RUSSIAN TWIST	0	0	1	15–30	303	0
4 PUSHUP HOLD, HANDS & FEET	0	0	1	10	5-sec holds	0
STRIP SET						
5 BARBELL WRIST CURL	1	10	1	10+10+10	311	0
TRICEPS TRISET						
6 EZ-BAR LYING TRICEPS EXTENSION	1	10	1	10	422	0
7 TRICEPS PUSHDOWN	1	10	1	10	422	0
8 DIP/BENCH DIP	1	10 (bench dip)	1	10	422	60–120
SUPERSET						
9 REVERSE DUMBBELL FLY	1	12	1	12	1.5s	0
10 DUMBBELL FLY	1	12	1	12	1.5s	60–120
SUPERSET						
11 SEATED CABLE ROW, NEUTRAL GRIP	1	10†	1	21	311	0
12 DUMBBELL BENCH PRESS, DECLINE	1	10†	1	21	311	60–120
SUPERSET						
13 SEATED CABLE ROW, WIDE GRIP, HIGH BAR	1	6 at 311 tempo	1	6	804	0
14 BARBELL BENCH PRESS, WIDE GRIP, HIGH BAR, FEET ON BENCH	1	6 at 311 tempo	1	6	804	60–120

† Normal range of motion

STAGE 1, WEEKS 4 THROUGH 6

Admit it: Weeks 1 through 3 were a lot harder than you thought they'd be. And now you're ready for something simpler. The next workouts are a lot simpler—just three or four exercises per workout, after you finish the ab circuit. Don't confuse "simple" with "easy," however.

You do either 5 or 10 sets of each exercise, as specified by the chart, trying to increase the weight slightly in each set, even though the repetitions stay the same.

Do high-repetition sets of the ab exercises; just try to establish a rhythmic tempo and knock out the reps without rushing through them.

The two arm exercises in workout B are paired in **ALTERNATED SETS, WITH FULL RECOVERIES BETWEEN SETS**. Do a set of one exercise, wait until you're fully recuperated, then do a set of another. Instead of doing them one right after the other, rest until your breathing is back to normal and you feel as strong as you did before your first set of your first exercise. Only then should you begin your first set of your second exercise.

STAGE 1
WEEKS 4–6
WORKOUT A

EXERCISE	WARMUP		WORK		TEMPO	REST (SEC)
	SETS	REPS	SETS	REPS		
ENDURANCE AB CIRCUIT						
1 THIN TUMMY, LIFT ONE LEG	0	0	1	10–30	313	0
2 CURLUP, HANDS ON OPPOSITE ELBOWS (NOT PICTURED)	0	0	1	10–30	311	0
3 RUSSIAN TWIST	0	0	1	10–30	202	0
4 MODIFIED V-SIT	0	0	1	10–30	301	0
STRAIGHT SETS						
5 DEADLIFT, WIDE GRIP	1	10	10	6	311	60
6 BARBELL SHRUG, WIDE GRIP	1	10	5	10	311	60
7 BARBELL SEATED SHOULDER PRESS, WIDE GRIP	1	10	5	6	311	60

STAGE 1
WEEKS 4–6
WORKOUT B

EXERCISE	WARMUP		WORK		TEMPO	REST (SEC)
	SETS	REPS	SETS	REPS		
ENDURANCE AB STRAIGHT SETS						
1 TOES TO SKY, ONE KNEE BENT	0	0	1	10–30	311	30
2 CURLUP, LEGS IN AIR, HANDS ON FOREHEAD, ELBOWS IN	0	0	1	10–30	311	30
3 SIDE RAISE, HANDS ON FOREHEAD, ELBOWS IN	0	0	1	10–30	311	30
4 WRIST-TO-KNEE CURLUP	0	0	1	10–30	311	30
STRAIGHT SETS						
5 SEATED CABLE ROW, WIDE GRIP, HIGH BAR	1	10	5	6–8	321	60
6 BARBELL BENCH PRESS, WIDE GRIP	1	10	5	6–8	321	60
ALTERNATED, WITH FULL RECOVERIES BETWEEN SETS						
7 DIP/BENCH DIP	1	10 (bench dip)	5	8–10	321	Full recovery
8 EZ-BAR BICEPS CURL, REVERSE GRIP	1	10	5	8–10	321	Full recovery

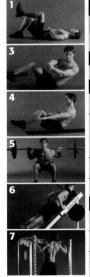

STAGE 1
WEEKS 4–6
WORKOUT C

EXERCISE	WARMUP		WORK		TEMPO	REST (SEC)
	SETS	REPS	SETS	REPS		
ENDURANCE AB CIRCUIT						
1 THIN TUMMY, LIFT ONE LEG	0	0	1	10–30	313	0
2 CURLUP, HANDS ON OPPOSITE ELBOWS (NOT PICTURED)	0	0	1	10–30	311	0
3 RUSSIAN TWIST	0	0	1	10–30	202	0
4 MODIFIED V-SIT	0	0	1	10–30	301	60–120
STRAIGHT SETS						
5 BARBELL SQUAT	1	10	10	10	311	60
6 STANDING CALF RAISE	1	15	5	15	311	60
7 PULLUP OR LAT PULLDOWN, WIDE-GRIP	1	10 (on lat-pulldown machine)	5	6–8	311	60

STAGE 2, WEEKS 8 THROUGH 10

Shift to fewer sets with more exercises and different loading schemes. Do two sets of six reps of the first two exercises in each workout, using heavy weights. Then do single sets with moderate reps, and finally single sets with high reps.

In workout B, note the explosive-tempo designation of 10* for the dynamic lunge. This indicates that you should take 1 second to lunge and then, without pausing, push back up as quickly as possible.

You'll do the abdominal exercises at the end of the workouts, and use weights as specified.

STAGE 2
WEEKS 8–10
WORKOUT A

EXERCISE	WARMUP		WORK		TEMPO	REST (SEC)
	SETS	REPS	SETS	REPS		
ALTERNATED, WITH FULL RECOVERIES BETWEEN SETS						
1 BARBELL BENT-OVER ROW, WIDE GRIP	2	Set 1:10 Set 2: 8	2	6	311	Full recovery
2 BARBELL BENCH PRESS, INCLINE, WIDE GRIP	2	Set 1: 10 Set 2: 8	2	6	311	Full recovery
ALTERNATED, WITH FULL RECOVERIES BETWEEN SETS						
3 BARBELL BENT-OVER ROW	0	0	1	10–12	311	Full recovery
4 BARBELL BENCH PRESS	0	0	1	10–12	311	Full recovery
ALTERNATED, WITH FULL RECOVERIES BETWEEN SETS						
5 DUMBBELL ONE-ARM BENT-OVER ROW	0	0	1	12–20	311	Full recovery
6 DUMBBELL BENCH PRESS, DECLINE	0	0	1	12–20	311	Full recovery
STRAIGHT SETS						
7 KNEE-UP, INCLINE	0	0	1	10–15	201	60
8 CURLUP, WEIGHTED (NOT PICTURED)	0	0	1	10–15	201	60
9 SIDE RAISE, HANDS ON FOREHEAD, ELBOWS OUT	0	0	1	10–15	201	60
10 SWISS-BALL ALTERNATE-LEG LIFT	0	0	1	10 (each leg)	5-sec holds	60

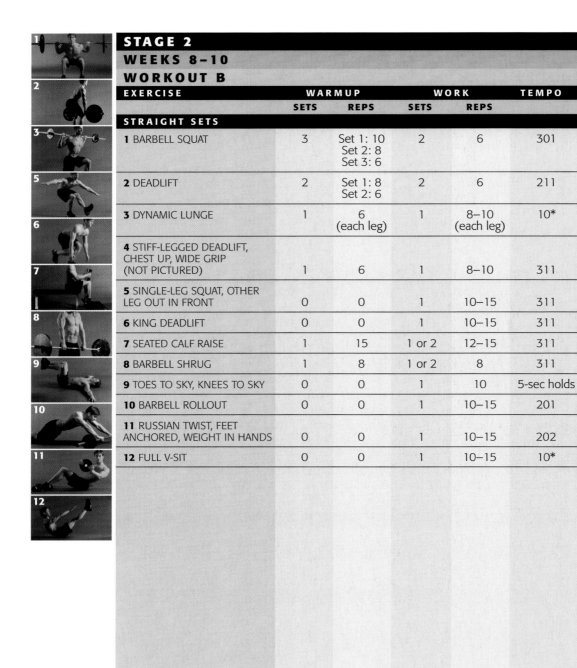

STAGE 2
WEEKS 8–10
WORKOUT B

EXERCISE	WARMUP		WORK		TEMPO	REST (SEC)
	SETS	REPS	SETS	REPS		
STRAIGHT SETS						
1 BARBELL SQUAT	3	Set 1: 10 Set 2: 8 Set 3: 6	2	6	301	180
2 DEADLIFT	2	Set 1: 8 Set 2: 6	2	6	211	180
3 DYNAMIC LUNGE	1	6 (each leg)	1	8–10 (each leg)	10*	120
4 STIFF-LEGGED DEADLIFT, CHEST UP, WIDE GRIP (NOT PICTURED)	1	6	1	8–10	311	120
5 SINGLE-LEG SQUAT, OTHER LEG OUT IN FRONT	0	0	1	10–15	311	60
6 KING DEADLIFT	0	0	1	10–15	311	60
7 SEATED CALF RAISE	1	15	1 or 2	12–15	311	60
8 BARBELL SHRUG	1	8	1 or 2	8	311	60
9 TOES TO SKY, KNEES TO SKY	0	0	1	10	5-sec holds	60
10 BARBELL ROLLOUT	0	0	1	10–15	201	60
11 RUSSIAN TWIST, FEET ANCHORED, WEIGHT IN HANDS	0	0	1	10–15	202	60
12 FULL V-SIT	0	0	1	10–15	10*	60

STAGE 2
WEEKS 8–10
WORKOUT C

EXERCISE	WARMUP		WORK		TEMPO	REST (SEC)
	SETS	REPS	SETS	REPS		
ALTERNATED, WITH FULL RECOVERIES BETWEEN SETS						
1 BARBELL SEATED SHOULDER PRESS	2	Set 1: 10 Set 2: 8	2	6	311	Full recovery
2 PULLUP	2	Set 1: 10 (on lat-pulldown machine) Set 2: 8 (on lat-pulldown machine)	2	6	311	Full recovery
ALTERNATED, WITH FULL RECOVERIES BETWEEN SETS						
3 BARBELL SEATED SHOULDER PRESS, TO FRONT	0	0	1	10–12	311	Full recovery
4 LAT PULLDOWN, WIDE GRIP, BEHIND NECK	0	0	1	10–12	311	Full recovery
ALTERNATED, WITH FULL RECOVERIES BETWEEN SETS						
5 DUMBBELL SEATED SHOULDER PRESS	0	0	1	12–20	311	Full recovery
6 LAT PULLDOWN, REVERSE GRIP	0	0	1	12–20	311	Full recovery
STRAIGHT SETS						
7 KNEE-UP, INCLINE	0	0	1	10–15	201	60
8 CURLUP, LEGS IN AIR, WEIGHT ON CHEST	0	0	1	10–15	201	60
9 RUSSIAN TWIST, LEG CYCLE	0	0	1	15–30	212	60
10 SWISS-BALL ALTERNATE-LEG LIFT	0	0	1	10 (each leg)	5-sec holds	60

STAGE 2, WEEKS 11 THROUGH 13

Lift more heavy weights, with a new twist: one or two **BACK-OFF SETS** on many of the exercises. For pullups and dips, you'll probably have to use lat pulldowns and bench dips for the warmups and final back-off sets. Here's how.

PULLUP: Do three warmup sets on the lat-pulldown machine. Then do two sets of 4 reps with weight (probably a belt with a chain for holding weight plates or a dumbbell between your legs). Try to do the first back-off set—8 reps—with your body weight. Even if you can manage only a few, you have 3 weeks to work your way up to 8. Then do the second back-off set—12 to 15 reps—on the lat-pulldown machine.

DIP: You may be able to do all the warmups—sets of 10, 8, and 6—on the parallel bars. Even if you can do that, you shouldn't. Ideally, do the first warmup set as triceps pushdowns, the second warmup as bench dips, and the final warmup as body-weight parallel-bar dips. Then you're ready for weighted dips in your work sets. Or, if you're really strong, you can the first warmup set as bench dips, the second warmup as body-weight parallel-bar dips, and the final warmup with a light weight. Another alternative is to do loaded bench dips—with a weight on your lap—for one of your warmup sets. The first back-off set should be lightly loaded or body-weight parallel-bar dips. And the second back-off set will almost certainly be bench dips.

Do your ab workouts three different ways: fast reps (workout A, with explosive tempos indicated by 10* or 20*); slow, controlled reps (workout B); and with some kind of external loading or gravitational disadvantage (workout C). Do each as a circuit, with no rest between exercises but a short rest between circuits if you do more than one.

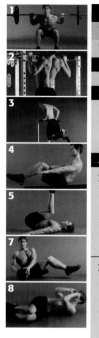

STAGE 2
WEEKS 11–13
WORKOUT A

EXERCISE	WARMUP		WORK		TEMPO	REST (SEC)
	SETS	REPS	SETS	REPS		
STRAIGHT SETS						
1 BARBELL SQUAT	3	Set 1: 10 Set 2: 8 Set 3: 6	3	Set 1: 4 Set 2: 4† Back-off set: 8	201	180
ALTERNATED, WITH FULL RECOVERIES BETWEEN SETS						
2 PULLUP	3	Set 1: 10 Set 2: 8 Set 3: 6	4	Set 1: 4 Set 2: 4† Back-off set 1: 8 Back-off set 2: 12–15	211	Full recovery
3 DIP	3	Set 1: 10 Set 2: 8 Set 3: 6	4	Set 1: 4 Set 2: 4† Back-off set 1: 8 Back-off set 2: 12–15	211	Full recovery
FAST AB CIRCUIT						
4 MODIFIED V-SIT	0	0	1 or 2	10–20	10*	0
5 KNEE-UP	0	0	1 or 2	10–20	20*	0
6 CURLUP, HANDS ON OPPOSITE SHOULDERS + TWIST (NOT PICTURED)	0	0	1 or 2	10–20	20*	0
7 RUSSIAN TWIST, MEDICINE BALL IN HANDS	0	0	1 or 2	15–25	101	0
8 SIDE RAISE, HANDS ON FOREHEAD, ELBOWS IN	0	0	1 or 2	10–15 (each side)	10*	60–120

† Use more weight

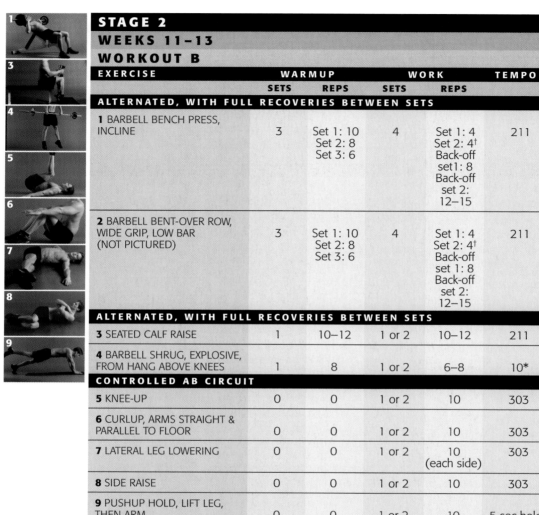

STAGE 2
WEEKS 11–13
WORKOUT B

EXERCISE	WARMUP		WORK		TEMPO	REST (SEC)
	SETS	REPS	SETS	REPS		
ALTERNATED, WITH FULL RECOVERIES BETWEEN SETS						
1 BARBELL BENCH PRESS, INCLINE	3	Set 1: 10 Set 2: 8 Set 3: 6	4	Set 1: 4 Set 2: 4† Back-off set1: 8 Back-off set 2: 12–15	211	Full recovery
2 BARBELL BENT-OVER ROW, WIDE GRIP, LOW BAR (NOT PICTURED)	3	Set 1: 10 Set 2: 8 Set 3: 6	4	Set 1: 4 Set 2: 4† Back-off set 1: 8 Back-off set 2: 12–15	211	Full recovery
ALTERNATED, WITH FULL RECOVERIES BETWEEN SETS						
3 SEATED CALF RAISE	1	10–12	1 or 2	10–12	211	Full recovery
4 BARBELL SHRUG, EXPLOSIVE, FROM HANG ABOVE KNEES	1	8	1 or 2	6–8	10*	Full recovery
CONTROLLED AB CIRCUIT						
5 KNEE-UP	0	0	1 or 2	10	303	0
6 CURLUP, ARMS STRAIGHT & PARALLEL TO FLOOR	0	0	1 or 2	10	303	0
7 LATERAL LEG LOWERING	0	0	1 or 2	10 (each side)	303	0
8 SIDE RAISE	0	0	1 or 2	10	303	0
9 PUSHUP HOLD, LIFT LEG, THEN ARM	0	0	1 or 2	10	5-sec holds	60–120

† Use more weight

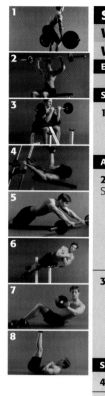

STAGE 2
WEEKS 11–13
WORKOUT C

EXERCISE	WARMUP		WORK		TEMPO	REST (SEC)
	SETS	REPS	SETS	REPS		
STRAIGHT SETS						
1 DEADLIFT	3	Set 1: 10 Set 2: 8 Set 3: 6	3	Set 1: 4 Set 2: 4† Back-off set: 8	211	180
ALTERNATED, WITH FULL RECOVERIES BETWEEN SETS						
2 BARBELL SEATED SHOULDER PRESS	3	Set 1: 10 Set 2: 8 Set 3: 6	4	Set 1: 4 Set 2: 4† Back-off set 1: 8 Back-off set 2: 12–15	211	Full recovery
3 EZ-BAR PREACHER CURL	2	Set 1: 10 Set 2: 8	4	Set 1: 4 Set 2: 4† Back-off set 1: 8 Back-off set 2: 12–15	211	Full recovery
STRENGTH AB CIRCUIT						
4 KNEE-UP, INCLINE	1	10	1	10–15	211	0
5 BARBELL ROLLOUT	1	10	1	10–15	201	0
6 SIDE RAISE, ON ROMAN CHAIR	1	10	1	10–15	201	0
7 RUSSIAN TWIST, FEET ANCHORED, WEIGHT IN HANDS	1	10	1	10–15	202	0
8 CURLUP, LEGS IN AIR, WEIGHT ON CHEST	1	10	1	10–15	201	60–120

† Use more weight

STAGE 3, WEEKS 15 THROUGH 17

Ready for a blast from the past? It's time to whipsaw back to a workout like the one you did in the first 3 weeks of the program. You use much heavier weights, but the concept is the same: Pre-exhaust smaller muscles before working your big muscles. In workout C, for example, do three triceps exercises before three different shoulder-press movements. Then, with your triceps and shoulders fried, do heavy chest work featuring three different bench-press variations.

Workout B is a little different from workouts A and C. The nine exercises start with the heavy strength movements—deadlift, squat, and shrug—and then progress to explosive variations of those exercises. Still, it's pre-exhaustion of sorts, in that it's much harder to generate power when muscles are exhausted from heavy lifts.

The ab exercises move back to the beginning of the workouts and also resurrect an earlier concept, focusing solely on control.

STAGE 3
WEEKS 15–17
WORKOUT A

EXERCISE	WARMUP		WORK		TEMPO	REST (SEC)
	SETS	REPS	SETS	REPS		
CONTROLLED AB CIRCUIT						
1 THIN TUMMY, LIFT & CYCLE OUT ONE LEG	0	0	1	10	313	0
2 CURLUP, ARMS STRAIGHT & PARALLEL TO FLOOR	0	0	1	10	515	0
3 RUSSIAN TWIST, LEG CYCLE	0	0	1	15–30	303	0
4 PUSHUP HOLD, LIFT LEG WITH OPPOSITE ARM	0	0	1	10	5-sec holds	60–120
STRAIGHT SETS						
5 DUMBBELL SEATED HAMMER CURL	2	Set 1: 10 Set 2: 8	2	Set 1: 5 Set 2: 5†	311	120
6 DUMBBELL SEATED BICEPS CURL	0	0	1	10	311	60–120
7 DUMBBELL SEATED BICEPS CURL, REVERSE GRIP (NOT PICTURED)	0	0	1	15	311	60
8 BARBELL BENT-OVER ROW	2	Set 1: 10 Set 2: 8	2	Set 1: 5 Set 2: 5†	311	120–180
9 BARBELL BENT-OVER ROW, REVERSE GRIP	0	0	1	10	311	120
10 BARBELL BENT-OVER ROW, WIDE GRIP	0	0	1	15	311	60–120
11 CHINUP	2 (on lat-pulldown machine)	Set 1:10 Set 2: 8	2	Set 1: 5 Set 2: 5†	311	120–180
12 PULLUP *OR* LAT PULLDOWN	0	0	1	5–10	311	120
13 WIDE-GRIP PULLUP *OR* LAT PULLDOWN	0	0	1	5–10	311	60–120

† Use more weight

STAGE 3
WEEKS 15–17
WORKOUT B

EXERCISE	WARMUP		WORK		TEMPO	REST (SEC)
	SETS	REPS	SETS	REPS		
CONTROLLED AB STRAIGHT SETS						
1 TOES TO SKY, ONE KNEE BENT	0	0	1	10	5-sec holds	30
2 CURLUP, LEGS IN AIR, HANDS ON FOREHEAD, ELBOWS IN	0	0	1	10–15	313	30
3 SIDE RAISE, HANDS ON FOREHEAD, ELBOWS IN	0	0	1	10–15	313	30
4 SEATED THIN TUMMY + CHEEK SQUEEZE	0	0	1	10	5-sec holds	30
STRAIGHT SETS						
5 DEADLIFT	2	Set 1: 10 Set 2: 8	2†	Set 1: 5 Set 2: 5	311	180
6 CLEAN PULL	1	5	1	5	10*	120–180
7 HIGH PULL	1	5	1	5	10*	120
8 BARBELL SQUAT	1	5	2†	5	301	180
9 BARBELL SQUAT, EXPLOSIVE	0	0	1	8	30*	120–180
10 BARBELL SQUAT, JUMP	0	0	1	10	10*	120
SHRUG TRISET						
11 BARBELL SHRUG	1	4	1	4	*	0
12 BARBELL SHRUG, EXPLOSIVE, FROM HANG ABOVE KNEES (NOT PICTURED)	1	4	1	4	*	0
13 BARBELL SHRUG, JUMP, FROM HANG ABOVE KNEES	1	4	1	4	*	60–120

† Use more weight on 2nd set

STAGE 3
WEEKS 15–17
WORKOUT C

EXERCISE	WARMUP		WORK		TEMPO	REST (SEC)
	SETS	REPS	SETS	REPS		
CONTROLLED AB CIRCUIT						
1 THIN TUMMY, LIFT CYCLE OUT ONE LEG	0	0	1	10	313	0
2 CURLUP, ARMS STRAIGHT & PARALLEL TO FLOOR	0	0	1	10	515	0
3 RUSSIAN TWIST, LEG CYCLE	0	0	1	15–30	303	0
4 PUSHUP HOLD, LIFT LEG WITH OPPOSITE ARM	0	0	1	10	5-sec holds	60–120
STRAIGHT SETS						
5 TRICEPS PUSHDOWN	2	Set 1: 10 Set 2: 8	2†	5	311	120
6 EZ-BAR LYING TRICEPS EXTENSION, WIDE GRIP	0	0	1	10	311	60–120
7 EZ-BAR OVERHEAD TRICEPS EXTENSION	0	0	1	15	311	60
8 BARBELL SEATED SHOULDER PRESS, TO FRONT	2	Set 1: 10 Set 2: 8	2†	5	311	120–180
9 BARBELL SEATED SHOULDER PRESS	0	0	1	10	311	120
10 BARBELL SEATED SHOULDER PRESS, WIDE GRIP	0	0	1	15	311	60–120
11 BARBELL BENCH PRESS	2 (on lat-pulldown machine)	Set 1: 10 Set 2: 8	2†	5	311	120–180
12 BARBELL BENCH PRESS, WIDE GRIP	0	0	1	10	311	120
13 BARBELL BENCH PRESS, WIDE GRIP, TO NECK, FEET ON BENCH (NOT PICTURED)	0	0	1	15	311	60–120

† Use more weight on 2nd set

STAGE 3, WEEKS 18 THROUGH 20

We think there's a good chance that these 3 weeks include the most aggressive strength workouts you've ever tried. The workouts feature two new techniques.

WAVE LOADING: Yes, you did one type of wave loading in the intermediate program (if you did that program before this one). Here we offer a different configuration. Do four sets of three reps, increasing and decreasing the weight you lift. Say you're doing barbell bench presses. Maybe you start with three reps at 185. Then you do three with 225, three with 205, and finally three with 245. Obviously, you want to bump up the numbers in each set of each workout so by the third workout you do, say, 205, 245, 225, and 265 in your four sets.

ECCENTRIC REPS: On three exercises—barbell bench presses, bent-over rows, and chinups—you do a set of three eccentric repetitions. This means load the bar— or in the case of the chinups, yourself—with 10 to 20 percent more weight than you used in your heaviest set. Take 5 seconds to lower the bar or your body. Then have spotters raise the bar off your chest or the floor (or climb back up to the chinup bar), and repeat for two more reps.

OFF BLOCKS/QUARTER REPS: For anyone other than elite lifters, it isn't wise or safe to do eccentric deadlifts or squats (often called *negative* deadlifts or squats). So to allow yourself to use more weight, you must use techniques that shorten your range of motion. To do a deadlift off blocks, set up the barbell on blocks or weight plates to raise it 6 or more inches off the floor. That should allow you to use 10 to 20 percent more weight than you did on your heaviest deadlift set. (If it doesn't, raise the blocks a bit for your next workout. And make sure to rest for the full 4 minutes between sets and exercises.)

For quarter reps on the squat, load the bar with 10 to 20 percent more weight than you used on your heaviest set, descend one-quarter of the way down, and then push back up.

When using either of these techniques, make sure you have great spotters, or work in a power rack with safety bars set at appropriate heights.

As for the ab exercises, they all use steady, rhythmic, high-repetition sets.

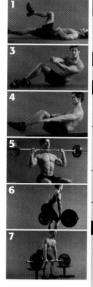

STAGE 3
WEEKS 18–20
WORKOUT A

EXERCISE	WARMUP		WORK		TEMPO	REST (SEC)
	SETS	REPS	SETS	REPS		
ENDURANCE AB CIRCUIT						
1 THIN TUMMY, BOTH LEGS UP, CYCLE OUT ONE LEG	0	0	1	10–30	313	0
2 CURLUP, HANDS ON OPPOSITE ELBOWS (NOT PICTURED)	0	0	1	10–30	311	0
3 RUSSIAN TWIST, FEET ANCHORED	0	0	1	10–30	202	0
4 MODIFIED V-SIT	0	0	1	10–30	301	60–120
WAVE SETS						
5 BARBELL SEATED SHOULDER PRESS, TO FRONT	3	Set 1: 10 Set 2: 8 Set 3: 5	5	Wave set 1: 3 Wave set 2: 3† Wave set 3: 3‡ Wave set 4: 3§ Back-off set: 10–20	211	240
6 DEADLIFT	3	Set 1: 8 Set 2: 5 Set 3: 3	4	Wave set 1: 3 Wave set 2: 3† Wave set 3: 3 ‡ Wave set 4: 3§	311	240
STRAIGHT SETS						
7 DEADLIFT, OFF BLOCKS	1	3	1	3	311	240

† Use more weight than in wave set 1
‡ Use more weight than in wave set 1, less than in wave set 2
§ Use more weight than in wave set 2

STAGE 3
WEEKS 18–20
WORKOUT B

EXERCISE	WARMUP		WORK		TEMPO	REST (SEC)
	SETS	REPS	SETS	REPS		
ENDURANCE AB STRAIGHT SETS						
1 TOES TO SKY, KNEES TO SKY	0	0	1	10–30	311	30
2 CURLUP, LEGS IN AIR, HANDS ON FOREHEAD, ELBOWS OUT	0	0	1	10–30	311	30
3 SIDE RAISE, ON ROMAN CHAIR	0	0	1	10–30	311	30
4 WRIST-TO-KNEE CURLUP, FULL LYING POSITION (NOT PICTURED)	0	0	1	10–30	311	30
WAVE SETS, ALTERNATED, WITH FULL RECOVERIES BETWEEN SETS						
5 BARBELL BENCH PRESS, TO LOWER CHEST, ARCHED BACK	3	Set 1: 10 Set 2: 8 Set 3: 5	4	Wave set 1: 3 Wave set 2: 3† Wave set 3: 3‡ Wave set 4: 3§	211	Full recovery
6 ECCENTRIC BARBELL BENCH PRESS, TO LOWER CHEST, ARCHED BACK	0	0	1	3	500	Full recovery
7 BARBELL BENCH PRESS	0	0	1	10–20	311	Full recovery
WAVE SETS, ALTERNATED, WITH FULL RECOVERIES BETWEEN SETS						
8 BARBELL BENT-OVER ROW, LOW BAR	3	Set 1: 10 Set 2: 8 Set 3: 5	4	Wave set 1: 3 Wave set 2: 3† Wave set 3: 3‡ Wave set 4: 3§	211	Full recovery
ALTERNATED, WITH FULL RECOVERIES BETWEEN SETS						
9 ECCENTRIC DUMBBELL ONE-ARM BENT-OVER ROW	0	0	1	3	500	Full recovery
10 BARBELL BENT-OVER ROW	0	0	1	10–20	311	Full recovery

† Use more weight than in wave set 1
‡ Use more weight than in wave set 1, less than in wave set 2
§ Use more weight than in wave set 2

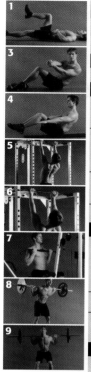

STAGE 3
WEEKS 18–20
WORKOUT C

EXERCISE	WARMUP		WORK		TEMPO	REST (SEC)
	SETS	REPS	SETS	REPS		
ENDURANCE AB CIRCUIT						
1 THIN TUMMY, BOTH LEGS UP, CYCLE OUT ONE LEG	0	0	1	10–30	313	0
2 CURLUP, HANDS ON OPPOSITE ELBOWS (NOT PICTURED)	0	0	1	10–30	311	0
3 RUSSIAN TWIST, FEET ANCHORED	0	0	1	10–30	202	0
4 MODIFIED V-SIT	0	0	1	10–30	301	0
WAVE SETS						
5 CHINUP	3 (use lat pulldown, reverse grip)	Set 1:10 Set 2: 8 Set 3: 5	4	Wave set 1: 3 Wave set 2: 3† Wave set 3: 3‡ Wave set 4: 3§	211	240
6 CHINUP, ECCENTRIC	0	0	1	3	500	240
7 LAT PULLDOWN, REVERSE GRIP	0	0	1	10–20	311	120–180
WAVE SETS						
8 SQUAT, LOW BAR	3	Set 1: 8 Set 2: 5 Set 3: 3	4	Wave set 1: 3 Wave set 2: 3† Wave set 3: 3‡ Wave set 4: 3§	201	240
9 SQUAT, LOW BAR, 1/4	1	3	1	3	201	240

† Use more weight than in wave set 1
‡ Use more weight than in wave set 1, less than in wave set 2
§ Use more weight than in wave set 2

STAGE 4, WEEKS 22 THROUGH 24

Now try another wave-loading pattern: Do a set of five reps, followed by a set of one with a heavier weight, followed by another set of five with a weight that's heavier than in the first set but lighter than in the second set, followed by another single with the heaviest weight yet.

For instance, when doing barbell bench presses, you could do your first set of five with 225. Then do a single rep with 265. Then do another set of 5 with 245, followed by a single rep with 285.

That's basically your program for these 3 weeks. Do 5-1-5-1 waves for six exercises, adding back-off sets to some and doing explosive versions of some others. Do weighted ab exercises at the end of each workout, then go home.

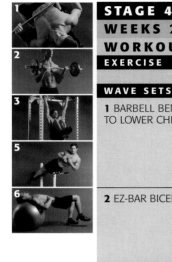

STAGE 4
WEEKS 22–24
WORKOUT A

EXERCISE	WARMUP		WORK		TEMPO	REST (SEC)
	SETS	REPS	SETS	REPS		
WAVE SETS, ALTERNATED, WITH FULL RECOVERIES BETWEEN SETS						
1 BARBELL BENCH PRESS, TO LOWER CHEST	3	Set 1: 10 Set 2: 8 Set 3: 5	5	Wave set 1: 5 Wave set 2: 1† Wave set 3: 5‡ Wave set 4: 1§ Back-off set: 10–20	211	Full recovery
2 EZ-BAR BICEPS CURL	3	Set 1: 10 Set 2: 8 Set 3: 5	5	Wave set 1: 5 Wave set 2: 1† Wave set 3: 5‡ Wave set 4: 1§ Back-off set: 10–20	211	Full recovery
STRAIGHT SETS						
3 KNEE-UP, VERTICAL	0	0	1	10–15	201	60
4 CURLUP, WEIGHTED (NOT PICTURED)	0	0	1	10–15	201	60
5 SIDE RAISE, ON ROMAN CHAIR, WEIGHT ON CHEST	0	0	1	10–15	201	60
6 SWISS-BALL ALTERNATE-LEG LIFT, LYING	0	0	1	10 (each leg)	5-sec holds	60

† Use more weight than in wave set 1
‡ Use more weight than in wave set 1, less than in wave set 2
§ Use more weight than in wave set 2

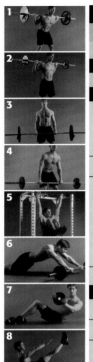

STAGE 4
WEEKS 22–24
WORKOUT B

EXERCISE	WARMUP		WORK		TEMPO	REST (SEC)
	SETS	REPS	SETS	REPS		
WAVE SETS						
1 BARBELL SQUAT, LOW BAR	3	Set 1:10 Set 2: 8 Set 3: 5	4	Wave set 1: 5 Wave set 2: 1† Wave set 3: 5‡ Wave set 4: 1§	201	180–240
2 BARBELL SQUAT, EXPLOSIVE	0	0	1	10	20*	180
3 DEADLIFT, ALTERNATING/MIXED GRIP	2	Set 1: 5 Set 2: 3	5	Wave set 1: 5 Wave set 2: 1† Wave set 3: 5‡ Wave set 4: 1§ Back-off set: 10	211	180–240
4 CLEAN PULL	1	5	1	5	10*	180
STRAIGHT SETS						
5 KNEE-UP, VERTICAL	0	0	1	10–15	201	60
6 BARBELL ROLLOUT	0	0	1	10–15	201	60
7 RUSSIAN TWIST, FEET ANCHORED, WEIGHT IN HANDS	0	0	1	10–15	202	60
8 FULL V-SIT	0	0	1	10–15	10*	60

† Use more weight than in wave set 1
‡ Use more weight than in wave set 1, less than in wave set 2
§ Use more weight than in wave set 2

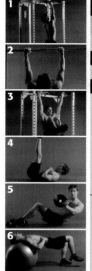

STAGE 4
WEEKS 22–24
WORKOUT C

EXERCISE	WARMUP		WORK		TEMPO	REST (SEC)
	SETS	REPS	SETS	REPS		
WAVE SETS, ALTERNATED, WITH FULL RECOVERIES BETWEEN SETS						
1 PULLUP, NEUTRAL GRIP	3 (on lat-pulldown machine)	Set 1: 10 Set 2: 8 Set 3: 5	5	Wave set 1: 5 Wave set 2: 1† Wave set 3: 5‡ Wave set 4: 1§ Back-off set: 10–20 (on lat-pulldown machine)	211	Full recovery
2 BARBELL BENCH PRESS, CLOSE GRIP	3	Set 1: 10 Set 2: 8 Set 3: 5	5	Wave set 1: 5 Wave set 2: 1† Wave set 3: 5‡ Wave set 4: 1§ Back-off set: 10–20	211	Full recovery
STRAIGHT SETS						
3 KNEE-UP, VERTICAL	0	0	1	10	201	60
4 CURLUP, LEGS IN AIR, WEIGHT ON CHEST	0	0	1	10–15	311	60
5 RUSSIAN TWIST, FEET ANCHORED, WEIGHT IN HANDS	0	0	1	10–15	212	60
6 SWISS-BALL ALTERNATE-LEG LIFT, LYING	0	0	1	10 (each leg)	5-sec holds	60

† Use more weight than in wave set 1
‡ Use more weight than in wave set 1, less than in wave set 2
§ Use more weight than in wave set 2

STAGE 4, WEEKS 25 THROUGH 27

Wrap up the advanced program with yet another wave pattern. Do two waves of three sets each (in other words, a total of six work sets). Each wave, do four repetitions in the first set, three reps in the second set, and two in the third set.

Let's use the barbell bench press yet again as an example. In the first wave, you might lift 235 pounds for four reps, 255 for three, and 275 for two. Then in the second wave, you might do 255 for four reps, 275 for three, and 295 for two. A key to this technique is using lighter weights than you ordinarily would for four, three, and two repetitions in the first wave. Working too hard in the first wave would exhaust your muscles, negating the neural boost the technique provides. So use submaximal weights the first time through in order to use heavier-than-normal weights the second time through.

Each workout, focus on one powerlift—barbell squat, barbell bench press, and deadlift—followed by eccentric or explosive work. On the eccentric bench presses, ¼ squats, and deadlifts off blocks, use 10 to 20 percent more weight than you used on your final wave set of two reps. So, using the above example, if you finish your final wave with two reps of 295 pounds, do your eccentric set with between 325 and 355 pounds. Don't forget to have a strong, vigilant spotter (or two) overseeing this great effort.

Your ab exercises again follow the heavy work, and you do three different circuits: fast, controlled, and weighted.

When you're finished, you should be the strongest you've ever been, and, depending on how strictly you've been watching your diet, your most muscular and/or buff.

Where you go from here is up to you. You could take a few days off and then test your maximum lifts in the bench press, deadlift, and squat, or go on a bodybuilding-type cutting program (higher overall volume of exercise, and more exercises for the smaller muscles) to take off whatever fat you have around the edges of your enlarged muscles.

Or you could just bask in the satisfaction of finishing an extremely challenging strength program, knowing your muscles are in the best shape ever.

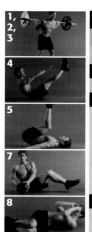

STAGE 4
WEEKS 25–27
WORKOUT A

EXERCISE	WARMUP		WORK		TEMPO	REST (SEC)
	SETS	REPS	SETS	REPS		
WAVE SETS						
1 SQUAT, LOW BAR (WEIGHT BELT OPTIONAL)	4	Set 1: 10 Set 2: 8 Set 3: 5 Set 4: 3	6	Wave set 1: 4 Wave set 2: 3† Wave set 3: 2† Wave set 4: 4‡ Wave set 5: 3§ Wave set 6: 2†	201	300
STRAIGHT SETS						
2 SQUAT, LOW BAR, 1/4 (BELT OPTIONAL)	1	4	1	4	201	300
3 BARBELL SQUAT, EXPLOSIVE, LOW BAR (BELT OPTIONAL)	0	0	1	10	20*	300
FAST AB CIRCUIT						
4 FULL V-SIT	0	0	1 or 2	10–20	10*	0
5 KNEE-UP	0	0	1 or 2	10–20	20*	0
6 CURLUP, HANDS ON FOREHEAD, ELBOWS OUT + TWIST (NOT PICTURED)	0	0	1 or 2	10–20	20*	0
7 RUSSIAN TWIST, MEDICINE BALL IN HANDS	0	0	1–2	15–25	101	0
8 SIDE RAISE, HANDS ON FOREHEAD, ELBOWS IN	0	0	1–2	10–15 (each side)	10*	0

† Use more weight than in previous set(s)
‡ Use same weight as in wave set 2
§ Use same weight as in wave set 3

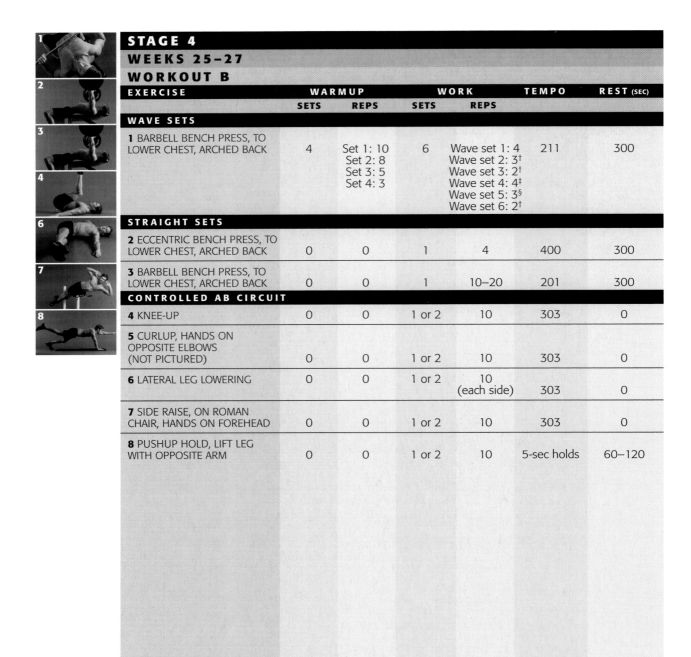

STAGE 4
WEEKS 25–27
WORKOUT B

EXERCISE	WARMUP		WORK		TEMPO	REST (SEC)
	SETS	REPS	SETS	REPS		
WAVE SETS						
1 BARBELL BENCH PRESS, TO LOWER CHEST, ARCHED BACK	4	Set 1: 10 Set 2: 8 Set 3: 5 Set 4: 3	6	Wave set 1: 4 Wave set 2: 3† Wave set 3: 2† Wave set 4: 4‡ Wave set 5: 3§ Wave set 6: 2†	211	300
STRAIGHT SETS						
2 ECCENTRIC BENCH PRESS, TO LOWER CHEST, ARCHED BACK	0	0	1	4	400	300
3 BARBELL BENCH PRESS, TO LOWER CHEST, ARCHED BACK	0	0	1	10–20	201	300
CONTROLLED AB CIRCUIT						
4 KNEE-UP	0	0	1 or 2	10	303	0
5 CURLUP, HANDS ON OPPOSITE ELBOWS (NOT PICTURED)	0	0	1 or 2	10	303	0
6 LATERAL LEG LOWERING	0	0	1 or 2	10 (each side)	303	0
7 SIDE RAISE, ON ROMAN CHAIR, HANDS ON FOREHEAD	0	0	1 or 2	10	303	0
8 PUSHUP HOLD, LIFT LEG WITH OPPOSITE ARM	0	0	1 or 2	10	5-sec holds	60–120

† Use more weight than in previous set(s)
‡ Use same weight as in wave set 2
§ Use same weight as in wave set 3

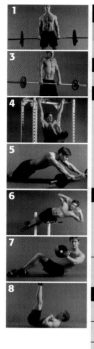

STAGE 4
WEEKS 25–27
WORKOUT C

EXERCISE	WARMUP		WORK		TEMPO	REST (SEC)
	SETS	REPS	SETS	REPS		
WAVE SETS						
1 DEADLIFT, ALTERNATING/ MIXED GRIP (WEIGHT BELT OPTIONAL)	4	Set 1: 10 Set 2: 8 Set 3: 5 Set 4: 3	6	Wave set 1: 4 Wave set 2: 3† Wave set 3: 2† Wave set 4: 4‡ Wave set 5: 3§ Wave set 6: 2†	211	300
STRAIGHT SETS						
2 DEADLIFT, ALTERNATING/ MIXED GRIP, OFF BLOCKS (WEIGHT BELT OPTIONAL) (NOT PICTURED)	1	4	1	4	211	300
3 CLEAN PULL, OFF FLOOR (WEIGHT BELT OPTIONAL)	1	6	1	6	10*	180–240
STRENGTH ABDOMINAL CIRCUIT						
4 KNEE-UP, VERTICAL	1	10	1	10–15	211	0
5 BARBELL ROLLOUT	1	10	1	10–15	201	0
6 SIDE RAISE, ON ROMAN CHAIR, HANDS ON FOREHEAD	1	10	1	10–15	201	0
7 RUSSIAN TWIST, FEET ANCHORED, WEIGHT IN HANDS	1	10	1	10–15	202	0
8 CURLUP, LEGS IN AIR, WEIGHT ON CHEST	1	10	1	10–15	201	60–120

† Use more weight than in previous set(s)
‡ Use same weight as in wave set 2
§ Use same weight as in wave set 3

INDEX

Underscored page references indicate tables. **Boldface** references indicate photographs or illustrations.